VOLUME **7**

DISEASE CONTROL PRIORITIES • THIRD EDITION

# Injury Prevention and Environmental Health

# DISEASE CONTROL PRIORITIES • THIRD EDITION

**Series Editors**

Dean T. Jamison

Rachel Nugent

Hellen Gelband

Susan Horton

Prabhat Jha

Ramanan Laxminarayan

Charles N. Mock

**Volumes in the Series**

Essential Surgery

Reproductive, Maternal, Newborn, and Child Health

Cancer

Mental, Neurological, and Substance Use Disorders

Cardiovascular, Respiratory, and Related Disorders

Major Infectious Diseases

Injury Prevention and Environmental Health

Child and Adolescent Health and Development

Disease Control Priorities: Improving Health and Reducing Poverty

# DISEASE CONTROL PRIORITIES

Budgets constrain choices. Policy analysis helps decision makers achieve the greatest value from limited available resources. In 1993, the World Bank published *Disease Control Priorities in Developing Countries* (*DCP1*), an attempt to systematically assess the cost-effectiveness (value for money) of interventions that would address the major sources of disease burden in low- and middle-income countries. The World Bank's 1993 *World Development Report* on health drew heavily on *DCP1*'s findings to conclude that specific interventions against noncommunicable diseases were cost-effective, even in environments in which substantial burdens of infection and undernutrition persisted.

*DCP2*, published in 2006, updated and extended *DCP1* in several aspects, including explicit consideration of the implications for health systems of expanded intervention coverage. One way that health systems expand intervention coverage is through selected platforms that deliver interventions that require similar logistics but deliver interventions from different packages of conceptually related interventions, for example, against cardiovascular disease. Platforms often provide a more natural unit for investment than do individual interventions. Analysis of the costs of packages and platforms—and of the health improvements they can generate in given epidemiological environments—can help to guide health system investments and development.

*DCP3* differs importantly from *DCP1* and *DCP2* by extending and consolidating the concepts of platforms and packages and by offering explicit consideration of the financial risk protection objective of health systems. In populations lacking access to health insurance or prepaid care, medical expenses that are high relative to income can be impoverishing. Where incomes are low, seemingly inexpensive medical procedures can have catastrophic financial effects. *DCP3* offers an approach to explicitly include financial protection as well as the distribution across income groups of financial and health outcomes resulting from policies (for example, public finance) to increase intervention uptake. The task in all of the *DCP* volumes has been to combine the available science about interventions implemented in very specific locales and under very specific conditions with informed judgment to reach reasonable conclusions about the impact of intervention mixes in diverse environments. *DCP3*'s broad aim is to delineate essential intervention packages and their related delivery platforms to assist decision makers in allocating often tightly constrained budgets so that health system objectives are maximally achieved.

*DCP3*'s nine volumes are being published in 2015, 2016, 2017, and 2018 in an environment in which serious discussion continues about quantifying the sustainable development goal (SDG) for health. *DCP3*'s analyses are well-placed to assist in choosing the means to attain the health SDG and assessing the related costs. Only when these volumes, and the analytic efforts on which they are based, are completed will we be able to explore SDG-related and other broad policy conclusions and generalizations. The final *DCP3* volume will report those conclusions. Each individual volume will provide valuable, specific policy analyses on the full range of interventions, packages, and policies relevant to its health topic.

More than 500 individuals and multiple institutions have contributed to *DCP3*. We convey our acknowledgments elsewhere in this volume. Here we express our particular gratitude to the Bill & Melinda Gates Foundation for its sustained financial support, to the InterAcademy Medical Panel (and its U.S. affiliate, the Institute of Medicine of the National Academy of Sciences), and to World Bank Publications. Each played a critical role in this effort.

*Dean T. Jamison*
*Rachel Nugent*
*Hellen Gelband*
*Susan Horton*
*Prabhat Jha*
*Ramanan Laxminarayan*
*Charles N. Mock*

VOLUME **7**

DISEASE CONTROL PRIORITIES • THIRD EDITION

# Injury Prevention and Environmental Health

EDITORS

Charles N. Mock
Rachel Nugent
Olive Kobusingye
Kirk R. Smith

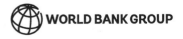 **WORLD BANK GROUP**

# Contents

# Foreword

The world continues to suffer from an enormous burden of morbidity, disability, and premature mortality from injuries and environmental health conditions. Much of this burden is unnecessary and can be prevented by evidence-based, high-impact interventions that can be implemented in all countries, irrespective of income.

Injuries are leading causes of death, responsible for an estimated 5 million deaths and around 9 percent of global mortality. Most of the deaths are in low- and middle-income countries (LMICs). More than 1.2 million people die too young each year because of road traffic injuries. According to the World Health Organization's (WHO) *Global Status Report 2015*, death rates in low-income countries are more than double those in high-income countries. The African region has the highest death rates.

The current situation presents a major challenge to socioeconomic development and has rightly been the focus of attention globally and within all countries. In 2010, a decade for action on road safety was established by the United Nations General Assembly; more recently, in 2015, as part of the Sustainable Development Goals, countries of the world made an ambitious commitment to halving the number of global deaths and injuries due to road traffic crashes by 2020.

There is, therefore, a pressing need for action. This volume of *Disease Control Priorities*, third edition provides an excellent evidence-based guide to policy makers on the approaches and rational choice of interventions to address this challenge. Many of the interventions included in the volume are among the most cost-effective interventions in public health and can make a substantial impact on reducing the health and socioeconomic burden due to injuries, particularly in LMICs. Yet, current progress is too slow. As highlighted in this volume and documented in the *Global Status Report*, implementation of the key public health measures is disappointingly low. Countries, particularly LMICs, need to do more. Policy makers should seriously consider the recommendations of this volume when they develop their own essential package of interventions, which is one of the three key pathways to achieve universal health coverage. International organizations and development agencies should increase their support to low-income countries to make this possible.

This volume focuses on another key challenge to public health across the globe. Environmental causes lead to more than 8 million deaths per year; outdoor and indoor air pollution accounts for more than 5 million of these deaths per year. Climate change, which results from unsustainable policies in many sectors, exacerbates air pollution threats and causes additional morbidity and mortality. Unsafe sanitation and lack of safe water and hygiene cause an estimated 1.4 million deaths, almost all in LMICs.

Although the enormous burden and serious health challenges caused by environmental risk factors are evident, surveillance and systematic monitoring of the magnitude of the risks and their health impacts are severely limited in many countries. The data gaps are particularly serious for air quality and air pollution levels. Increasing awareness among high-level government officials and policy makers on the seriousness of environmental risks and the pressing need to take effective multisectoral action should be a key priority for all countries. This volume makes a strong case for advocacy and for strengthening commitment, and it provides clear policy advice on strategic directions to consider.

Despite the fact that there are limited economic analysis studies on some environmental health conditions, there is clear evidence for a range of interventions recommended in the volume that are cost-effective or supported by favorable cost-benefit ratios. Implementing them will have a considerable impact on reducing environmental health risks and preventing a broad range of common communicable and noncommunicable conditions responsible for a major proportion of global disease burden and premature mortality. In addition to their desirable health effects, many of these interventions will also have important non-health outcomes that may be part of the priorities of the non-health sectors involved.

An important challenge to health and development is climate change. Although the importance of climate change challenges is increasingly recognized, and tackling them is becoming a global priority, addressing the health consequences is not receiving adequate attention. Policy makers at the highest levels of government and in different sectors need to be made fully aware of the seriousness of the health dimensions and the effective approaches to mitigate them.

Finally, making a difference in addressing injuries and environmental health risks will require solid commitments from all parts of governments, particularly sectors such as transport, energy, industry, agriculture, housing, and waste management. The health sector will have to demonstrate leadership in evidence-based advocacy, governance, technical support, and surveillance. The need to act is highlighted by a range of goals and targets included in the sustainable development agenda. Countries that initiate effective action now will benefit from improved health and realize considerable health care savings.

Ala Alwan, MD, FRCP, FFPH
*Regional Director Emeritus,*
*WHO Eastern Mediterranean Region*

# Preface

The fields of injury prevention and environmental health address diverse health problems that arise from exposure to outside forces, such as chemicals and other toxins, infectious agents, kinetic energy, and thermal energy. The health problems addressed by these fields include the following:

- Unintentional injuries, such as road traffic accidents, falls, burns, and drowning
- Intentional injuries, such as interpersonal violence
- Diseases, such as those caused or aggravated by exposure to airborne and waterborne pollutants
- Occupational hazards, such as injuries and diseases caused or aggravated by workplace toxins,
- Effects of climate change due to human greenhouse emissions, such as enhancement of waterborne infectious diseases.

The conditions and risks encompassed in these fields account for more than 12 million deaths per year—21 percent—of the annual global total of 56 million deaths.

Most of these conditions and risks have not been effectively addressed globally; in recent years, however, some have received increased attention. This *Injury Prevention and Environmental Health* volume of *Disease Control Priorities*, third edition (*DCP3*), contributes to the understanding of how to address these health problems in the following ways:

- Elucidating the health burden of these conditions
- Documenting trends in the health burden at different phases of national development
- Identifying the most cost-effective and cost-beneficial interventions
- Describing policies and platforms that can widely and effectively deliver these interventions.

This volume looks at several types of policy approaches to reduce the burden of ill health from environmental and occupational risks and injuries. Unlike the other *DCP3* volumes, most of the actions proposed in this volume speak directly to non-health sectors, where a substantial portion of disease and injury prevention policies and programs needs to occur. These actions include fiscal and intersectoral policies, such as taxes and subsidies; regulations; and policies that affect infrastructure, the built environment, and product design. Also included are information, education, and communication initiatives to promote behavioral changes; these initiatives leverage a range of vehicles, from mass media campaigns to one-on-one counseling. A second major difference from other *DCP3* volumes is that the economic evidence supporting the actions described in this volume is primarily benefit-cost analyses—the benefits and costs may occur outside of the health sector and must be accounted for in common monetized units. We include two extended cost-effectiveness analyses (ECEAs) that indicate policies that provide strong financial risk protection for individuals and households.

Most of the policies and interventions discussed in this volume have not been fully implemented in high-income countries (HICs); their implementation in low- and middle-income countries (LMICs) is substantially more incomplete. More complete implementation would help to reduce the disproportionately high rates of death and disability from these conditions in LMICs. Doing so could avert over seven million premature deaths annually from environmental and occupational exposures and injuries in LMICs.

The goal of the editors and authors of *Injury Prevention and Environmental Health* is to provide the requisite evidence-based rationale and guidance to increase implementation of effective strategies to prevent injuries and lower environmental risks in countries at all economic levels. We hope to stimulate increased implementation of proven effective strategies that have not yet been applied widely, let alone universally. We also seek to focus attention on the need to identify new strategies that would be particularly effective in LMICs. Finally, we wish to highlight the potentially substantial health hazards of climate change. This particular environmental issue will likely become increasingly preeminent in the 21st century. The resultant health problems, including food and water insecurity, may rival those of other major risk factors. The toll could be especially tragic among the world's poorest people. Enhancing the understanding of climate change and identifying effective interventions are likely to become major challenges in the next generation.

We thank the following individuals who provided valuable comments and assistance to this effort: Elizabeth Brouwer, Kristen Danforth, Mary Fisk, Rumit Pancholi, Jinyuan Qi, Shamelle Richards, and Carlos Rossel. The authors also thank the reviewers organized by the National Academy of Medicine and the InterAcademy Medical Panel listed separately in this volume. We especially thank Brianne Adderley for her hard work in keeping this large endeavor well organized.

*Charles N. Mock*
*Rachel Nugent*
*Olive Kobusingye*
*Kirk R. Smith*

# Abbreviations

| | |
|---|---|
| ALRI | acute lower respiratory infection |
| BCA | benefit-cost analysis |
| BCR | benefit-cost ratio |
| BPL | below poverty line |
| CAMx | Comprehensive Air Quality Model with Extensions (Eulerian photochemical dispersion model) |
| CATS | Community Approach to Total Sanitation |
| CCT | conditional cash transfer |
| CDD | community-driven development |
| CEA | cost-effectiveness analysis |
| CERC | Central Electricity Regulatory Authority |
| CI | confidence interval |
| CIRCLE | Climate Impact Research and Response Coordination for a Larger Europe |
| CLTS | community-led total sanitation |
| CO | carbon monoxide |
| COPD | chronic obstructive pulmonary disease |
| CPLS | cost per life saved |
| CRA | comparative risk assessment |
| CTC | Communities that Care |
| CVD | cardiovascular disease |
| DALY | disability-adjusted life year |
| DHS | Demographic and Health Survey |
| ECEA | extended cost-effectiveness analysis |
| ESI | Economics of Sanitation Initiative |
| EU | European Union |
| FGD | flue-gas desulfurization |
| GACC | Global Alliance for Clean Cookstoves |
| GBD | Global Burden of Disease |
| GDP | gross domestic product |
| GIU | Give It Up |
| GNI | gross national income |
| GNP | gross national product |

| | |
|---|---|
| GPOBA | Global Program for Output-Based-Aid |
| GRP | gross regional product |
| GW | gigawatt |
| | |
| HAP | household air pollution |
| HAPIT | Household Air Pollution Intervention Tool |
| HICs | high-income countries |
| HLY | healthy life-year |
| HRTWS | Human Right to Safe Drinking Water and Sanitation |
| HWTS | household water treatment and storage |
| | |
| IAQG | Indoor Air Quality Guidelines |
| ICER | incremental cost-effectiveness ratio |
| IER | integrated-exposure response |
| IHD | ischemic heart disease |
| IHDS | Indian Human Development Survey |
| IHME | Institute for Health Metrics and Evaluation |
| IMAGE | Intervention with Microfinance for AIDS and Gender Equity |
| IOM | Institute of Medicine |
| IPV | intimate partner violence |
| ISBI | International Society for Burn Injuries |
| | |
| JMP | Joint Monitoring Programme |
| | |
| kWh | kilowatt-hour |
| | |
| LC | lung cancer |
| LICs | low-income countries |
| LMICs | low- and middle-income countries |
| LPG | liquefied petroleum gas |
| | |
| MDGs | Millennium Development Goals |
| mg/m$^3$ | milligrams per cubic meter |
| MHM | menstrual hygiene management |
| MICS | Multiple Indicator Cluster Survey |
| MICs | middle-income countries |
| MW | megawatt |
| | |
| NCAP | New Car Assessment Program |
| NCDs | noncommunicable diseases |
| NGO | nongovernmental organization |
| NISP | National Improved Stove Program |
| NOx | oxides of nitrogen |
| | |
| OBA | output-based aid |
| OECD | Organisation for Economic Co-operation and Development |
| OOP | out of pocket |
| OR | odds ratio |
| OSH | occupational safety and health |
| | |
| PFD | personal flotation device |
| PIC | products of incomplete combustion |
| PM | particulate matter |
| PPPHW | Global Public-Private Partnerships for Handwashing |
| PRB | Powder River Basin |
| | |
| QALY | quality-adjusted life year |

| | |
|---|---|
| RCT | randomized controlled trial |
| RHS | Reproductive Health Survey |
| RTI | road traffic injury |
| | |
| SDGs | Sustainable Development Goals |
| SERC | State Electricity Regulatory Commission |
| SFU | solid fuel use |
| SLTS | School-Led Total Sanitation |
| $SO_2$ | sulfur dioxide |
| SPA | Service Provision Assessment |
| STHs | soil-transmitted helminths |
| STIs | sexually transmitted infections |
| SV | Smokeless Village |
| swFGD | seawater flue-gas desulfurization |
| | |
| TSSM | Total Sanitation and Sanitation Marketing |
| | |
| UMICs | upper-middle-income countries |
| UN | United Nations |
| UNICEF | United Nations Children's Fund |
| UNRSC | United Nations Road Safety Collaboration |
| | |
| VSL | value per statistical life |
| | |
| WASH | water, sanitation, and hygiene |
| WASH-BAT | Water, Sanitation, and Hygiene-Bottleneck Analysis Tool |
| wFGD | wet limestone flue-gas desulfurization |
| WHO | World Health Organization |
| WTP | willingness to pay |
| | |
| YLDs | years lived with disability |
| YLLs | years of life lost |

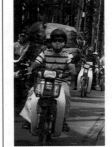

# Chapter 1

# Injury Prevention and Environmental Health: Key Messages from *Disease Control Priorities*, Third Edition

Charles N. Mock, Kirk R. Smith, Olive Kobusingye, Rachel Nugent, Safa Abdalla, Rajeev B. Ahuja, Spenser S. Apramian, Abdulgafoor M. Bachani, Mark A. Bellis, Alexander Butchart, Linda Cantley, Claire Chase, Mark Cullen, Nazila Dabestani, Kristie L. Ebi, Xiagming Fang, G. Gururaj, Sarath Guttikunda, Jeremy J. Hess, Connie Hoe, Guy Hutton, Adnan A. Hyder, Rebecca Ivers, Dean T. Jamison, Puja Jawahar, Lisa Keay, Carol Levin, Jiawen Liao, David Mackie, Kabir Malik, David Meddings, Nam Phuong Nguyen, Robyn Norton, Zachary Olson, Ian Partridge, Margie Peden, Ajay Pillarisetti, Fazlur Rahman, Mark L. Rosenberg, John A. Staples, Stéphane Verguet, Catherine L. Ward, and David A. Watkins

## VOLUME SUMMARY

*Injury Prevention and Environmental Health* identifies essential prevention strategies and related policies that address substantial population health needs, are cost-effective, and are feasible to implement. This chapter summarizes and critically assesses the volume's four key findings.

- There is a large burden of death and disability from injuries and environmental health conditions. Worldwide, injuries result in more than 5 million premature deaths per year out of a global total of 56 million deaths (based on widely used estimates). There are also large numbers of deaths attributable to risk factors related to noninjury occupational exposures (560,000); inadequate access to clean water, sanitation, and hygiene (1.4 million); and air pollution (5.5 million). The vast majority of these deaths are in low- and middle-income countries.

- Risk factors for deaths from these diseases vary with stages of national development in ways that can be understood and used in designing prevention strategies.

- A range of interventions could effectively address these problems; many of these interventions are among the most cost-effective and cost-beneficial of all interventions used to prevent disease.

- This chapter synthesizes the volume's prevention strategies to identify an effective essential package of interventions and policies, most of which have been inadequately applied on a global scale. Better implementation of these interventions and policies would help bring down the high rates of death and disability

Corresponding author: Charles N. Mock, Departments of Surgery and Global Health, University of Washington, Seattle, Washington, United States; cmock@uw.edu.

from injury and environmental and occupational risks in low- and middle-income countries (LMICs) toward the lower rates in high-income countries. Doing so could avert more than 7 million deaths annually from environmental and occupational exposures and injuries.

## INTRODUCTION

*Injury Prevention and Environmental Health* identifies essential prevention strategies and related policies that address substantial population health needs and that are cost-effective and feasible to implement. This volume addresses diverse conditions that arise from exposure to outside forces, such as chemicals and toxins, kinetic energy, or thermal energy. These conditions require similar policy approaches to reducing risk and mandate involvement of multiple sectors. Included in this group of conditions are injuries attributable to unintentional mechanisms (road traffic crashes, falls, burns, and drowning); injuries attributable to intentional mechanisms (interpersonal violence); disorders caused by or aggravated by exposure to airborne toxins (air pollution); occupational issues (injuries and disorders caused by or aggravated by toxins in the workplace); and waterborne infectious diseases. This volume focuses exclusively on interventions to prevent these conditions. Treatment for health conditions resulting from injury and environmental risk factors is covered in other volumes of the third edition of *Disease Control Priorities* (*DCP3*), as are immunizations and prevention of suicide (Black, Laxminarayan, and others 2016; Black, Levin, and others 2016; Bundy and others 2017; Debas and others 2015; Mock and others 2015; Patel and others 2015; Patel and others 2016; Prabhakaran and others 2017).

In this review, we identify several key messages. First, there is a large health burden from injury, occupational risk factors, air pollution, unclean water, and poor sanitation. These conditions are major global health problems to which inadequate attention has been directed. Second, these disorders and the risk factors that cause them have predictable patterns across stages of national development. Understanding these patterns can assist with the planning of prevention efforts. Third, cost-effective and cost-beneficial interventions that can address these conditions already exist and are in established use in most high-income countries (HICs). In most low- and middle-income countries (LMICs), these interventions have been implemented only to a modest extent or not at all. On the basis of these interventions' cost-effectiveness and their potential to lower the disease burden, we propose a package of policy interventions (box 1.1).

---

**Box 1.1**

### From the Series Editors of *Disease Control Priorities*, Third Edition

Budgets constrain choices. Policy analysis helps decision makers achieve the greatest value from limited resources. In 1993, the World Bank published *Disease Control Priorities in Developing Countries* (*DCP1*), which sought to assess systematically the cost-effectiveness (value for money) of interventions addressing the major sources of disease burden in low- and middle-income countries (Jamison and others 1993). The World Bank's *World Development Report* 1993 drew heavily on *DCP1*'s findings to conclude that specific interventions to combat noncommunicable diseases were cost-effective, even in environments with substantial burdens of infection and undernutrition (World Bank 1993).

*Disease Control Priorities in Developing Countries,* second edition (*DCP2*) published in 2006, updated and extended *DCP1* in several respects, giving explicit consideration to the implications for health systems of expanded intervention coverage (Jamison and others 2006). One way to expand coverage of health interventions is through platforms for interventions that require similar logistics but that address heterogeneous health problems. Platforms often provide a more natural unit for investment than do individual interventions, but conventional health economics has offered little understanding of how to make choices across platforms. Analysis of the costs of packages and platforms—and of the

*box continues next page*

**Box 1.1** (continued)

health improvements they can generate in given epidemiological environments—can help guide health system investments and development.

*DCP3* introduces the notion of packages of interventions. Whereas platforms contain logistically related sets of interventions, packages contain conceptually related ones. The 21 packages developed in the nine volumes of *DCP3* include those for surgery and cardiovascular disease, for example. In addition, *DCP3* explicitly considers health systems' objective of financial risk protection. In populations lacking access to health insurance or prepaid care, medical expenses that are high relative to income can be impoverishing. Where incomes are low, seemingly inexpensive medical procedures can have catastrophic financial effects. *DCP3* considers financial protection and the distribution across income groups as outcomes resulting from policies (for example, public finance) to increase intervention uptake and improve delivery quality. All of the volumes seek to combine the available science about interventions implemented in specific locales and conditions with informed judgment to reach reasonable conclusions about the impact of intervention mixes in diverse environments. *DCP3*'s broad aim is to delineate essential intervention packages—such as those for injury prevention and environmental health in this

volume—and their related delivery platforms. This information is intended to assist decision makers in allocating often tightly constrained budgets and in achieving health system objectives.

Four of *DCP3*'s nine volumes were published in 2015 and 2016, and the remaining five will appear in 2017 and 2018. The volumes appear in an environment in which serious discussion continues about quantifying and achieving the Sustainable Development Goal (SDG) for health (United Nations 2015). *DCP3*'s analyses are well placed to assist in choosing the means with which to attain the health SDG and assessing the related costs. These volumes, and the analytic efforts on which they are based, will enable researchers to explore SDG-related and other broad policy conclusions and generalizations. The final volume will report those conclusions. Each individual volume provides specific policy analyses on the full range of interventions, packages, and policies relevant to its health topic.

*Dean T. Jamison*
*Rachel Nugent*
*Hellen Gelband*
*Susan Horton*
*Prabhat Jha*
*Ramanan Laxminarayan*
*Charles N. Mock*

## KEY MESSAGES

### Disease Burden Addressable by Injury Prevention and Environmental Health

The different topics examined take advantage of one or more widely used data sources, such as the World Health Organization (WHO) Global Health Estimates or the Global Burden of Disease (GBD) study.

Other global datasets may show slightly different relationships, but the patterns would be similar.[1]

### Injury

Injuries include those arising from unintentional causes (such as road traffic crashes, falls, and burns) and intentional causes (such as suicide and violence). In 2012, injuries altogether caused more than 5 million premature deaths globally (table 1.1).[2]

The vast majority (85 percent) of these deaths were in LMICs. The annual incidence of mortality from injury is considerably higher in LMICs (76 per 100,000) compared with HICs (58 per 100,000) (WHO 2016). In most LMICs, half or more of road traffic crash deaths happen to vulnerable road users, such as motorcyclists, bicyclists, and especially pedestrians. Injuries to vehicle occupants predominate in most HICs. Other leading causes of unintentional injury are falls, drowning, and burns. The leading cause of intentional injury deaths is suicide. Homicide is the next leading cause, followed at a distant third by deaths directly due to war and other forms of collective violence (Watkins, Dabestani, Mock, and others 2017; WHO 2016). Interpersonal violence is also an important yet under-recognized risk factor for high-risk behaviors, such as unsafe sex, smoking, and substance abuse, and, through these behaviors, for some

**Table 1.1** Injuries: Deaths by Cause, All Ages, Both Sexes, 2012

| | Low- and Middle-Income Countries 2012 | | High-Income Countries 2012 | |
| --- | --- | --- | --- | --- |
| | Total deaths (thousands) | Percent of all deaths | Total deaths (thousands) | Percent of all deaths |
| All causes | 44,200 | 100 | 11,700 | 100 |
| Injuries (unintentional and intentional) | 4,400 | 10 | 750 | 6 |
| *Unintentional injuries* | **3,220** | **7** | **510** | **4** |
| Road traffic injuries | 1,140 | 3 | 120 | 1 |
| Other unintentional injuries | 750 | 2 | 180 | 2 |
| Falls | 580 | 1 | 120 | 1 |
| Drowning | 340 | 1 | 40 | 0 |
| Fire, heat, and hot substances | 250 | 1 | 20 | 0 |
| Poisoning | 160 | 0 | 30 | 0 |
| Exposure to forces of nature | 2 | 0 | 0 | 0 |
| *Intentional injuries* | **1,190** | **3** | **240** | **2** |
| Self-harm | 610 | 1 | 200 | 2 |
| Interpersonal violence | 460 | 1 | 40 | 0 |
| Collective violence and legal intervention | 120 | 0 | 0 | 0 |

*Source:* WHO Global Health Estimates 2012 (WHO 2016).
*Note:* Not all totals are exact due to rounding.

communicable and noncommunicable diseases, as well as for mental health conditions, including anxiety disorders, depression, and suicidal ideation.

## Occupational Risks

Occupational and environmental (water and air) risks lead to a substantial health burden. In the usual estimates of global disease burden, this burden is reflected in disease-specific estimates; for example, unsafe water leads to deaths from diarrhea, which are reported in the main global disease burden estimates (Watkins, Dabestani, Mock, and others 2017; WHO 2016). Additional analyses discussed later show the burden from the risk factors themselves.

Occupationally related deaths and disabilities include on-the-job injuries and exposure to chemicals (such as pesticides, solvents, and heavy metals); heat; and noise; among other risk factors. An estimated 720,000 deaths occur annually from occupational exposures globally, 79 percent of which are in LMICs. The largest contributors to this burden are injuries and exposure to particulate matter, gases, and fumes (which contribute to respiratory and cardiovascular disease and cancers) (table 1.2). Occupational ergonomic factors and exposure to noise do not cause mortality, but they contribute significantly to disability.

Notwithstanding the global estimates in table 1.2, estimates and sources of overall burden of occupational deaths and disabilities are not well known for many countries. Part of the problem is lack of reporting on occupational issues, which is aggravated by the fact that most people in LMICs work in the informal sector, for which accurate, or sometimes any, statistics are not kept. Occupational health problems encompass some that are long-standing, such as agricultural injuries. Others arise or are aggravated by changes in manufacturing and supply chain practices globally as more dangerous jobs are transferred to LMICs, especially to locations with limited environmental and safety safeguards, and are performed by people with lower levels of training and who usually have limited or no access to protective equipment (Watkins, Dabestani, Mock, and others 2017).

## Water, Sanitation, and Hygiene

Inadequate access to safe water, sanitation, and hygiene (WASH) was estimated to result in about 1.4 million deaths globally in 2013, virtually all (more than 99 percent) in LMICs (table 1.3). WASH-related deaths account for a large proportion of diarrheal disease and intestinal infectious diseases, almost all among children. The major attribual factors are unsafe water sources (1,240,000 deaths globally), unsafe sanitation (820,000 deaths), and lack of hygiene (especially availability of handwashing with soap: 520,000 deaths), with an uncertain degree of overlap in attributable deaths among

**Table 1.2** Occupational Risks: Attributable Deaths by Cause, All Ages, Both Sexes, 2013

| | Deaths (Thousands) | |
| --- | --- | --- |
| | Low- and middle-income countries 2013 | High-income countries 2013 |
| *Total attributable deaths* | 23,800 | 7,000 |
| *Total environmental and occupational risks* | 7,420 | 760 |
| *Occupational risks* | **570** | **140** |
| Occupational asthmagens | 50 | 0 |
| Occupational carcinogens | 190 | 110 |
| Occupational ergonomic factors | 0 | 0 |
| Occupational injuries | 140 | 20 |
| Occupational noise | 0 | 0 |
| Occupational particulate matter, gases, and fumes | 200 | 10 |

*Source:* Global Burden of Disease (GBD) 2013 Study (IHME 2016).
*Note:* Each of the six major occupational hazards is listed as a subcategory of "occupational risks," which are a subset of "total environmental and occupational risks," which are a subset of "total attributable deaths." Data from GBD 2013 were used because similar data were unavailable from the WHO Global Health Estimates. GBD 2010 and GBD 2015 estimates are somewhat different from GBD 2013. Not all totals are exact due to rounding.

**Table 1.3** Environmental Risks: Attributable Deaths by Cause, All Ages, Both Sexes, 2013

| | Deaths (Thousands) | |
| --- | --- | --- |
| | Low- and middle-income countries 2013 | High-income countries 2013 |
| *Total attributable deaths* | 23,800 | 7,000 |
| *Total environmental and occupational risks* | 7,420 | 760 |
| *Unsafe water, sanitation, and handwashing* | **1,390** | **10** |
| No handwashing with soap | 510 | 10 |
| Unsafe sanitation | 820 | 0 |
| Unsafe water source | 1,240 | 10 |
| *Air pollution* | **4,990** | **540** |
| Ambient ozone pollution | 180 | 40 |
| Ambient particulate matter pollution | 2,430 | 500 |
| Household air pollution from solid fuels | 2,880 | 10 |

*Source:* Global Burden of Disease (GBD) 2013 Study (IHME 2016).
*Note:* Each of the major environmental hazards is listed as a subcategory of the bolded categories. Data from GBD 2013 were used because similar data were unavailable from the WHO Global Health Estimates. There is an unknown degree of overlap between the impacts across the air pollution and unsafe water categories, which is not addressed here.

these causes. Water and sanitation were the topics of Millennium Development Goal 7 and have received considerable attention over the past several decades. As a result, there have been significant advances in access to clean water and improved sanitation, with related decreases in burden. In addition, better nutrition and rehydration therapy have reduced case fatality substantially. The total number of deaths estimated as attributable to inadequate WASH has declined by 49 percent, from 2.7 million deaths in 1990 to 1.4 million deaths in 2013 (Watkins, Dabestani, Mock, and others 2017). Despite these improvements, inadequate access to WASH remains a major health problem, accounting for approximately 43 percent of under-five mortality in South and South-East Asia and Sub-Saharan Africa (Humphrey 2009; Petri and Miller 2008).

**Air Pollution**
Exposure to airborne pollutants in ambient and household settings was estimated to result in more than

5 million deaths globally in 2013 (table 1.3). In disease burden estimates, air pollution contributes a significant proportion of deaths attributable to respiratory infections; chronic obstructive pulmonary disease; cerebrovascular disease; ischemic heart disease; and cancers of the trachea, bronchus, and lung. The forms of air pollution evaluated were ambient particulate matter pollution (approximately 2.9 million deaths globally) and household air pollution from solid fuels (approximately 2.9 million deaths globally) in the form of particle and ozone pollution, although there are other categories that have not yet been assessed globally. Overall, 90 percent of air pollution deaths are in LMICs. However, because use of solid cooking fuels in households is confined almost entirely to LMICs, essentially all impacts occur there. Ambient particulate matter air pollution occurs in rural and urban areas and is related to a variety of emissions sources, including motorized transport, power plants, industry, road and construction dust, brick kilns, and garbage burning. Household air pollution occurs primarily in less urbanized areas and is related to use of solid fuels for cooking and heating. It also is a major source of ambient pollution, causing at least a quarter of ambient pollution exposures in India and China, for example (Chafe and others 2014; Lelieveld and others 2015). Thus, perhaps 16 to 31 percent of the burden attributed to ambient pollution actually started in households, although this burden is not yet well characterized. Ambient air pollution is estimated to account for a larger proportion of cardiovascular and cerebrovascular diseases, while household air pollution accounts for a larger proportion of chronic and acute respiratory disease, the latter affecting children (Watkins, Dabestani, Mock, and others 2017).

Taken together, the conditions and risks covered in this review comprise more than 12 million deaths per year, not accounting for possible overlaps among different categories of attributable causes. Climate change contributes a small portion of the current burden of climate-sensitive health outcomes but, given its trajectory, will become increasingly important in future decades.

## Environmental and Injury Risk Transitions

All comparisons in this section rely on the widely used GBD 2015 dataset—other global datasets may show slightly different absolute levels and relationships, but the patterns will be similar.[3,4] A classic portrayal of mortality trends during the national development process is the "mortality transition" that documents shifts over time in causes of death (figure 1.1) (Omran 1971).

This portrayal gives the false impression, however, that the impact of noncommunicable disease increases with development, which is not the case at large scale. For comparisons of the health status of populations, the correct calculation is the age-standardized version. The age-standardized version is the true *epidemiological transition*, which takes account of the younger age structure in poor countries, as shown in figure 1.2 (Smith and Ezzati 2005). Age-standardized data provide a more accurate illustration of the comparative health of someone going through the life course in each region, what most people consider the important comparison of health status across populations. In contrast to what is shown in the mortality transition (figure 1.1), in figure 1.2 all general disease categories—communicable (category I), noncommunicable (category II), and injuries (category III)—actually decline across income groups after age standardization, substantially so in categories I and III (communicable and injuries), but definitively for noncommunicable as well. Thus, as is uncomfortably true for many of life's conditions, it is generally better to live in a richer rather than a poorer society.

Many factors other than income affect health, and many of these are amenable to policy. Policy, in turn, is affected by factors other than income, although income remains one primary determinant. All analyses in this section use age-standardized deaths per capita to normalize across the four World Bank income regions and aggregate large categories of disease and risk that tend to obfuscate individual differences. It should be noted that higher resolution by more subregions, specific diseases, or even by country might show subtleties not revealed by comparison across only four income regions. Mortality trends are not reflective of the entire picture of health because nonfatal injury and illness also affect health status. The aggregated patterns shown in this section, however, show similar trends when disability-adjusted life years (DALYs) are used.

As shown in figure 1.3, the overall health impacts from environmental and occupational exposures and from injuries tend to decline across country income groups after age standardization. Examined in more detail, however, the trends for environmental risks can be divided into three categories in what has been termed the *environmental risk transition* (Smith 1990).

### Traditional Environmental Health Risks

Traditional environmental health risks (poor food, air, water, and sanitation at the household level) tend to decline with economic development, but they do so at varying rates depending on policy and the degree of income and education equity in societies. This link to income is observed in figure 1.4, which shows the

**Figure 1.1** Crude Death Rates across Income Categories for All Category I, II, and III Diseases, All Ages, 2015

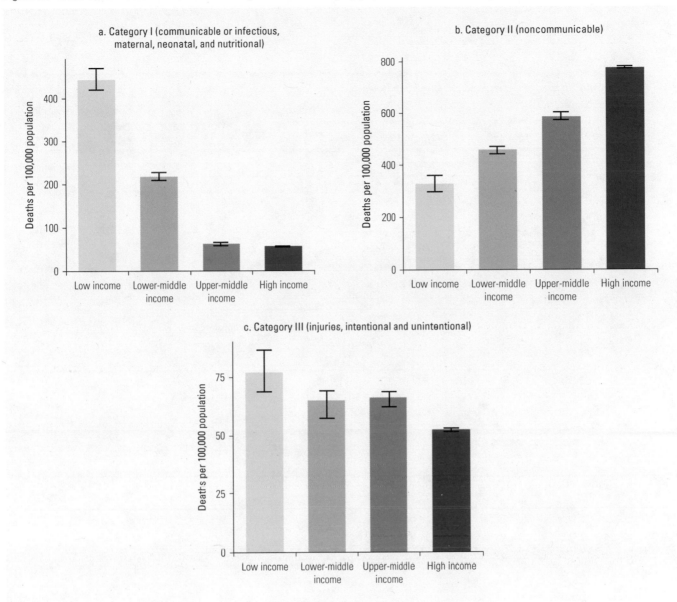

burden from household air pollution and from poor water, sanitation, and hygiene steadily declining across income groups. Although much diminished in rich countries, these risks still dominate global environmental health burdens today.

**Modern Environmental Health Risks**
Modern environmental health risks from industrialization, urbanization, vehicularization, and agricultural modernization tend to rise at first during the development process, then peak and fall at higher levels of income and education. Again, the height these risks

reach and the point at which they turn downward are strongly determined by preventive policy. Figure 1.5 illustrates how the burdens from ambient particle pollution, environmental tobacco smoke, and ambient ozone air pollution rise and then fall with development.

**Global Environmental Health Risks**
The imposition of a set of global environmental risks—exemplified by release of greenhouse pollutants and including other global environmental stressors, such as biodiversity loss—has risen with development. The notable exception is reductions of stratospheric

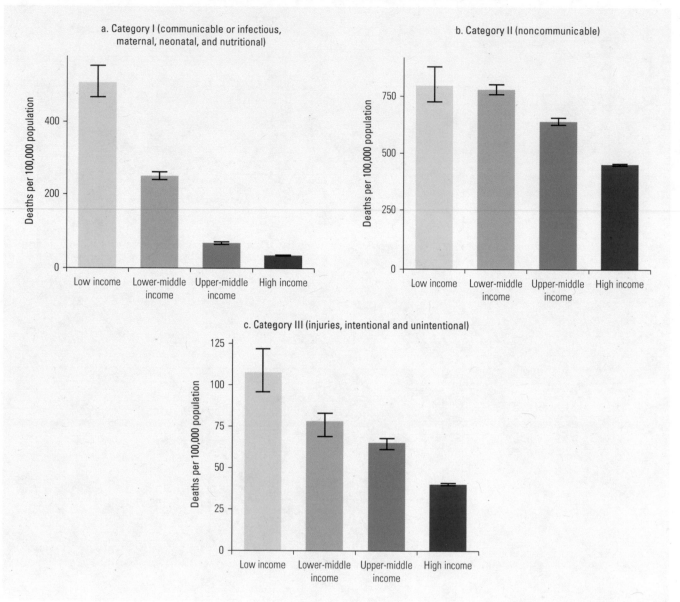

ozone–depleting pollutants under the Montreal Protocol, which is one of the major examples of successful international policy. Such global hazards do not dominate current environmental health burdens, but as these threats continue to rise, they may dominate health burdens later in the century unless strong actions are implemented. The trends for risks from greenhouse gas emissions are illustrated in figure 1.6 for the two most important gases, carbon dioxide and methane (Smith, Desai, and others 2013).

In summary, as shown in figure 1.7, all environmental risk factors taken together declined over the development spectrum because of the strong decline in traditional risks. In general, traditional risks are faced mostly at the household level in lower-income countries, where required behavioral changes and low access to resources are barriers to interventions. Modern risks are commonly seen at the community level because they derive from larger-scale social organization, including industrialization and urban design. Global risks arise at larger geographic and organizational scales, with most health impacts generally occurring in populations that have contributed little to concentrations of greenhouse gases in the atmosphere.

*Is there an injury risk transition?* Panel c of figure 1.2 illustrates that the impact of all forms of injuries declines with development. A question, however, is whether

examination of individual injury categories reveals different patterns, recognizing that reporting bias is present for many types of injury. Mortality from, in declining number, road traffic injuries, falls, drowning, fires, occupational injuries, and snakebites (surprisingly prevalent in poor areas) appears generally to follow the classic traditional risk form, declining steadily with development (figure 1.8). Mortality from interpersonal violence and poisoning may also follow the traditional form, but trends are not clear at this resolution (four income groups only; figure 1.9). Thus, there is no clear transition from one to another type of injury with development, but rather a steady decline across essentially all categories examined here as protective policies and infrastructure are put in place and daily work and living environments evolve.

Transition frameworks are common in development discussion (for example, demographic, nutrition, and inequality transitions) but should primarily be considered tools for parsing observed patterns rather than generating normative predictions of what will happen. They provide a structure for categorizing changes that occur during development and for designing policies that avoid the worst trends and enhance the best ones. They are not destiny but analytic tools.

It is important to be aware that the relationships in this chapter are cross-sectional and thus cannot take into account the different world situation in place when currently developed regions were developing as compared with poor countries today. Nevertheless, they provide instructive ways to understand and organize current risk patterns.

**Figure 1.3** Age-Standardized Mortality, 2015, from All Occupational and Environmental Risk Factors Examined in the Global Burden of Disease Study 2015

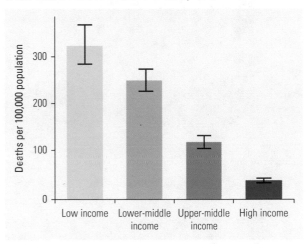

*Note:* This figure is based on summed impacts from estimates of the impacts of separate risk factors. It thus includes contributions from communicable diseases (category I), noncommunicable diseases (category II), and injuries (category III). This figure contains no contribution from global risks, but as shown in the vertical axis of figure 1.6, global risks are relatively small at present.

**Figure 1.4** Age-Standardized Trends in Mortality Risk for Household Air Pollution and for Poor Water, Sanitation, and Hygiene, 2015

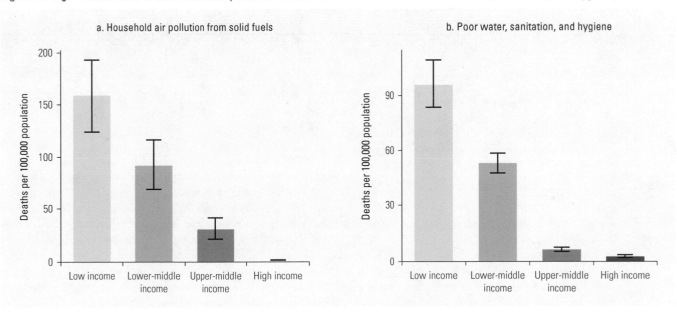

**Figure 1.5** Age-Standardized Trends in Mortality Risk for Ambient Particle Pollution, Environmental (Secondhand) Tobacco Smoke, and Ambient Ozone Pollution, 2015

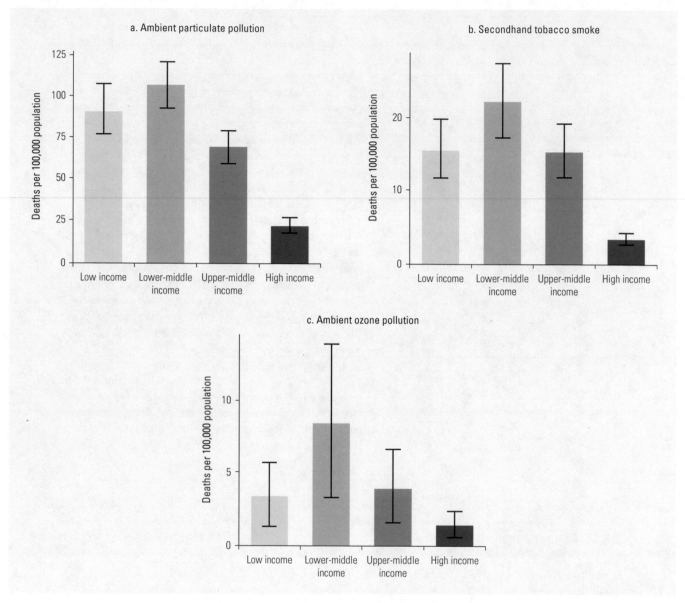

## ECONOMIC EVALUATION OF INJURY PREVENTION AND ENVIRONMENTAL INTERVENTIONS

Economic evaluation aims to inform decision making by quantifying tradeoffs between resource inputs required for alternative strategies and resulting outcomes. Four main approaches are discussed in box 1.2.

Economic evaluation of the interventions that address the conditions in this review has not been conducted to the same extent as for many other health problems (Watkins, Dabestani, Nugent, and Levin 2017), in part because many of the interventions are population-based policies and regulations that use multisectoral approaches, which are inherently less straightforward to study using economic methods that are more readily applied to individual-level health interventions. In addition, several of the environmental interventions have notable non-health outcomes that are often difficult to cost, such as time savings, reduction in black carbon emissions, and lower pressure on forests from shifts in household fuels.

Nevertheless, there is an accumulating body of evidence that many of the interventions addressing injury and environmental health are very cost-effective

**Figure 1.6** Trends of Global Environmental Health Risk by Income Using WHO Regions

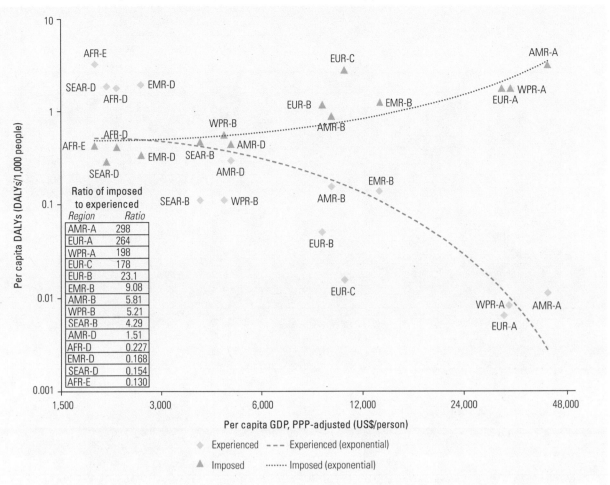

| Region | Ratio |
|--------|-------|
| AMR-A | 298 |
| EUR-A | 264 |
| WPR-A | 198 |
| EUR-C | 178 |
| EUR-B | 23.1 |
| EMR-B | 9.08 |
| AMR-B | 5.81 |
| WPR-B | 5.21 |
| SEAR-B | 4.29 |
| AMR-D | 1.51 |
| AFR-D | 0.227 |
| EMR-D | 0.168 |
| SEAR-D | 0.154 |
| AFR-E | 0.130 |

*Source:* Smith, Desai, and others 2013.
*Note:* DALY = disability-adjusted life year; GDP = gross domestic product; PPP = purchasing power parity. In key, AFR = African Region; AMR = American Region; EMR = Eastern Mediterranean Region; EUR = European Region; SEAR = South-East Asia Region; WPR = Western Pacific Region. A–E refer to specific groupings of countries by mortality strata within each region. The trend for "experiencing" the risk is inverse to the trend for "imposing the risk." The latter is based on parsing the total estimated global burden from climate change according to each region's contribution to emissions of carbon dioxide and methane over time—its natural debt.

**Figure 1.7** Deaths from All Environmental Risk Factors, Age Standardized, 2015

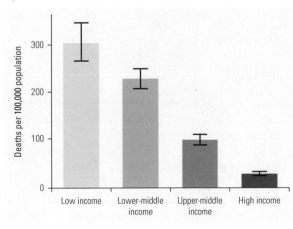

in LMICs. For example, studies in LMICs have shown that speed bumps at high-risk junctions cost US$12 per DALY averted (in 2012 US$), improved enforcement of traffic laws costs US$84 per DALY averted, and enforcing motorcycle helmet use costs US$615 per DALY averted (Bishai and Hyder 2006; Ditsuwan and others 2013; Watkins, Dabestani, Nugent, and Levin 2017). Swimming lessons and improved supervision of children to prevent drowning cost US$27 and US$256 per DALY averted, respectively (Rahman and others 2012; Watkins, Dabestani, Nugent, and Levin 2017).

In general, an intervention with a cost-effectiveness ratio of one to three times the per capita gross domestic product of a country is considered cost-effective (Newall, Jit, and Hutubessy 2014; Watkins, Dabestani, Nugent, and Levin 2017). Thus, for almost all countries, the examples

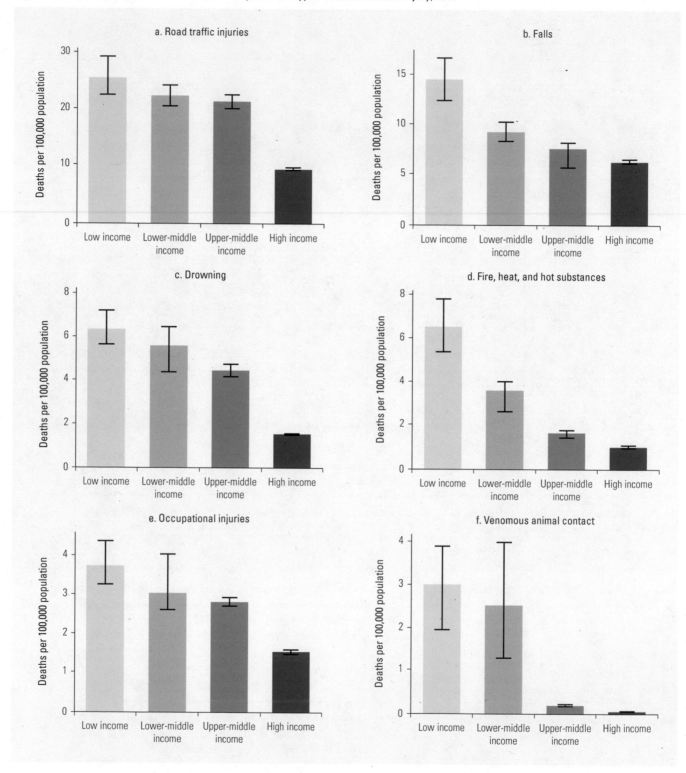

**Figure 1.9** Age-Standardized Trends in Mortality Risk for Interpersonal Violence and Poisoning, 2015

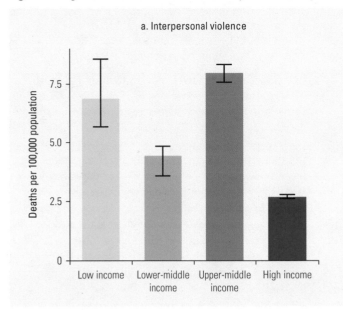

a. Interpersonal violence

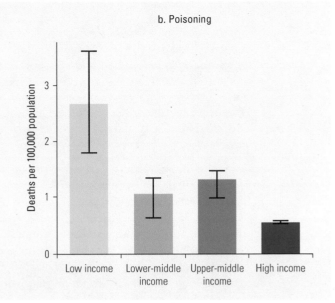

b. Poisoning

---

**Box 1.2**

## Economic Evaluation of Investments in Injury Prevention and Environmental Health

Economic evaluation aims to inform decision making by quantifying tradeoffs between resource inputs required for alternative investments and resulting outcomes. Four main approaches are relevant to this chapter:

- Assessing how much of a *specific health outcome*—for example, serious injuries averted—can be attained for a given level of resource input.
- Assessing how much of an *aggregate measure of health*—such as deaths or disabilities or disability-adjusted life years (DALYs) averted—can be attained from a given level of resource inputs applied to alternative interventions. This approach (cost-effectiveness analysis, or CEA) allows comparisons of the attractiveness of interventions addressing different health outcomes (for example, motorcycle helmet use versus cesarean section) to be made.
- Assessing how much *health and financial risk protection* and its distribution across population subgroups can be attained for a given policy

(for example, public sector finance of a given intervention, such as regulation of helmets for motorcyclists). This approach, extended cost-effectiveness analysis (ECEA), enables assessment not only of efficiency in improving the health of a population but also of efficiency in achieving the other major goal of a health system—protecting the population from financial risk of medical impoverishment—along with the distributional consequences of the given policy, such as equity.

- Assessing the *economic benefits*, measured in monetary terms, from investment in a health intervention and weighing that benefit against its cost (benefit-cost analysis, or BCA). BCA enables comparison of the attractiveness of interventions in the same sector and across different sectors. Benefit-cost ratios greater than 1 identify interventions that represent net positive returns on investment.

CEAs predominate among economic evaluations in injury prevention. Three recent overviews of CEA findings for injury prevention in low- and

*box continues next page*

**Box 1.2** (continued)

middle-income countries (one in this volume) have especially focused on road safety and drowning prevention. These studies underpin this chapter's conclusion that many injury prevention modalities are highly cost-effective even in resource-constrained environments (Ditsuwan and others 2013; Rahman and others 2012; Watkins, Dabestani, Nugent, and Levin 2017).

BCAs predominate among economic evaluations in environmental health, especially for air pollution and for water, sanitation, and hygiene. BCAs are especially suitable for these topics because they are able to consider the benefits of nonhealth outcomes, such as time savings in procuring water or fuels. These BCAs have consistently identified interventions with benefit-cost ratios greater than 1, and

many greater than 10 (Hutton and Chase 2017; Watkins, Dabestani, Nugent, and Levin 2017).

ECEAs are still a relatively new evaluation approach. This volume presents two new ECEAs. One is on the impact of motorcycle helmet regulation on health, equity, and medical impoverishment in Vietnam (Olson and others 2017). The other found that a public-private subsidy for poor Indian households to receive clean fuels could avert 44,000 deaths for US$825 each and about 1.5 million DALYs for US$25 each. This result was far cheaper than cookstove alternatives, and the subsidy for clean fuels provided greater health benefits to all income groups. The greatest health benefit is achieved when the clean fuel subsidy is targeted to the poor (Pillarisetti, Jamison, and Smith 2017).

---

cited earlier for injury prevention would be considered cost-effective. Likewise, the cost-effectiveness of the interventions is similar to that of many widely implemented health interventions, for example, treatment of severe malaria (US$5–US$220 per DALY averted), micronutrient supplementation (US$20–US$100 per DALY averted), oral rehydration solution (US$150 per DALY averted), and treatment of pneumonia (US$300–US$500 per DALY averted) (Black, Laxminarayan, and others 2016).

The area of WASH has undergone extensive economic analysis, primarily using benefit-cost analysis. A benefit-cost ratio (BCR) greater than 1 is generally considered a good investment. Favorable BCRs (1.9–5.1) have been identified for a range of interventions: filters, piped water, boreholes, and private latrines. Combinations of interventions have shown even higher BCRs (2–45) for improved water, sanitation, and universal basic access (Hutton 2013; Hutton and Chase 2016; Hutton and Chase 2017; Watkins, Dabestani, Nugent, and Levin 2017).

Air pollution control has been subjected to limited economic analysis in LMICs. Two studies on ambient air pollution in Mexico found that retrofitting vehicles to reduce emissions produced net benefits of US$100–US$11,000 per vehicle, corresponding to BCRs of 1.1–7.0. Measures to decrease pollution from brick kilns, including filtration systems, switching to natural gas, and relocating kilns to less densely populated areas, produced net benefits corresponding to BCRs of 38 and higher (Blackman and others 2000; Stevens, Wilson, and Hammitt 2005; Watkins, Dabestani, Nugent, and Levin 2017).

For household air pollution control, a limited but growing literature evaluates cost-effectiveness and BCRs associated with transitions to cleaner cooking. Hutton and others performed global cost-benefit analyses of scenarios in which households made the transition away from solid fuels to either clean fuels or clean biomass stoves and found the transition to clean fuel and the transition to improved stoves had BCRs of 4.3 and approximately 60, respectively (Hutton and others 2006; Hutton, Rehfuess, and Tediosi 2007). Benefit-cost analysis has been applied in other specific geographies, including in Nepal (Malla and others 2011; Pant 2011), China (Aunan and others 2013), the Western Pacific Region (Arcenas and others 2010), and in Kenya and Sudan (Malla and others 2011).

Similarly, the few occupational safety and health interventions that have been studied in LMICs do appear cost-effective or cost-beneficial. Simulation studies using the WHO-CHOICE methodology found engineering controls that decrease the release of silica into the air at the workplace to be a cost-effective method for preventing silicosis in several industries in LMICs; these were found to be more cost-effective than the use of masks and respirators (but all with cost-effectiveness ratios in the range of several hundred U.S. dollars per DALY averted) (Lahiri and others 2005). Similar methodology identified training programs to prevent back injury to be a cost-effective method for preventing back pain in LMICs globally; these training programs were found to be more cost-effective than engineering controls (but all with cost-effectiveness ratios of less than US$1,000) (Lahiri, Markkanen, and Levenstein 2005). Ergonomic changes in footwear manufacturing in Brazil had a BCR of 7.2 (Guimarães, Ribeiro, and Renner 2012; Watkins, Dabestani, Nugent, and Levin 2017).

In summary, although the literature on economic evaluation of injury prevention and environmental health in LMICs is small, consistent evidence is emerging that a range of interventions are cost-effective, cost-beneficial, or both. One particular environmental issue will likely become increasingly preeminent in the twenty-first century: climate change. The economic consequences of the resulting health problems and food and water insecurity will potentially rival those of other major risk factors. In addition to lowering greenhouse gas emissions, a range of countermeasures have been considered, such as establishing occupational heat exposure standards and enhancing surveillance for water- and vector-borne infections. Economic analyses of such measures are in their infancy but have nonetheless suggested that not addressing climate change will be very costly to health systems in less than two decades (Ebi, Hess, and Watkiss 2017).

## Essential Interventions to Address Injury and Environmental Health

On the basis of their cost-effectiveness or cost-benefit, feasibility, and potential to lower the burden of these conditions, a package of policy interventions can be recommended (tables 1.4 and 1.5). These interventions include policies in the health sector and in other sectors, including taxes and regulations that affect infrastructure and the built environment—especially interventions that have proven cost-effectiveness in LMICs.

**Table 1.4** Essential Injury and Occupational Health Policies

| | Fiscal and Intersectoral Policy | | | |
| | | | | |
| Domain of action | Taxes and subsidies | Infrastructure, built environment, and product design | Regulation | Information, education, and communication |
|---|---|---|---|---|
| *Road safety* | | | | |
| Overall | Subsidized public transportation | Mass transport infrastructure and land use (bus rapid transit, rail) | Adoption and enforcement of harmonized motor vehicle safety standards | |
| Pedestrian safety | | Increased visibility, areas for pedestrians separate from fast motorized traffic | | Increased supervision of children walking to school |
| Motorcycle safety | | Exclusive motorcycle lanes | Mandatory use of daytime running lights for motorcycles | |
| | | | Mandatory motorcycle helmet laws | |
| Bicycle safety | | Increased visibility, lanes for cyclists separate from fast motorized traffic | | Social marketing to promote helmet use by child bicyclists |
| Child passenger safety | | | Legislation for and enforcement of child restraints (including seats) | |
| Speed control | | Traffic-calming infrastructure (for example, speed bumps), especially at dangerous road segments | Setting and enforcement of speed limits appropriate to function of roads | |
| Driving under the influence of alcohol | | | Setting and enforcement of blood alcohol concentration limits | |
| Seatbelt use | | | Mandatory seatbelt use laws for all occupants | Social marketing to promote seatbelt use |

*table continues next page*

**Table 1.4** Essential Injury and Occupational Health Policies (continued)

| Domain of action | Fiscal and Intersectoral Policy | | | |
| --- | --- | --- | --- | --- |
| | Taxes and subsidies | Infrastructure, built environment, and product design | Regulation | Information, education, and communication |
| *Other unintentional injury* | | | | |
| Drowning | | | Legislation and enforcement of use of personal flotation devices for recreational and other high-risk boaters | Parental or other adult supervision (for example, use of crèches) in high-risk areas<br><br>Swimming lessons for children |
| Burns | | Safer stove design | | |
| Poisoning | | Child-resistant containers | | Information, education, and communication for safe storage of hazardous substances |
| *Violence* | | | | |
| Child maltreatment | | | Corporal punishment ban | Parent training, including nurse home visitation, for high-risk families |
| Youth violence | | | | Social development programs that teach social skills and incorporate training for parents<br><br>Information sharing between police and hospital emergency departments |
| Gender-based violence and intimate partner violence | Microfinance combined with gender equity training | | | School-based programs to address gender norms and attitudes<br><br>Interventions for problem drinkers (who are also abusive partners)<br><br>Advocacy support programs (for example, to increase availability and use of shelters for at-risk women) |
| Cross cutting for multiple types of injury | Reducing availability and harmful use of alcohol through increased taxation and decreased availability of outlets | Dispensing alcohol in plastic rather than glass that could be used as a weapon | Stricter licensing laws and reduced availability of firearms | |
| *Occupational safety and health* | | | | |
| | | Engineering controls to decrease release of silica and other toxins<br><br>Safe injection devices, such as blunt-tip suture needles | Enforcement of safety standards<br><br>Formalization of large informal sectors in low- and middle-income countries | Training in hazard recognition and control relevant to the work performed (for example, task-based training for hazardous tasks)<br><br>Effective use of available personal protective equipment<br><br>Occupational health workforce development |

*Note:* Interventions for treatment—for example, trauma care for injured people—are covered in other *DCP3* volumes and are not addressed here.

**Table 1.5** Essential Environmental Policies

| Domain of action | Fiscal and Intersectoral Policy | | | Information, education, and communication |
| | Taxes and subsidies | Infrastructure and built environment | Regulation | |
|---|---|---|---|---|
| *Water and sanitation* | Targeted subsidies to poor and vulnerable groups<br><br>Incentives for private sector to become more involved with WASH for supply chain and service provision | Quality WASH facilities in schools, workplaces, public spaces, and health care facilities | Defined WASH standards per setting (household, outside household) | National awareness campaigns (for example, on handwashing)<br><br>WASH behavior-change interventions, such as community-led total sanitation |
| *Outdoor air pollution* | Fuel taxes<br><br>Fines for residential trash burning<br><br>Fines for not controlling construction dust<br><br>Tax polluters<br><br>Cap and trade policies for specific pollutants (for example, SO$_2$)<br><br>No more subsidies for coal | Relocation of industrial sources, such as brick kilns<br><br>Municipal trash collection<br><br>Diesel to CNG transition for fleets<br><br>Movement toward banning solid fuels in cities<br><br>Regular street cleaning to control dust | Diesel retrofits<br><br>Coal to natural gas transition<br><br>Brick kiln retrofits for emissions control<br><br>PM, SO$_2$, and NO$_2$ emissions control<br><br>Acceleration of Euro standards for vehicles<br><br>National regulation to reduce household emissions to outdoors<br><br>Construction and road dust controls<br><br>Adoption of European Union fuel standards | Updated health information systems to include vulnerability, adaptation, and capacity assessment |
| *Household air pollution* | Advanced biomass stove subsidies<br><br>Targeted and expanded LPG and other clean fuel subsidies to the poor<br><br>Subsidies for clean alternatives to kerosene<br><br>Campaigns for middle class to give up subsidies intended for poor | Improved ventilation as part of building codes and norms<br><br>Enhanced clean fuel distribution networks<br><br>Electrification as a health measure<br><br>Application of modern digital technology to enhance access to household clean fuel | Lower barriers and expanded licensure requirements for clean fuel distribution<br><br>Kerosene ban<br><br>National regulation on clean household fuels to match UN SE4ALL goals<br><br>Smoke-free communities | Ventilation<br><br>HAP health effects education<br><br>Promotion of kitchen retrofits to encourage HAP-reducing interventions and behaviors |
| *Chemical contamination* | | Regulations on hazardous waste disposal covering land, air, and water | Arsenic: monitoring of groundwater supplies and provision of alternatives if needed<br><br>Asbestos: banning of import, export, mining, manufacture, and sale<br><br>Mercury: monitoring and reduction or elimination of use in artisanal mining, large-scale smelting, and cosmetics<br><br>Established and enforced toxic element emissions limits for air and water<br><br>Restricted access to contaminated sites<br><br>Strict control and movement to selective bans of highly hazardous pesticides | Notification of public of locations of contaminated sites |

*table continues next page*

**Table 1.5** Essential Environmental Policies (continued)

| Domain of action | Fiscal and Intersectoral Policy | | | Information, education, and communication |
| | Taxes and subsidies | Infrastructure and built environment | Regulation | |
|---|---|---|---|---|
| *Lead exposure* | Concessionary financing for remediation of worst conditions | Minimization of occupational and environmental exposures in maintaining, renovating, and demolishing buildings and other structures with lead paint | Ban on lead paint and leaded fuels<br><br>Ban on lead in water pipes, cookware, drugs, food supplements, and cosmetics<br><br>Reduction in corrosiveness of drinking water<br><br>National take-back requirements for collecting used lead batteries<br><br>Regulations governing land-based waste disposal<br><br>Risk-based limits for lead in air, water, soil, and dust | Lead poisoning training for health care providers |
| *Global climate change* | Carbon tax or cap and trade (mitigation)<br><br>Subsidies to renewable energy | Mitigation policies and incentives, including land-use plans, building design, transportation, to reduce GHGs<br><br>Resilient design in buildings and infrastructure (adaptation)<br><br>Consideration of climate change in public health infrastructure (mitigation and adaptation) | Energy efficiency and fuel efficient vehicles (mitigation)<br><br>Mainstreaming of climate change into public health planning and programs, and into health system policies and plans<br><br>Methane control regulations | Early warning and emergency response systems |

*Note:* CNG = compressed natural gas; GHG = greenhouse gas; HAP = household air pollution; LPG = liquefied petroleum gas; $NO_2$ = nitrogen dioxide; PM = particulate matter; $SO_2$ = sulfur dioxide; UN SE4ALL = United Nations Sustainable Energy for All program; WASH = water, sanitation, and hygiene. Interventions for treatment (for example, oral rehydration solution for diarrhea) or other individual-level medical services (for example, deworming, growth monitoring) are covered in other *DCP3* volumes and are not addressed here. Interventions in this table include those that have been shown to be cost-effective or cost-beneficial in low- and middle-income countries or for which such cost-effectiveness or cost-benefit can be logically concluded from high-income or other data. For water and sanitation, many of the policy-level interventions mentioned do not have such evidence; however, the individual items promoted by these policies (for example, filters, piped water, boreholes, private latrines) do have a strong evidence base. Unlike interventions with only health benefits, however, many if not most interventions in environmental health bring a range of other benefits lying outside the health sector, for example, time savings, property values, IQ enhancement, and so on. Cost-effectiveness measured solely in health terms, therefore, can be misleading with regard to total social benefit-cost relationships.

The package also includes interventions with proven cost-effectiveness in HICs with high likelihood of transferability to LMICs. Finally, the package also includes interventions that are logical and feasible, but for which there is currently little empirical evidence on cost-effectiveness. Details of these policies, including the evidence for them, are addressed in the chapters of this volume.

We acknowledge that the list is not exhaustive. Other policies might be considered essential. For many countries, tables 1.4 and 1.5 provide a reasonable starting point for an essential policy package to comprehensively address injury prevention and environmental health, although there will be country-specific variations.

Examples from injury prevention include promoting safer forms of transportation. In general, the individual automobile (especially two- and three-wheeled motorized vehicles) is one of the least safe modes of transportation. The overall field of transport safety would be considerably advanced by government policies (including taxes and subsidies) that promote alternative safer and more energy-efficient forms of transportation, such as mass transport, especially rail, as well as by promoting and ensuring the safety of walking and cycling. For road traffic crashes themselves, promoting safer infrastructure is a key intervention. For example, traffic-calming infrastructure such as speed bumps, especially at dangerous intersections, is a very cost-effective method for protecting pedestrians. In similar fashion, safety-related product design, such as child-resistant containers for poisons and medicines, has played a major role in injury prevention. Safety-related product design encompasses engineering (as do infrastructure and the built environment) as well as regulation because safer products are often best promoted by mandating them in legislation. Other key injury prevention regulations include mandating the use of restraints for automobile occupants and helmets for motorcycle riders.

Within the public health sector, information and communication strategies can be successfully delivered through mass media, as with strategies to promote safe driving behaviors such as seatbelt and helmet use. Such strategies usually do not work well in isolation but are best combined with legislation and effective enforcement. Information and communication strategies can also be delivered in smaller group settings and individually, as with many of the violence prevention strategies. For example, home visiting programs using skills training to promote better parenting skills, especially to high-risk groups such as young first-time parents from lower socioeconomic status, have been found to be very effective in preventing child maltreatment in HICs.

Occupational safety and health overlap with injury prevention. However, interventions in this field primarily target the worksite and thus are distinct from those described earlier that target the general population. Key strategies in promoting occupational safety and health include regulations such as setting appropriate limits on work hours. Given higher risks faced by those in the informal work sector, formalizing this sector, including encompassing it within appropriate and context-specific regulatory and organized labor systems, is a key measure that needs to be promoted globally. On an individual basis, better application of known safe practices and known effective personal protective equipment, such as masks and respirators to prevent inhalation of silica and other airborne toxins, is needed.

Many of the individual WASH interventions, such as filters, piped water, boreholes, and private latrines, have been documented to be very cost-effective and cost-beneficial (table 1.5). However, access to these interventions can be difficult for the poor, especially in rural areas. Policies to ensure that these interventions reach everyone include financing strategies (such as targeted subsidies to poor and vulnerable groups), strengthening supply chains for water and sanitation products and services, and developing national standards on universal access.

Pollution-related interventions include those addressing air pollution (household and ambient, both of which are primarily related to combustion-derived particulate matter) as well as a number of chemical contaminants, such as lead, asbestos, arsenic, and pesticides. The range of policy levers can be used for these issues: taxes and subsidies (such as targeting clean fuel subsidies to the poor); infrastructure and built environment (such as relocating industrial sources such as brick kilns); regulation and international agreements (such as banning the import, export, mining, manufacture, and sale of asbestos); and actions within the health sector (such as establishing environmental lead surveillance). Among these, awareness of the health impacts of household air pollution is relatively recent, and understanding of the true scale of the impact of other issues, such as lead, has recently been greatly enhanced. Thus, actions in the health sector have lagged the knowledge of potential benefits.

Some of the interventions, although listed for one condition, have beneficial effects for other conditions. For example, promoting alternatives to private automobiles decreases both injury rates and pollutant emissions. Improved stoves and fuels decrease air pollution and rates of household burns. Violence prevention strategies (such as home visiting and life and social skills training) reduce substance abuse, mental health problems, and subsequent crime and violence, and increase positive outcomes, including academic attainment and employment.

A set of policies for a specific subset of pollution, climate change, is presented in table 1.5. Many of these policies have been widely considered and are straightforward and logical (such as promoting active transport and early warning and emergency response systems). As noted above, economic analysis of their impact has just recently begun.

Implementation of many of the interventions requires intersectoral collaboration. For example, road safety involves law enforcement, ministries of transport, government agencies that regulate manufacturing, and public health agencies. Likewise, surveillance plays a key role. Surveillance includes not only monitoring of trends for disease burden, but also surveillance for risk factors. For example, a key element for managing air pollution is monitoring of air quality. Such monitoring, which is especially important for lead control, includes such activities as examining sample surveys of blood in children and monitoring of levels from hot spots such as lead battery manufacturing and recycling sites. Similarly, a key component of improving WASH is a strengthened monitoring and rapid feedback system for the coverage and quality of water and sanitation services.

## CONCLUSIONS

Injury and occupational and environmental risks result in a large health burden. Some of this burden tends to decrease with economic development (for example, risks from unsafe water and sanitation), whereas some tends to initially increase with economic development before declining at high-income levels (for example, ambient air pollution and transport injuries). A range of interventions can speed the decrease in burden for the former or mitigate the rises for the latter. Many of these interventions have been shown to be among the most cost-effective or cost-beneficial of all interventions used to prevent or treat disease. The interventions summarized in this chapter include these as well as other similar interventions that are reasonable but have not yet been subjected to sufficient economic analysis. Given their potential to lower this significant health burden, these interventions are high priorities for future population, policy, and implementation research.

Implementation of most of the interventions that address the conditions in this volume (tables 1.4 and 1.5) has been far less than optimal, especially in LMICs. For example, the WHO's *Global Status Report on Road Safety* (WHO 2015) assessed 180 countries for the status of key road safety interventions. Although the majority of countries (105) implemented best practice standards for seatbelt laws (such as mandatory seatbelts for all occupants), far fewer had best practice standards for laws on speed control (47), mandatory motorcycle helmet use (44), and drunk driving (34) (WHO 2015). Formal health-based intervention programs for household air pollution have not shown major worldwide implementation success to date, although local progress during the relatively short period that they have been implemented is occasionally seen. Nevertheless, clean fuels, through nonhealth actions and economic growth, have brought major health benefits to hundreds of millions of people. Finding ways to expand the rate of these improvements to cover populations that would not benefit otherwise is clearly a high priority.

Many of the interventions considered herein need to be better applied in HICs, but most have been implemented to a lesser extent in LMICs, which has contributed to the higher health burden from injury and from occupational and environmental risk factors in LMICs. To assess the potential gains from more widespread implementation of these interventions, we estimated the deaths that could be averted if the age-adjusted mortality rates for these conditions in HICs pertained in LMICs. This assessment was straightforward for injury deaths. However, for deaths from occupational and environmental exposures, we considered "attributable deaths" (tables 1.2 and 1.3). These are not mutually exclusive, with overlap of some of the categories. For example, deaths from unsafe water and lack of handwashing partly overlap. Hence, differences in mortality rates were considered for the overall categories of WASH, air pollution, and occupational health, not by subcategory. There is likely minimal overlap between air pollution and unsafe WASH. For simplicity and lack of systematic analysis of these overlaps, they are ignored in this analysis.

Within these caveats, it can be estimated that more widespread implementation of the package of interventions and policies covered in this review could avert about 2 million deaths from injury (not including suicide, which is not addressed in this volume); 200,000 deaths from occupational risk factors (not including injury); 1.4 million deaths from unsafe water and sanitation; and about 4 million deaths from air pollution (the larger component of which is attributable to household fuels). A total of more than 7 million deaths could be averted (table 1.6).

Several factors might cause the real number of potentially avertable deaths to be lower or higher. For example, the differences in death rates between countries at different economic levels is in part attributable to better prevention, but also to better medical treatment, which is not addressed in the policy package considered in this volume. Therefore, the estimates of deaths averted by improved prevention alone might be overstated. However, these estimates do not take into account the lives that could be saved by addressing some of the other nonoccupational toxins, such as lead and arsenic. Finally, the interventions considered here have not been fully applied in many HICs, and many deaths could be averted there as well. Even within these caveats and limitations, it is apparent that a large number of deaths could be

**Table 1.6** Disease Burden Avertable by Improved Injury Prevention, Occupational Safety and Health, and Environmental Policy in Low- and Middle-Income Countries

| | Total Deaths (Thousands) | | |
|---|---|---|---|
| | Current scenario | Hypothetical scenario | Avertable |
| Injury (excluding suicide) | 3,790 | 1,730 | 2,060 |
| Occupational risks (excluding injury) | 430 | 220 | 210 |
| Unsafe water, sanitation, and handwashing | 1,390 | 20 | 1,370 |
| Air pollution | 4,990 | 950 | 4,040 |
| Total | | | 7,680 |

*Source:* Global Burden of Disease (GBD) 2013 Study (IHME 2016); WHO Global Health Estimates 2012 (WHO 2016).
*Note:* Hypothetical scenario is the disease burden that would occur if age-specific rates for these conditions in high-income countries applied in low- and middle-income countries. Avertable burden is the difference between current and hypothetical scenarios. Three levels of significance are kept to reduce rounding errors, but true uncertainty is possibly higher. Even so, totals may not add due to rounding.

averted by better implementation of the low-cost and feasible interventions considered in this volume.

## ACKNOWLEDGMENTS

The Bill & Melinda Gates Foundation provides financial support for the Disease Control Priorities Network project, of which this volume is a part. Brianne Adderley, Kristen Danforth, and Shamelle Richards provided valuable comments and assistance on this chapter.

Members of the *DCP3* Injury Prevention and Environmental Health Author Group wrote the chapters on which this chapter draws. The Group includes those listed as coauthors of this chapter, as well as Maureen Cropper, Susan D. Hillis, James A. Mercy, and Paul Watkiss.

## NOTES

World Bank Income Classifications as of July 2014 are as follows, based on estimates of gross national income (GNI) per capita for 2013:

- Low-income countries (LICs) – US$1,045 or less
- Middle-income countries (MICs) are subdivided:
  a) lower-middle-income = US$1,046 to US$4,125
  b) upper-middle-income (UMICs) = US$4,126 to US$12,745
- High-income countries (HICs) = US$12,746 or more.

1. This chapter cites the source of burden estimates at each use, but these estimates change regularly as new data become available and modeling tools improve. There are some discrepancies between the estimates done by different organizations, namely, the Institute for Health Metrics and Evaluation and the WHO, because of different assumptions and methods. The precision is generally kept at three places of significance to avoid rounding errors, but in reality true uncertainties are much larger.
2. Note on terminology: Some definitions of *premature deaths* involve those deaths below a certain age, for example, younger than age 70 years. This table and the other tables in this chapter consider all of the deaths to be premature but not relative to a specific threshold for age.
3. Except for figure 1.1, all analyses in this section are presented with age-standardized deaths per capita to normalize across the four World Bank income regions using GBD 2015 data. Results are similar if using age-standardized DALYs, however. Only environmental risks examined in the GBD 2015 were included. It should be noted that conducting the analysis using more subregions or by country might show subtleties not revealed by comparison across only four income regions.
4. Like the environmental risk factors, the occupational injury category was examined in a comparative risk assessment framework, that is, with a nonzero

counterfactual based on what is considered feasible to obtain. The estimates shown for all the other injury categories, however, here assume that 100 percent of the impact can be avoided.

## REFERENCES

Arcenas, A., J. Bojö, B. Larsen, and F. Ruiz Ñunez. 2010. "The Economic Costs of Indoor Air Pollution: New Results for Indonesia, the Philippines, and Timor-Leste." *Journal of Natural Resources Policy Research* 2 (1): 75–93.

Aunan, K., L. W. H. Alnes, J. Berger, Z. Dong, L. Ma, and others. 2013. "Upgrading to Cleaner Household Stoves and Reducing Chronic Obstructive Pulmonary Disease among Women in Rural China—A Cost-Benefit Analysis." *Energy for Sustainable Development* 17 (5): 489–96.

Bishai, D. M., and A. A. Hyder. 2006. "Modeling the Cost Effectiveness of Injury Interventions in Lower and Middle Income Countries: Opportunities and Challenges." *Cost Effectiveness and Resource Allocation* 4: 2.

Black, R. E., R. Laxminarayan, M. Temmerman, and N. Walker, editors. 2016. *Disease Control Priorities* (third edition): Volume 2, *Reproductive, Maternal, Newborn, and Child Health*. Washington, DC: World Bank.

Black, R. E., C. Levin, N. Walker, D. Chou, L. Liu, and others. 2016. "Reproductive, Maternal, Newborn, and Child Health: Key Messages from *Disease Control Priorities*, 3rd Edition." *The Lancet* 388 (10061): 2713–836.

Blackman, A., S. Newbold, J. Shih, and J. Cook. 2000. "The Benefits and Costs of Informal Sector Pollution Control: Mexican Brick Kilns." Discussion Paper 00-46, Resources for the Future, Washington, DC.

Bundy, D. A. P., N. de Silva, S. Horton, D. T. Jamison, and G. C. Patton, editors. 2017. *Disease Control Priorities* (third edition): Volume 8, *Child and Adolescent Health and Development*. Washington, DC: World Bank.

Chafe, Z. A., M. Brauer, Z. Klimont, R. Van Dingenen, S. Mehta, and others. 2014. "Household Cooking with Solid Fuels Contributes to Ambient PM2.5 Air Pollution and the Burden of Disease." *Environmental Health Perspectives* 122 (12): 1314–20.

Debas, H. T., P. Donkor, A. Gawande, D. T. Jamison, M. E. Kruk, and C. N. Mock, editors. 2015. *Disease Control Priorities* (third edition): Volume 1, *Essential Surgery*. Washington, DC: World Bank.

Ditsuwan, V., J. L. Veerman, M. Bertram, and T. Vos. 2013. "Cost-Effectiveness of Interventions for Reducing Road Traffic Injuries Related to Driving under the Influence of Alcohol." *Value in Health* 16 (1): 23–30.

Ebi, K., J. Hess, and P. Watkiss. 2017. "Health Risks and Costs of Climate Variability and Change." In *Disease Control Priorities* (third edition): Volume 7, *Injury Prevention and Environmental Health*, edited by C. N. Mock, R. Nugent, O. Kobusingye, and K. R. Smith. Washington, DC: World Bank.

Guimarães, L. D., J. L. Ribeiro, and J. S. Renner. 2012. "Cost-Benefit Analysis of a Socio-Technical Intervention in a Brazilian Footwear Company." *Applied Ergonomics* 43 (5): 948–57.

Humphrey, J. 2009. "Child Undernutrition, Tropical Enteropathy, Toilets, and Handwashing." *The Lancet* 3754 (9694): 1032–35.

Hutton, G. 2013. "Global Costs and Benefits of Reaching Universal Coverage of Sanitation and Drinking-Water Supply." *Journal of Water and Health* 11 (1): 1–12.

Hutton, G., and C. Chase. 2016. "The Knowledge Base for Achieving the Sustainable Development Goal Targets on Water Supply, Sanitation and Hygiene." *International Journal of Environmental Research and Public Health* 13 (6): E536.

———. 2017. "Water Supply, Sanitation, and Hygiene." In *Disease Control Priorities* (third edition): Volume 7, *Injury Prevention and Environmental Health*, edited by C. N. Mock, R. Nugent, O. Kobusingye, and K. R. Smith. Washington, DC: World Bank.

Hutton, G., E. Rehfuess, and F. Tediosi. 2007. "Evaluation of the Costs and Benefits of Interventions to Reduce Indoor Air Pollution." *Energy for Sustainable Development* 11 (4): 34–43.

Hutton, G., E. Rehfuess, F. Tediosi, and S. Weiss. 2006. *Evaluation of the Costs and Benefits of Household Energy and Health Interventions at Global and Regional Levels.* Geneva: World Health Organization.

Jamison, D. T., J. G. Breman, A. R. Measham, G. Alleyne, M. Claeson, D. B. Evans, P. Jha, A. Mills, and P. Musgrove, editors. 2006. *Disease Control Priorities in Developing Countries* (second edition). Washington, DC: Oxford University Press and World Bank.

Jamison, D. T., W. Mosley, A. R. Measham, and J. Bobadilla, editors. 1993. *Disease Control Priorities in Developing Countries* (first edition). New York: Oxford University Press.

Lahiri, S., C. Levenstein, D. I. Nelson, and B. J. Rosenberg. 2005. "The Cost Effectiveness of Occupational Health Interventions: Prevention of Silicosis." *American Journal of Industrial Medicine* 48 (6): 503–14.

Lahiri, S., P. Markkanen, and C. Levenstein. 2005. "The Cost Effectiveness of Occupational Health Interventions: Preventing Occupational Back Pain." *American Journal of Industrial Medicine* 48 (6): 515–29.

Lelieveld, J., J. S. Evans, M. Fnais, D. Giannadaki, and A. Pozzer. 2015. "The Contribution of Outdoor Air Pollution Sources to Premature Mortality on a Global Scale." *Nature* 525: 367–71.

Malla, M. B., N. Bruce, E. Bates, and E. Rehfuess. 2011. "Applying Global Cost-Benefit Analysis Methods to Indoor Air Pollution Mitigation Interventions in Nepal, Kenya and Sudan: Insights and Challenges." *Energy Policy* 39 (12): 7518–29.

Mock, C. N., P. Donkor, A. Gawande, D. T. Jamison, M. E. Kruk, and others. 2015. "Essential Surgery: Key Messages from *Disease Control Priorities*, 3rd Edition." *The Lancet* 385 (9983): 2209–19.

Newall, A. T., M. Jit, and R. Hutubessy. 2014. "Are Current Cost-Effectiveness Thresholds for Low- and Middle-Income Countries Useful? Examples from the World of Vaccines." *Pharmacoeconomics* 32 (6): 525–31.

Olson, Z., J. Staples, C. N. Mock, N. P. Nguyen, A. Bachani, and others. 2017. "Helmet Regulation in Vietnam: Impact on Health, Equity and Medical Impoverishment." In *Disease Control Priorities* (third edition): Volume 7, *Injury Prevention and Environmental Health*, edited by C. N. Mock, R. Nugent, O. Kobusingye, and K. R. Smith. Washington, DC: World Bank.

Omran, A. R. 1971. "The Epidemiologic Transition: A Theory of the Epidemiology of Population Change." *The Milbank Quarterly* 83 (4): 731–57.

Pant, K. P. 2011. "Cheaper Fuel and Higher Health Costs among the Poor in Rural Nepal." *AMBIO* 41 (3): 271–83.

Patel, V., D. Chisholm, T. Dua, R. Laxminarayan, and M. E. Medina-Mora, editors. 2015. *Disease Control Priorities* (third edition): Volume 4, *Mental, Neurological, and Substance Use Disorders.* Washington, DC: World Bank.

Patel, V., D. Chisholm, R. Parikh, F. J. Charlson, L. Degenhardt, and others. 2015. "Addressing the Burden of Mental, Neurological, and Substance Use Disorders: Key Messages from *Disease Control Priorities*, 3rd Edition." *The Lancet* 387 (10028): 1672–85.

Petri, W., and M. Miller. 2008. "Enteric Infections, Diarrhea, and Their Impact on Function and Development." *Journal of Clinical Investigation* 118 (4): 1277–90.

Pillarisetti, A., D. T. Jamison, and K. Smith. 2017. "Household Energy Interventions and Health and Finances in Haryana, India: An Extended Cost-Effectiveness Analysis." In *Disease Control Priorities* (third edition): Volume 7, *Injury Prevention and Environmental Health*, edited by C. N. Mock, R. Nugent, O. Kobusingye, and K. R. Smith. Washington, DC: World Bank.

Prabhakaran, D., T. Gaziano, J.-C. Mbanya, Y. Wu, and Rachel Nugent, editors. 2017. *Disease Control Priorities* (third edition): Volume 5, *Cardiovascular, Respiratory, and Related Disorders.* Washington, DC: World Bank.

Rahman, F., S. Bose, M. Linnan, A. Rahman, S. Mashreky, and others. 2012. "Cost-Effectiveness of an Injury and Drowning Prevention Program in Bangladesh." *Pediatrics* 130 (6): e1621–28.

Smith, K. 1990. "Indoor Air Quality and the Pollution Transition." In *Indoor Air Quality*, edited by H. Kasuga. Berlin, Heidelberg: Springer-Verlag.

Smith, K., M. A Desai, J. V. Rogers, and R. A. Houghton. 2013. "Joint $CO_2$ and $CH_4$ Accountability for Global Warming." *Proceedings of the National Academy of Sciences* 110 (31): E2865–74.

Smith, K., and M. Ezzati. 2005. "How Environmental Health Risks Change with Development: The Epidemiologic and Environmental Risk Transitions Revisited." *Annual Review of Environment and Resources* 30: 291–333.

Stevens, G., A. Wilson, and J. K. Hammitt. 2005. "A Benefit-Cost Analysis of Retrofitting Diesel Vehicles with Particulate Filters in the Mexico City Metropolitan Area." *Risk Analysis* 25 (4): 883–99.

United Nations. 2015. *Transforming Our World: The 2030 Agenda for Sustainable Development.* New York: United Nations.

Watkins, D., N. Dabestani, C. Mock, M. Cullen, K. Smith, and others. 2017. "Trends in Morbidity and Mortality Attributable to Injuries and Selected Environmental

Hazards." In *Disease Control Priorities* (third edition): Volume 7, *Injury Prevention and Environmental Health*, edited by C. N. Mock, R. Nugent, O. Kobusingye, and K. R. Smith. Washington, DC: World Bank.

Watkins, D., N. Dabestani, R. Nugent, and C. Levin. 2017. "Interventions to Prevent Injuries and Reduce Environmental and Occupational Hazards: A Review of Economic Evaluations from Low- and Middle-Income Countries." In *Disease Control Priorities* (third edition): Volume 7, *Injury Prevention and Environmental Health*, edited by C. N. Mock, R. Nugent, O. Kobusingye, and K. R. Smith. Washington, DC: World Bank.

WHO (World Health Organization). 2015. *Global Status Report on Road Safety 2015*. Geneva: WHO.

———. 2016. "Global Health Estimates (2012)." WHO, Geneva.

World Bank. 1993. *World Development Report 1993: Investing in Health*. New York: Oxford University Press.

Chapter **2**

# Trends in Morbidity and Mortality Attributable to Injuries and Selected Environmental Hazards

David A. Watkins, Nazila Dabestani, Charles N. Mock,
Mark R. Cullen, Kirk R. Smith, and Rachel Nugent

## INTRODUCTION

The effects of globalization on low- and middle-income countries (LMICs) have led to major changes in the disease burden attributable to injuries and environmental risks. On the one hand, rapidly developing regions face a rising number of road traffic injuries (RTIs) and fatalities, as well as health effects from increasingly polluted air. On the other hand, economic development has led to greater availability of water, sanitation, and hygiene (WASH) services and a reduced burden of diarrheal and helminthic illness in many settings. These trends are heterogeneous, however, and very poor countries, and regions within populous countries such as India, exhibit slower progress.

This chapter presents an overview of trends in the burden of injuries and environmental health issues in LMICs. We focus on five major groups of conditions, presented as they appear in this volume and not in order of importance:

- Unintentional injuries, which include RTIs and those resulting from other causes
- Interpersonal and collective violence
- Occupational hazards
- WASH-related illnesses
- Health effects of air pollution.

Self-harm is not covered in detail in this chapter because it is covered in volume 4, chapter 9, of *Disease Control Priorities* (third edition) (Vijayakumar and others 2015). Although the conditions presented above are seemingly very different, a common feature links them: they can all be addressed through multisectoral interventions, including legal and regulatory frameworks and public works investments. These interventions are assessed further in the subsequent chapters of this volume.

This chapter presents two types of burden estimates. For injuries, we present deaths and disability-adjusted life years (DALYs). For occupational and environmental hazards, we present attributable deaths and DALYs. The distinction between these two types of estimates is that the former are related to specific causes of death, such as RTIs, whereas the latter are related to risk factors, such as unimproved water, for specific causes of death, such as diarrheal disease. Attributable deaths and DALYs are estimated using the comparative risk assessment (CRA) methodology rather than mortality analysis. They often total greater or less than 100 percent owing to multiple risk factors (or no known risk factors) for various causes of death. Hence, estimates of the burden of environmental and occupational risk factors cannot be directly compared to estimates of the burden of injuries.

Corresponding author: David A. Watkins, Department of Medicine, University of Washington, Seattle, Washington, United States; davidaw@uw.edu.

This chapter presents estimates from two sources of data. Mortality and morbidity data on injuries are taken from the World Health Organization's (WHO) Global Health Estimates database, most recently updated in 2014 (WHO 2016). Details on the methods for estimating cause-specific mortality and DALYs—including calculation of years of life lost and disability weights—are available in the relevant documentation from the WHO. Attributable mortality and morbidity data on occupational and environmental risks are taken from the Global Burden of Disease 2013 Study (GBD 2013) because similar data were not available from the WHO. Details on the methods for estimating attributable mortality and DALYs using CRA are provided in Forouzanfar and others (2015).

We compare trends in total deaths with trends in age-standardized mortality rates. For injuries, we calculated age-standardized rates based on the global population structure in 2012 and compared mortality in 2000 to mortality in 2012. For occupational and environmental risks, we used age-standardized attributable rates from GBD 2013, which based calculations on the global population structure in 2013 and compared attributable mortality in 1990 to attributable mortality in 2013.

## UNINTENTIONAL INJURIES

### Road Traffic Injuries

Among unintentional injuries, RTIs remain the most common cause of deaths and DALYs. RTIs cause the single-highest number of injuries worldwide in any category, and their number continues to increase. RTIs caused 1.1 million deaths and 70 million DALYs in 2012, accounting for 3 percent of total deaths and DALYs in LMICs. RTIs rank among the top 10 causes of death globally, and LMICs constitute a higher proportion of deaths. Most deaths occur among vulnerable road users, such as pedestrians, motorcyclists, and cyclists. Poor design, traffic congestion, and lack of road maintenance and safety systems in many LMICs make prevention more challenging (Peden and others 2004).

The United Nations Road Safety Collaboration has highlighted the unequal effect of RTIs by socioeconomic status, age, and gender. In general, adolescent and younger working-age adult males are most affected by RTIs, and the increase in deaths between 2000 and 2012 has been largest in this group (table 2.1). Yet many countries do not regularly collect data on RTIs, thereby limiting awareness of the problem and potential interventions, such as speed limits, seat belt enforcement, and impaired-driving laws (WHO 2013).

The number of RTI-related deaths and DALYs in LMICs increased by 36 percent and 23 percent, respectively, between 2000 and 2012 (table 2.1). This increasing burden of RTIs is independent of demographic changes and is related to increasing age-specific mortality rates: the age-standardized mortality rate from RTIs increased 17 percent from 18 per 100,000 persons to 21 per 100,000 persons in LMICs (table 2.2). Notably, no

**Table 2.1** Road Traffic Injuries: Deaths and DALYs in LMICs by Age and Gender, 2000–12

| Gender | Age | Deaths | | Change (%) | DALYs | | Change (%) |
|---|---|---|---|---|---|---|---|
| | | 2000 | 2012 | | 2000 | 2012 | |
| Both genders | Total | 836,500 | 1,134,800 | 36 | 57,241,000 | 70,385,200 | 23 |
| (percentage of total deaths or DALYs) | | (2.0) | (2.6) | | (2.3) | (3.0) | |
| Male | 0–27 days | 1,300 | 1,300 | 0 | 120,000 | 117,000 | –3 |
| | 1–59 months | 30,800 | 27,100 | –12 | 2,820,000 | 2,485,000 | –12 |
| | 5–14 years | 48,600 | 50,200 | 3 | 4,453,000 | 4,532,000 | 2 |
| | 15–29 years | 199,700 | 232,800 | 17 | 15,664,000 | 18,038,200 | 15 |
| | 30–49 years | 197,200 | 260,200 | 32 | 13,289,000 | 16,760,000 | 26 |
| | 50–59 years | 53,900 | 102,900 | 91 | 2,808,000 | 4,948,000 | 76 |
| | 60–69 years | 42,400 | 73,400 | 73 | 1,655,000 | 2,626,000 | 59 |
| | 70+ years | 41,800 | 78,500 | 88 | 952,000 | 1,600,000 | 68 |
| | Total | 615,700 | 826,400 | 34 | 41,761,000 | 51,106,200 | 22 |

*table continues next page*

**Table 2.1** Road Traffic Injuries: Deaths and DALYs in LMICs by Age and Gender, 2000–12 (continued)

| Gender | Age | Deaths 2000 | Deaths 2012 | Change (%) | DALYs 2000 | DALYs 2012 | Change (%) |
|--------|-----|------|------|------|------|------|------|
| Female | 0–27 days | 1,400 | 1,300 | –7 | 128,000 | 120,000 | –6 |
| | 1–59 months | 23,400 | 20,200 | –14 | 2,137,000 | 1,847,000 | –14 |
| | 5–14 years | 29,500 | 30,500 | 3 | 2,680,000 | 2,751,000 | 3 |
| | 15–29 years | 49,900 | 61,000 | 22 | 4,351,000 | 5,264,000 | 21 |
| | 30–49 years | 50,300 | 70,900 | 41 | 3,820,000 | 5,160,000 | 35 |
| | 50–59 years | 20,000 | 37,900 | 90 | 1,066,000 | 1,905,000 | 79 |
| | 60–69 years | 20,700 | 36,900 | 78 | 768,000 | 1,289,000 | 68 |
| | 70+ years | 25,600 | 49,700 | 94 | 530,000 | 943,000 | 78 |
| | Total | 220,800 | 308,400 | 40 | 15,480,000 | 19,279,000 | 25 |

*Source:* WHO 2016.
*Note:* DALYs = disability-adjusted life years; LMICs = low- and middle-income countries. Estimates and percentage changes may vary slightly because of rounding.

**Table 2.2** Injuries: Deaths and Mortality Rates by Cause in LMICs, All Ages and Both Genders, 2000–12

| Cause | 2000 Total deaths (thousands) | 2000 ASMR per 100,000 persons | 2012 Total deaths (thousands) | 2012 ASMR per 100,000 persons | Change (%) Deaths | Change (%) ASMR |
|-------|------|------|------|------|------|------|
| All causes | 41,800 | 1,050 | 44,200 | 880 | 6 | –16 |
| Injuries (unintentional and intentional) | 4,130 | 93 | 4,410 | 81 | 7 | –13 |
| Unintentional injuries | 2,920 | 66 | 3,220 | 60 | 10 | –9 |
| Road traffic injuries | 800 | 18 | 1,140 | 21 | 43 | 17 |
| Poisonings | 220 | 5 | 160 | 3 | –27 | –40 |
| Falls | 440 | 12 | 580 | 12 | 32 | 0 |
| Burns (fire, heat, and hot substances) | 240 | 5 | 250 | 4 | 4 | –20 |
| Drownings | 390 | 8 | 340 | 6 | –13 | –25 |
| Exposures to forces of nature | 0 | 0 | 0 | 0 | 0 | 100 |
| Other unintentional injuries | 830 | 18 | 750 | 14 | –10 | –22 |
| Intentional injuries | 1,210 | 27 | 1,190 | 21 | –2 | –22 |
| Self-harm | 680 | 16 | 610 | 11 | –10 | –30 |
| Interpersonal violence | 420 | 9 | 460 | 8 | 10 | –11 |
| Collective violence and legal intervention | 110 | 2 | 120 | 2 | 9 | 0 |

*Source:* WHO 2016.
*Note:* ASMR = age-standardized mortality rate; LMICs = low- and middle-income countries. Percentages may vary slightly because of rounding.

apparent age-specific peak occurred in female deaths from RTIs. Finally, although RTIs frequently lead to premature mortality, nonfatal outcomes contribute a substantial proportion of total DALYs (Peden and others 2004). The majority of RTI-related DALYs occurs among males ages 15–49.

## Other Unintentional Injuries

Although RTIs are the single leading cause of death by injury, nontransport unintentional injuries collectively—including poisonings, falls, burns, and drownings—account for twice the number of deaths and DALYs as do RTIs (tables 2.2 and 2.3). The proportion of deaths and DALYs as a result of unintentional injuries is higher in LMICs than in high-income countries. Nontransport unintentional injuries account for more than 6,700 deaths per day and 2.4 million deaths annually—almost twice the number of deaths from transport injuries and twice the number of deaths from intentional injuries. Nontransport unintentional injuries also account for over 128 million DALYs annually—almost twice the number from transport injuries and from intentional injuries. Trends across individual causes vary: deaths from falls and burns are increasing, while deaths from poisonings and drownings are decreasing (table 2.2). At the same time, age-standardized mortality

rates for nontransport unintentional injuries are all declining substantially with the exception of falls.

## Poisonings

The burden of unintentional poisoning is declining, with age-standardized mortality rates declining 40 percent from 2000 to 2012. In 2012, LMICs experienced an estimated 163,000 deaths and 9.3 million DALYs. Most poisoning cases continue to occur among children who have unintentionally gained access to toxic chemicals (Balan and Lingam 2012).

## Falls

After RTIs, falls are the most frequent cause of death and DALYs owing to unintentional injury, resulting in 577,000 deaths and 33.5 million DALYs in LMICs in 2012. Age-standardized mortality rates from falls have stagnated since 2000 in contrast to other unintentional injuries. A high incidence of falls has been observed in South-East Asia. Most falls occur among the elderly, even in LMICs (Kalula and others 2011; Ranaweera and others 2013). The burden of falls is also being driven by population aging and is exacerbated by lack of treatment for cognitive problems and by unsafe living environments (Lau and others 2001). Work-related falls and other injuries are also a major problem in LMICs.

**Table 2.3** Injuries: DALYs by Cause in LMICs, All Ages and Both Genders, 2000–12

| | 2000 | | 2012 | | |
|---|---|---|---|---|---|
| Cause | Total DALYs (thousands) | Percentage of all DALYs | Total DALYs (thousands) | Percentage of all DALYs | Change (%) |
| All causes | 2,486,000 | 100 | 2,355,000 | 100 | –5 |
| Injuries (unintentional and intentional) | 266,000 | 11 | 264,000 | 11 | –1 |
| Unintentional injuries | 197,000 | 8 | 197,000 | 8 | 0 |
| Road traffic injuries | 57,000 | 2 | 70,000 | 3 | 23 |
| Poisonings | 13,000 | 1 | 9,000 | 0 | –31 |
| Falls | 28,000 | 1 | 33,000 | 1 | 18 |
| Burns (fire, heat, and hot substances) | 17,000 | 1 | 17,000 | 1 | 0 |
| Drownings | 28,000 | 1 | 22,000 | 1 | –21 |
| Exposures to forces of nature | 0 | 0 | 0 | 0 | 0 |
| Other unintentional injuries | 54,000 | 2 | 46,000 | 2 | –15 |
| Intentional injuries | 69,000 | 3 | 67,000 | 3 | –3 |
| Self-harm | 36,000 | 1 | 31,000 | 1 | –14 |
| Interpersonal violence | 26,000 | 1 | 29,000 | 1 | 12 |
| Collective violence and legal intervention | 7,000 | 0 | 7,000 | 0 | 0 |

*Source:* WHO 2016.

*Note:* DALYs = disability-adjusted life years; LMICs = low- and middle-income countries. Percentages may vary slightly because of rounding.

**Burns**

In 2012, an estimated 245,000 deaths and 16.8 million DALYs in LMICs were attributable to burns. Deaths from burns have remained stable since 2000, especially in Sub-Saharan Africa, South-East Asia, Europe, and the Eastern Mediterranean. Age-standardized mortality rates from burns declined 20 percent, suggesting that increases in numbers of deaths are being driven by population growth or increases in death rates in specific groups only. Among injuries, burns are uniquely more prevalent among females. This pattern is due to differential exposure to unsafe cooking appliances and other hazards in households in LMICs (Ahuja and Bhattacharya 2002; Ahuja, Bhattacharya, and Rai 2009; Ahuja, Dash, and Shrivastava 2011; Hyder and others 2009; Mabrouk, El Badawy, and Sherif 2000). Another important etiology of burns among women is acid attacks, which have received particular media attention in the past few years and seem to be more frequent in South Asia (Acid Survivors Foundation 2014).

**Drownings**

Drowning-related deaths (337,000) and DALYs (21.8 million) in LMICs are decreasing. Death rates declined by 13 percent and age-standardized mortality rates by 25 percent. Drowning continues to be most common among children, adolescents, and young adult males. It often occurs as a result of risky behaviors and the exacerbating effects of harmful alcohol use (Peden and McGee 2003). Drowning among children under age five occurs most frequently in settings where swimming education and child supervision are inadequate, such as rural areas (Rahman and others 2012).

**Other Causes**

Exposures to forces of nature and other unintentional injuries (not elsewhere classified) account for a substantial additional fraction of total deaths and DALYs. Because interventions for these conditions are not specifically addressed in *Disease Control Priorities* (third edition), they are not discussed further here.

## INTERPERSONAL AND COLLECTIVE VIOLENCE

In 2012, LMICs experienced 461,000 deaths and 29 million DALYs related to interpersonal violence. Although deaths from interpersonal violence, which is the major cause of intentional injury covered in chapter 5 of this volume (Mercy and others 2017), are increasing worldwide, the rate of increase was 9 percent in LMICs from 2000 to 2012, which was faster than the global average (table 2.2). At the same time, age-standardized mortality rates from interpersonal violence in LMICs remained stable, suggesting that the increase in violence-related deaths was due to demographic changes. A significant proportion of cases in LMICs are gender based (Jan and others 2010). Female infant deaths among infanticide victims are far more common. The mortality rates among males ages 15–29 are approximately five times those among females in the same age group. Collective violence, which tends to be episodic, accounts for a smaller fraction of total deaths and DALYs (less than 1 percent) compared with interpersonal violence.

## OCCUPATIONAL HEALTH RISKS

Occupational health encompasses numerous issues, including chemical, biological, physical, and psychosocial hazards. Relatively more is known about occupational injuries because most countries track these in the aggregate, although some LMICs do not separate serious events and fatalities in the workplace from those of other origin. Substantially less information is available from LMICs regarding occupational health for many of the same reasons that control remains problematic: knowledge is limited; regulations are either nonexistent or unenforceable because of lack of trained personnel; and the research community has focused on more salient health issues, such as infectious diseases or the emerging epidemic of noncommunicable chronic diseases. Noncommunicable diseases may well have a workplace contribution, but this is unstudied. Infectious diseases, such as tuberculosis, have been linked to workplace exposures or living conditions, including migrant labor practices.

Existing estimates of occupational risks in LMICs suggest that they are generally increasing in parallel with global trends (table 2.4). From 1990 to 2013, attributable deaths and DALYs from occupational risks increased by 27 percent. They constituted 2.4 percent of total attributable deaths and 5.7 percent of total attributable DALYs in LMICs in 2013. The single-largest causes of attributable deaths were occupational particulate matter, gases, and fumes (196,000), occupational carcinogens (189,000), and occupational injuries (135,000). Health loss from carcinogens in particular increased dramatically from 1990 to 2013. However, age-standardized mortality rates from occupational risks decreased for all causes except occupational carcinogens, which increased 33 percent. This suggests that most of the increase in the number of attributable deaths is due to demographic changes, but that a real increase in exposure to carcinogens occurs independent of demographic patterns. Although occupational ergonomic

**Table 2.4** Occupational Risks: Estimated Attributable Deaths, Mortality Rates, and DALYs in LMICs by Cause, All Ages and Both Genders, 1990–2013

| Cause | Deaths (thousands) 1990 | Deaths (thousands) 2013 | Deaths (thousands) Change (%) | ASMR per 100,000 persons 1990 | ASMR per 100,000 persons 2013 | ASMR per 100,000 persons Change (%) | DALYs (thousands) 1990 | DALYs (thousands) 2013 | DALYs (thousands) Change (%) |
|---|---|---|---|---|---|---|---|---|---|
| Total | 18,700 | 23,800 | 27 | 729 | 597 | −18 | 880,000 | 837,000 | −5 |
| Total environmental and occupational risks | 7,600 | 7,400 | −3 | 280 | 188 | −33 | 378,000 | 271,000 | −28 |
| Occupational risks | 460 | 580 | 26 | 17 | 13 | −24 | 37,000 | 47,000 | 27 |
| Occupational asthmagens | 60 | 50 | −17 | 3 | 1 | −67 | 2,600 | 2,500 | −4 |
| Occupational carcinogens | 80 | 190 | 138 | 3 | 4 | 33 | 1,800 | 4,000 | 122 |
| Occupational ergonomic factors | — | — | — | — | — | — | 13,000 | 18,000 | 38 |
| Occupational injuries | 130 | 140 | 8 | 3 | 2 | −33 | 8,000 | 8,100 | 1 |
| Occupational noise | — | — | — | — | — | — | 4,000 | 6,500 | 63 |
| Occupational particulate matter, gases, and fumes | 190 | 200 | 5 | 8 | 5 | −38 | 6,600 | 8,200 | 24 |

*Source:* IHME 2015.

*Note:* ASMR = age-standardized mortality rate; DALYs = disability-adjusted life years; LMICs = low- and middle-income countries; — = not available. Each of the six major occupational hazards is listed as a subcategory of "occupational risks," which are a subset of "total environmental and occupational risks," which are a subset of "total" attributable deaths and DALYs. Data from the Global Burden of Disease Study 2013 (IHME 2015) were used because similar data were unavailable from the World Health Organization's Global Health Estimates database. Percentages may vary slightly because of rounding.

factors and occupational noise were not attributable to any deaths, they were substantial contributors to DALYs and appear to be a growing problem.

In congruence with these estimates, the handful of empirical studies on occupational health hazards in LMICs that appear annually suggest an acceleration in risks as more dangerous trades move in the global marketplace to regions of lower training and regulation. In particular, the emerging global supply chain in electronics, toys, and textiles is replete with chemical and physical hazards, including heavy metals, solvents, plastics, noise, and heat (see chapter 6 in this volume, Abdalla and others 2017). Further, a major factor driving occupational injury trends in LMICs is the export of hazardous industries to these countries because of lower wages. Workers in these hazardous positions number 1.52 billion—an increase of 23 million since 2009 (ILO 2012).

The gender and age distributions of occupational injuries are noteworthy. Women are at higher risk for injuries and experience more severe injuries than men in many high-income workplaces, after accounting for job tasks. Women also appear to be more severely affected by occupational risks in the Middle East and North Africa, although the data are less satisfactory (Abdalla and others 2017). However, many occupational injuries appear to implicate high-hazard sectors that tend to employ males, such as construction, fishing, and mining. These industries often lack safety equipment, training,

and regulations. Decreasing gender gaps in many professions are leading to more women being injured in the workplace (Kelsh and Sahl 1996; Nordander 2008; Turgoose, Carter, and Stride 2006). Children are also at much greater risk in many LMICs: between 3 and 75 percent of children ages 7–14 years are informally employed, depending on the country and occupation (World Bank 2014). Child workers are at especially high risk because of growing bodies that are more susceptible to toxic and carcinogenic substances. Most child workers are employed in agriculture, where they are exposed to strenuous labor and pesticides (ILO 2011).

Finally, the number of people working in the informal sector worldwide is increasing, and such work is fraught with poor regulations, inadequate standards, and insufficient availability of protective equipment (Charmes 2012; ILO 2002). Although research on the informal sector is challenging, it clearly shows that informal workers frequently live in poverty, routinely face adverse working conditions (Muntaner and others 2010), and generally have limited access to health care (Noe and others 2004). Strategies for prevention and control of disease are generally very limited for this population of globally staggering proportion. Occupational health and safety are generally viewed as an area within the broad province of primary health care, rather than the focus of specialized, separate strategies, as in high-income countries. Expanded training of the health care workforce in this domain is essential.

## WATER, SANITATION, AND HYGIENE–RELATED ILLNESSES

Health loss owing to unsafe water, poor sanitation, and poor handwashing practices is an important indicator of overall population health and poverty in LMICs. The Millennium Development Goal target for improved drinking water was met in 2010. However, many LMICs still lack WASH intervention coverage because countries have set different standards for improved water supply and sanitation (Roaf and Khalfan 2005). Disparities within countries persist, particularly in rural areas. In rural Sub-Saharan Africa, for example, many individuals must walk long distances to collect adequate drinking water, while piped water is readily available in urban areas.

Although the rate of open defecation has decreased globally, it is still common practice in many rural areas. Poor hygiene practices, such as infrequent use of soap for handwashing, exacerbate the spread of pathogens (Strickland 2000). Helminths are commonly transmitted through feces and drinking water sources and are particularly problematic for agricultural workers and children in rural areas (Lozano and Naghavi 2010). As a consequence, diarrheal illnesses are responsible for approximately 43 percent of under-five mortality in South and South-East Asia and Sub-Saharan Africa (Humphrey 2009; Petri

and Miller 2008). Nonfatal enteric infections can have long-term health consequences as well: pathogenic bacteria can cause inflammation in children's intestines, reducing proper absorption of nutrition. This process generates a cycle of malnutrition and enteropathy, which then contributes further to under-five mortality and to chronic nutritional deficiency that can extend into adulthood (Black and others 2008; Black and Victora 2013).

The social and psychological disadvantages of having poor access to WASH services are also noteworthy. Significant stress can be traced to lack of improved water sources and sanitation among the poor (Hutton and others 2014). Women generally bear the burden of collecting water. Children who have difficulty accessing water or practice open defecation can readily spread waterborne diseases to others. Infected children are less likely to attend school. Further, low WASH intervention coverage has a large environmental effect: elimination in bodies of water negatively affects ecosystems and disrupts natural resources (Corcoran and Nellemann 2011; Rabalais and Turner 2013).

Table 2.5 provides estimates of morbidity and mortality attributable to lack of WASH services. These estimates represent a lower bound, because many other health effects that are not easily measured but are nonetheless linked to WASH likely exist. The estimates demonstrate the effect of having met the Millennium

**Table 2.5** Environmental Risks: Estimated Attributable Deaths, Mortality Rates, and DALYs in LMICs by Cause, All Ages and Both Genders, 1990–2013

| Cause | Deaths (thousands) | | | ASMR per 100,000 persons | | | DALYs (thousands) | | |
|---|---|---|---|---|---|---|---|---|---|
| | 1990 | 2013 | Change (%) | 1990 | 2013 | Change (%) | 1990 | 2013 | Change (%) |
| Total | 18,700 | 23,800 | 27 | 729 | 597 | –18 | 880,000 | 837,000 | –5 |
| Total environmental and occupational risks | 7,600 | 7,400 | –3 | 280 | 188 | –33 | 378,000 | 271,000 | –28 |
| Air pollution | 4,100 | 5,000 | 22 | 179 | 132 | –26 | 145,000 | 133,000 | –8 |
| Ambient ozone pollution | 100 | 180 | 80 | 6 | 6 | 0 | 2,000 | 4,000 | 100 |
| Ambient particulate matter air pollution | 1,600 | 2,400 | 50 | 68 | 62 | –9 | 56,000 | 62,000 | 11 |
| Household air pollution from solid fuels | 2,800 | 2,900 | 4 | 122 | 79 | –35 | 101,000 | 81,000 | –20 |
| Unsafe water, sanitation, and handwashing | 2,700 | 1,400 | –48 | 69 | 30 | –57 | 190,000 | 83,000 | –56 |
| No handwashing with soap | 1,000 | 500 | –50 | 26 | 11 | –58 | 70,000 | 31,000 | –56 |
| Unsafe sanitation | 1,700 | 800 | –53 | 45 | 17 | –62 | 124,000 | 49,000 | –60 |
| Unsafe water source | 2,400 | 1,200 | –50 | 62 | 27 | –56 | 169,000 | 75,000 | –56 |

*Source:* IHME 2015.

*Note:* ASMR = age-standardized mortality rate; DALYs = disability-adjusted life years; LMICs = low- and middle-income countries. Each of the major environmental hazards is listed as a subcategory. Data from the Global Burden of Disease Study 2013 (IHME 2015) were used because similar data were unavailable from the World Health Organization's Global Health Estimates database. Percentages may vary slightly because of rounding.

Development Goal target; attributable deaths and DALYs have decreased by 48 percent and 56 percent, respectively, and age-standardized mortality rates have decreased by 57 percent. Nevertheless, the health effect remains significant: 6 percent of deaths and 10 percent of DALYs in LMICs in 2013 were attributable to WASH-related illnesses.

## HEALTH EFFECTS OF AIR POLLUTION

Air pollution continues to have significant health effects in LMICs, where it accounted for nearly 21 percent of attributable deaths and 16 percent of attributable DALYs in 2013. Total attributable deaths from air pollution have increased 22 percent since 1990, while DALYs have decreased 8 percent. Further, age-standardized attributable mortality rates have decreased 26 percent (IHME 2015).

Table 2.5 shows recent estimates that about 2.5 million deaths in LMICs in 2013 were attributable to airborne pollutants in public settings. In the disease burden estimates, air pollution contributes a significant proportion of deaths as a result of respiratory infections; chronic obstructive pulmonary disease; cerebrovascular disease; ischemic heart disease; and cancers of the trachea, bronchus, and lung. The forms of air pollution that have been evaluated are (1) ambient particulate matter air pollution (approximately 2.6 million attributable deaths in LMICs) in the form of particle and ozone pollution and (2) household air pollution from solid fuels (approximately 2.9 million deaths in LMICs), although other categories have not yet been assessed globally. (Because of a degree of overlap, totals are less than the sum of individual components.)

Overall, 90 percent of air pollution deaths are in LMICs. However, because household solid cookfuel use is essentially confined entirely to LMICs, essentially all effects occur in these settings. Ambient particulate matter air pollution occurs in both rural and urban areas and is related to a variety of emission sources, including motorized transport, power plants, industry, road and construction dust, brick kilns, garbage burning, and the like. Household air pollution occurs primarily in less urbanized areas and is related to the use of solid fuels for cooking and heat in homes. It is also a major source of ambient pollution, causing at least one-fourth of ambient pollution exposures in India and China, for example. Thus, perhaps 15 percent of the burden accounted to ambient pollution actually began in households in LMICs.

Ambient particulate matter air pollution accounts for a relatively larger proportion of cardiovascular and cerebrovascular diseases. Household air pollution accounts for a relatively larger proportion of chronic and acute respiratory disease, the latter affecting children.

Of all LMICs, India experiences the most significant effect from air pollution because of population size, weak regulation, and rapid industrialization; two-thirds of the population still uses solid fuels (Smith 2015). At the same time, the major source of air pollution in less urbanized areas is household air pollution, which results from the use of solid fuels for cooking and heat in homes (Smith 2015). In contrast to outdoor air pollution, morbidity from household air pollution appears to be decreasing in LMICs, as is suggested by a 20 percent reduction in DALYs from 1990 to 2013. However, most of this reduction is due to the decline in background child pneumonia rates related to improvements in health care and nutrition.

Surveillance of air pollution is challenging for several reasons. Measurement devices are typically located in urban areas, so less is known about air pollution in rural areas. Satellite observations combined with modeling, however, are becoming a major source of information on ambient air quality in rural and other unmonitored areas (Brauer and others 2016). Linking production, exposure, and health effects is problematic, because dispersion of particulate matter can be widespread. Health effects per unit of pollution emitted are thought to be greatest among people living close to household sources and roads (Smith 2015).

Integrated exposure-response relationships are now used to determine health burdens and suggest policies. These relationships link results from epidemiological studies across a wide range of exposures to combustion particles—from ambient air pollution, secondhand tobacco smoke, household air pollution, and active smoking (Burnett and others 2014). These are linked, in turn, to global models of population exposure based on a wide range of data sources. The analyses suggest that outdoor air pollution accounts for a relatively larger proportion of cardiovascular disease and cancer, while household air pollution accounts for acute (children only) and chronic respiratory disease (IHME 2015).

## CONCLUSIONS

Recent decades have seen dramatic shifts in the patterns of health loss from injuries and occupational and environmental hazards in LMICs:

- The burden of RTIs and falls, in particular, is increasing substantially, resulting in a net increase in the overall burden of injuries despite a decline in the burden of drownings and poisonings.

- In keeping with trends in economic development in LMICs, health loss from occupational hazards is increasing. The rapid growth in the effect of occupational carcinogens in these settings is of particular concern.
- As a group, environmental risks are declining, in particular, risks related to unsafe water and poor sanitation.
- Household air pollution also appears to be declining, but it is being replaced by ambient particulate matter air pollution from vehicles and industrial sources, particularly in urban areas in populous countries such as India and China.

Designing interventions and policies to address injuries and occupational and environmental hazards requires up-to-date information on the relative magnitude of these conditions and their trends over time. Surveillance for many of these conditions is politically and technically challenging, so the estimates presented in this chapter likely reflect a lower bound on their total burden in LMICs. The need to set priorities around each of these conditions should be explicitly linked to efforts to improve information systems, both within the health sector and elsewhere, for example, in the labor and environment sectors.

The conditions presented in this volume are important contributors to the overall burden of disease in LMICs. Injuries are responsible for about 9 percent of deaths and 7 percent of DALYs, whereas occupational and environmental risks are responsible for about 29 percent of attributable deaths and 31 percent of attributable DALYs. With some notable exceptions, their importance continues to increase in parallel with economic development, urbanization, and the epidemiological transition. Hence, policies that focus on these conditions must also account for and attempt to address the complex social, demographic, and economic factors that are driving health trends.

## NOTE

World Bank Income Classifications as of July 2014 are as follows, based on estimates of gross national income (GNI) per capita for 2013:

- Low-income countries (LICs) = US$1,045 or less
- Middle-income countries (MICs) are subdivided:
  a) Lower-middle-income countries = US$1,046 to US$4,125
  b) Upper-middle-income countries (UMICs) = US$4,126 to US$12,745
- High-income countries (HICs) = US$12,746 or more.

## REFERENCES

Abdalla, S., S. S. Apramian, L. F. Cantley, and M. R. Cullen. 2017. "Occupation and Risk for Injuries." In *Disease Control Priorities* (third edition): Volume 7, *Injury Prevention and Environmental Health*, edited by C. N. Mock, R. Nugent, O. Kobusingye, and K. R. Smith. Washington, DC: World Bank.

Acid Survivors Foundation. 2014. *Annual Report 2014*. Dhaka, Bangladesh. http://www.acidsurvivors.org /images/frontImages/Annual_Report-2014.pdf.

Ahuja, R., and S. Bhattacharya. 2002. "An Analysis of 11,196 Burn Admissions and Evaluation of Conservative Management Techniques." *Burns* 28 (6): 555–61.

Ahuja, R., S. Bhattacharya, and A. Rai. 2009. "Changing Trends of an Endemic Trauma." *Burns* 35 (5): 650–56.

Ahuja, R., K. Dash, and P. Shrivastava. 2011. "A Comparative Analysis of Liquefied Petroleum Gas (Lpg) and Kerosene Related Burns." *Burns* 37 (8): 1403–10.

Balan, B., and L. Lingam. 2012. "Unintentional Injuries among Children in Resource Poor Settings: Where Do the Fingers Point?" *Archives of Disease in Childhood* 97 (1): 35–38.

Black, R., L. Allen, Z. Bhutta, L. Caulfield, M. de Onis, and others. 2008. "Maternal and Child Undernutrition: Global and Regional Exposures and Health Consequences." *The Lancet* 371 (9608): 243–60.

Black, R., and C. Victora. 2013. "Maternal and Child Undernutrition and Overweight in Low-Income and Middle-Income Countries." *The Lancet* 382: 427–51.

Brauer, M., G. Freeman, J. Frostad, A. von Donkelaar, R. V. Martin, and others. 2016. "Ambient Air Pollution Exposure Estimation for the Global Burden of Disease 2013." *Environmental Science and Technology* 50 (1): 79–88.

Burnett, R. T., C. A. Pope III, M. Ezzati, C. Olives, S. S. Lim, and others. 2014. "An Integrated Risk Function for Estimating the Global Burden of Disease Attributable to Ambient Fine Particulate Matter Exposure." *Environmental Health Perspectives* 122 (4). doi:10.1289/ehp.1307049.

Charmes, J. 2012. "The Informal Economy Worldwide: Trends and Characteristics." *Margin: the Journal of Applied Economic Research* 6 (2): 103–32.

Corcoran, E., and C. Nellemann. 2011. *Sick Water? The Central Role of Wastewater Management in Sustainable Development: A Rapid Response Assessment*. Arendal, Norway: United Nations Environment Programme, United Nations Human Settlements Programme, GRID-Arendal.

Forouzanfar, M., L. Alexander, H. R. Anderson, V. F. Bachman, S. Biryukov, and others. 2015. "Global, Regional, and National Comparative Risk Assessment of 79 Behavioural, Environmental and Occupational, and Metabolic Risks or Clusters of Risks in 188 Countries, 1990–2013: A Systematic Analysis for the Global Burden of Disease Study 2013." *The Lancet* 386 (10010): 2287–323.

Humphrey, J. 2009. "Child Undernutrition, Tropical Enteropathy, Toilets, and Handwashing." *The Lancet* 3754: 1032–35.

Hutton, G., U. Rodriguez, A. Winara, N. Anh, K. Phyrum, and others. 2014. "Economic Efficiency of Sanitation Interventions in Southeast Asia." *Journal of Water, Sanitation and Hygiene for Development* 4 (1): 23–36.

Hyder, A., D. Sugerman, P. Puvanachandra, J. Razzak, and H. El Sayed. 2009. "Global Childhood Unintentional Injury Surveillance in Four Cities in Developing Countries: A Pilot Study." *Bulletin of the World Health Organization* 87 (5): 345–52.

IHME (Institute for Health Metrics and Evaluation). 2015. *Global Burden of Disease 2013 Study.* Seattle, WA: IHME.

ILO (International Labour Organization). 2002. *Women and Men in the Informal Economy: A Statistical Picture.* Geneva: ILO.

———. 2011. *Children in Hazardous Work: What We Know, What We Need to Do.* International Programme on the Elimination of Child Labour. Geneva: ILO.

———. 2012. "Global Employment Trends 2012: World Faces a 600 Million Jobs Challenge, Warns ILO." Press release, ILO, Geneva, January 24.

Jan, S., G. Ferrari, C. Watts, J. Hargreaves, J. Kim, and others. 2010. "Economic Evaluation of a Combined Microfinance and Gender Training Intervention for the Prevention of Intimate Partner Violence in Rural South Africa." *Health Policy and Planning* 26: 366–72.

Kalula, S., V. Scott, A. Dowd, and K. Brodrick. 2011. "Falls and Fall Prevention Programmes in Developing Countries: Environmental Scan for the Adaptation of the Canadian Falls Prevention Curriculum for Developing Countries." *Journal of Safety Research* 42 (6): 461–72.

Kelsh, M., and J. Sahl. 1996. "Sex Differences in Work-Related Injury Rates among Electric Utility Workers." *American Journal of Epidemiology* 143 (10): 1050–58.

Lau, E., P. Suriwongpaisal, J. Lee, S. Das De, and M. Festin. 2001. "Risk Factors for Hip Fracture in Asian Men and Women: The Asian Osteoporosis Study." *Journal of Bone and Mineral Research* 16 (3): 572–80.

Lozano, R., and M. Naghavi. 2010. "Global and Regional Mortality from 235 Causes of Death for 20 Age Groups in 1990 and 2010: A Systematic Analysis for the Global Burden of Disease Study 2010." *The Lancet* 380: 2095–128.

Mabrouk, A., A. El Badawy, and M. Sherif. 2000. "Kerosene Stove as a Cause of Burns Admitted to the Ain Shams Burn Unit." *Burns* 26 (5): 474–77.

Mercy, J., S. D. Hillis, A. Butchart, M. A. Bellis, C. L. Ward, and others. 2017. "Interpersonal Violence: Global Impact and Paths to Prevention." In *Disease Control Priorities* (third edition): Volume 7, *Injury Prevention and Environmental Health,* edited by C. N. Mock, R. Nugent, O. Kobusingye, and K. R. Smith. Washington, DC: World Bank.

Muntaner, C., O. Solar, C. Vanroelen, J. Martinez, M. Vergara, and others. 2010. "Unemployment, Informal Work, Precarious Employment, Child Labor, Slavery, and Health Inequalities: Pathways and Mechanisms." *International Journal of Health Services* 40 (2): 281–95.

Noe, R., J. Rocha, C. Clavel-Arcas, C. Aleman, M. Gonzales, and others. 2004. "Occupational Injuries Identified by an Emergency Department Based Injury Surveillance System in Nicaragua." *Injury Prevention* 10 (4): 227–32.

Nordander, C. 2008. "Gender Differences in Workers with Identical Repetitive Industrial Tasks: Exposure and Musculoskeletal Disorders." *International Archives of Occupational and Environmental Health* 81 (8): 939–47.

Peden, M., and K. McGee. 2003. "The Epidemiology of Drowning Worldwide." *Injury Control and Safety Promotion* 10 (4): 195–99.

Peden, M., R. Scurfield, D. Sleet, D. Mohan, A. Hyder, and others. 2004. *World Report on Road Traffic Injury Prevention.* Geneva: World Health Organization.

Petri, W., and M. Miller. 2008. "Enteric Infections, Diarrhea, and Their Impact on Function and Development." *Journal of Clinical Investigation* 118 (4): 1277–90.

Rabalais, N., and E. Turner. 2013. *Coastal Hypoxia: Consequences for Living Resources and Ecosystems.* Coastal and Estuarine Studies 58. Washington, DC: American Geophysical Union.

Rahman, F., S. Bose, M. Linnqn, A. Rahman, S. Mashreky, and others. 2012. "Cost-Effectiveness of an Injury and Drowning Prevention Program in Bangladesh." *Pediatrics* 130 (6): 1–10.

Ranaweera, A., P. Fonseka, A. Pattiya, and S. Siribaddana. 2013. "Incidence and Risk Factors of Falls among the Elderly in the District of Colombo." *Ceylon Medical Journal* 58: 100–6.

Roaf, V., and A. Khalfan. 2005. "Monitoring Implementation of the Right to Water: A Framework for Developing Indicators." Global Issue Papers 14, Heinrich Boll Foundation, Berlin.

Smith, K. R. 2015. "Report of the Steering Committee on Air Pollution and Health Related Issues." Ministry of Health and Family Welfare, Government of India, New Delhi.

Strickland, G. 2000. *Hunter's Tropical Medicine and Emerging Infectious Diseases,* sixth edition. Philadelphia, PA: WB Saunders.

Turgoose, L., A. Carter, and C. Stride. 2006. "Encouraging an Increase in the Employment of Women Returners in Areas of Skill Shortage in Traditionally Male Industries." DoTaI University of Sheffield and Institute of Work Psychology, Sheffield, U.K.

Vijayakumar, L., M. R. Phillips, M. M. Silverman, D. Gunnell, and V. Carli. 2015. "Suicide." In *Disease Control Priorities* (third edition): Volume 4, *Mental, Neurological, and Substance Use Disorders,* edited by V. Patel, D. Chisholm, T. Dua, R. Laxminarayan, and M. E. Medina-Mora. Washington, DC: World Bank. http://www.dcp-3.org/mentalhealth.

WHO (World Health Organization). 2013. "Road Safety: Basic Facts." Fact Sheet #1, WHO, Geneva.

———. 2016. Global Health Estimates 2012 (database). WHO, Geneva. http://www.who.int/healthinfo/global _burden_disease/en/.

World Bank. 2014. *World Development Indicators: Children at Work.* Washington, DC: World Bank.

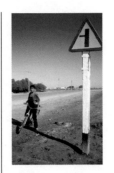

Chapter **3**

# Road Traffic Injuries

Abdulgafoor M. Bachani, Margie Peden, G. Gururaj,
Robyn Norton, and Adnan A. Hyder

## INTRODUCTION

Road traffic injuries (RTIs) are the leading cause of unintentional injuries, accounting for the greatest proportion of deaths from unintentional injuries. They are the leading cause of injury-related disability-adjusted life years (DALYs), and they pose a significant economic and societal burden. Despite this burden, RTIs remain a largely neglected public health problem, especially in low- and middle-income countries (LMICs), where urbanization and motorization are rapidly increasing. Unfortunately, reliable data on the burden of RTIs and cost-effective interventions in LMICs are sorely lacking. In 2010, global efforts to reduce the burden of road safety injuries received a major boost when the United Nations (UN) General Assembly launched the Decade of Action for Road Safety 2011–2020, with a goal of saving 5 million lives worldwide by 2020 (United Nations Road Safety Collaboration 2010). Since then, awareness of road safety and its close relationships to economic and social development has grown significantly, and activities that promote road safety at international and national levels have gained new momentum.

This chapter uses the latest global and regional estimates to characterize the burden of RTIs, including their mortality; morbidity; and economic and social impacts on individuals, families, and society. It summarizes economic evidence on proven and promising interventions that address the burden. The goal of this chapter is to further inform the global discourse on reducing RTIs worldwide, with a special focus on LMICs, where 90 percent of fatal RTIs occurred yet only 54 percent of global vehicles were registered (WHO 2015a).

## HEALTH BURDEN OF ROAD TRAFFIC INJURIES

Each day, more than 3,400 people die on the world's roads (1.25 million people each year), making RTIs the ninth leading cause of death globally (WHO 2014). The global rate of mortality resulting from RTIs has increased 46 percent since 1990 (Lozano and others 2012). Latest estimates from the Global Health Estimates (WHO 2014) show that road traffic crashes were responsible for 24 percent of all injury-related deaths globally (figure 3.1)—and a total of 78.7 million DALYs lost in 2012, up from 69.1 million in 2000 (WHO 2014). Current trends suggest that RTIs will become the seventh leading cause of death by 2030 unless action is taken (WHO 2015a).

Across World Health Organization (WHO) regions, the highest road traffic mortality rate was in Africa (26.6 per 100,000 population); the lowest was Europe (9.3 per 100,000) (WHO 2015a). Over the past two decades, in the absence of effective road safety programs, mortality resulting from RTIs has increased steadily in East Asia, South Asia, and Eastern and Western Sub-Saharan Africa

Corresponding author: Abdulgafoor M. Bachani, Department of International Health, Johns Hopkins International Injury Research Unit, Johns Hopkins Bloomberg School of Public Health, Baltimore, MD, United States; abachani@jhu.edu.

(Odero, Khayesi, and Heda 2003; WHO 2014). This trend contrasts with that in high-income countries (HICs), where road traffic fatalities are on a downward trajectory following the implementation of safety programs over the past decade (table 3.1) (Garcia-Altes, Suelves, and Barberia 2013; WHO 2013a, 2014).Importantly, within the same region, considerable disparity exists in death rates across countries of different income status. In Europe, for example, low-income countries (LICs) had RTI mortality rates more than twice those for HICs (18.8 per 100,000 versus 8.3 per 100,000, respectively) (WHO 2015a).[1]

LMICs overall bear a disproportionally high burden of RTIs (Hyder, Labinjo, and Muzaffar 2006; Hyder, Muzaffar, and Bachani 2008; Hyder and others 2013; Hyder and Peden 2003; WHO 2013a). They have a little more than 50 percent of the world's vehicles but more than 90 percent of the road traffic deaths (WHO 2015a). More than twice as many individuals per 100,000 population die from RTIs in LMICs compared to HICs (WHO 2014, 2015a) (table 3.1). Even within HICs, individuals from lower socioeconomic backgrounds are more likely to be involved in road traffic crashes than their more affluent counterparts (WHO 2015b).

All types of road users are at risk of RTIs, but marked differences exist in the fatality rates. In particular, *vulnerable road users* (such as pedestrians and users of two-wheelers) are at greater risk compared to motor-vehicle occupants, and they usually bear the greatest

**Figure 3.1** Global Mortality from All Injuries, 2012

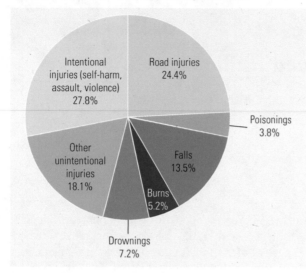

*Source:* WHO 2014.

**Table 3.1** Death Rates and Rates of DALY Losses Resulting from Road Traffic Injuries, by Gender and Income, 2012 and 2000

| | 2012 | | | | | | | | |
| | Global | | | LMICs | | | HICs | | |
| | Total | Men | Women | Total | Men | Women | Total | Men | Women |
|---|---|---|---|---|---|---|---|---|---|
| *Deaths (per 100,000 population)* | | | | | | | | | |
| All unintentional injuries | 52.5 | 67.0 | 37.8 | 55.6 | 70.6 | 40.1 | 39.0 | 50.3 | 28.0 |
| RTIs | 17.7 | 25.6 | 9.7 | 19.6 | 28.2 | 10.8 | 9.2 | 13.9 | 4.8 |
| *DALY losses (per 100,000 population)* | | | | | | | | | |
| All unintentional injuries | 3,211.4 | 4,216.2 | 2,190.2 | 3,434.0 | 4,477.8 | 2,361.6 | 2,216.5 | 3,011.7 | 1,446.4 |
| RTIs | 1,112.6 | 1,603.8 | 613.5 | 1,217.3 | 1,744.2 | 676.0 | 644.8 | 957.3 | 342.1 |
| | 2000 | | | | | | | | |
| *Deaths (per 100,000 population)* | | | | | | | | | |
| All unintentional injuries | 57.7 | 74.6 | 40.4 | 60.1 | 76.4 | 43.3 | 47.5 | 66.9 | 29.0 |
| RTIs | 16.7 | 24.3 | 8.9 | 17.0 | 24.7 | 9.1 | 15.4 | 22.9 | 8.3 |
| *DALY losses (per 100,000 population)* | | | | | | | | | |
| All unintentional injuries | 3,772.6 | 4,942.0 | 2,585.8 | 4,008.3 | 5,152.6 | 2,830.0 | 2,807.4 | 4,047.0 | 1,621.7 |
| RTIs | 1,129.0 | 1,636.1 | 614.3 | 1,163.0 | 1,672.4 | 638.4 | 989.9 | 1,481.8 | 519.4 |

*Source:* WHO 2014.
*Note:* DALY = disability-adjusted life year; HICs = high-income countries; LMICs = low- and middle-income countries; RTIs = road traffic injuries.

burden of injury (Peden and others 2004). For example, almost 50 percent of the global road traffic deaths occur among vulnerable road users—motorcyclists (23 percent), pedestrians (22 percent), and cyclists (4 percent) (WHO 2015a). In many LMICs, where the proportion of vulnerable road users is as high as 57 percent, few, if any, interventions are in place to protect these road users; pedestrian deaths account for almost 40 percent of all road injury fatalities in LICs and about 20 percent in middle-income countries (Bachani, Koradia, and others 2012; Bachani, Zhang, and others 2014; Hyder and Bishai 2012; Hyder, Ghaffar, and Masood 2000; WHO 2013a).

Definite data on the number of people who survive RTIs but live with disabilities are almost nonexistent. However, estimates suggest that for every one RTI-related death, an additional 20–50 more individuals suffer some disability (Peden and others 2004). The WHO estimates that RTIs accounted for a total of almost 14 million life years lost annually due to disability in 2012 globally; RTIs represented 30 percent of the injury-related disability burden (WHO 2014).

Empirical evidence in LMICs (although limited and with varied quality) supports these estimates. For example, a study in Arkhangelsk, the Russian Federation, that investigated trends in traffic crashes between 2005 and 2010 found 217 fatalities and 5,964 non-fatal injuries. The study used police data, which was considered the most reliable existing data source for this purpose (Kudryavtsev and others 2013). Another study in China (using a national disability survey) estimated the prevalence of RTI-related disability to be 1.12 per 1,000 population in 2006 (Lin and others 2013). Given the high burden of disability associated with RTIs, better measurement of this disability is necessary not only to highlight but also to develop appropriate strategies for addressing this burden. Recent applications of approaches to obtaining empirical population-level data on the prevalence and impact of disability in LMICs is a step in the right direction (Bachani, Galiwango, and others 2014, 2015; Madans and Loeb 2013; Madans, Loeb, and Altman 2011).

The significant burden of RTIs in terms of both premature mortality and disability is attributable to the fact that young adults (ages 15–44 years) are among the most affected age group. More than 460,000 young people under age 30 years die in road traffic crashes each year—about 1,262 a day (WHO 2007, 2013b, 2014). Among them, more than 75 percent of the deaths occur among young men (WHO 2015b). The rates of both injury-related death and DALY losses were about three times higher among men than women in both LMICs and HICs in 2012, and the gender disparity has persisted over the past decade (table 3.1) (WHO 2014).

## ECONOMIC AND SOCIETAL BURDEN OF ROAD TRAFFIC INJURIES

### Economic Burden

In addition to the health burden, RTIs account for profound economic costs to individuals, families, and societies. In resource-constrained settings, assessing RTI-related costs would help policy makers and health planners to prioritize and choose the most appropriate interventions to control and prevent RTIs (Bishai and Bachani 2012). However, accurately quantifying these costs is not easy. The tangible costs—direct costs, such as medical costs, and indirect costs, including lost productivity and economic opportunity—can be estimated in economic terms; the intangible costs associated with suffering and pain, however, often are more difficult to assess.

Three approaches have been developed to estimate costs of injury: the human capital, willingness-to-pay, and general equilibrium frameworks (Bishai and Bachani 2012).

- *The human capital approach* estimates the aggregated injury costs at societal, national, and regional levels as the sum of the costs at the individual level, including direct medical costs, indirect lost productivity costs, and intangible psychological costs of pain and suffering. The strategies for measuring pain and suffering in this model are not fully developed, and most studies using this approach exclude this component. Because of its structured nature and the ability to compartmentalize costs into different categories, the human capital framework remains the most common approach to value RTI-related injury and death, especially in LMICs (Bishai and Bachani 2012).
- *The willingness-to-pay approach* estimates the value of pain and suffering by asking what people would be willing to pay to live in a world with a lower risk of injuries. By placing monetary values on injuries that are grounded in the consumers' own preferences, this approach provides an option for including estimates of the value of pain and suffering to determine the cost of injuries.
- *The general equilibrium approach* provides strategies for actually measuring the costs from a broader macroeconomic perspective using simulation-modeling techniques. The estimates using this approach are a dynamic assessment of the present value of forgone consumption opportunities resulting from injuries. However, this approach has not been applied to estimating costs of injuries.

Comparisons across these approaches are not appropriate because of the different methodologies and different level of data (micro versus macro) used in the three measures.

Because of the demand for epidemiologic data on the number and nature of RTIs, as well as the challenges of measuring intangible costs, few studies have attempted to estimate RTI-related costs, but this has been changing over the past decade. One large 21-country study estimated that the global cost of RTIs was US$518 billion; the costs of RTIs at the national level in most cases exceeded 1 percent of the gross national product (GNP) (Jacobs, Aeron-Thomas, and Astrop 2000). Another study that used the human capital approach in 11 HICs gave an average cost equivalent to 1.3 percent of the GNP in the 1990s—ranging from 0.5 percent for the United Kingdom to 2.8 percent for Italy (Elvik 2000). More recent studies in Australia (Connelly and Supangan 2006), the Republic of Korea (Lim, Chung, and Cho 2011), New Zealand (O'Dea and Wren 2010), and the United States (Blincoe and others 2015) have also highlighted the significant burden that RTIs impose on a nation's economy. A WHO analysis reveals similar economic burden of RTIs across countries—ranging from 0.2 percent of the gross domestic product (GDP) in Chile and Jamaica to 7.8 percent in South Africa (WHO 2015a).

Cost studies on RTIs in LMICs often are scant because of the poor capacity of health information systems in these settings (WHO 2013a). Studies show that RTIs cost approximately US$89.6 billion a year (in 2012 US$) in LMICs, or 1–2 percent of their GNPs (Jacobs, Aeron-Thomas, and Astrop 2000). The high RTI-related costs as a share of GNP have also been shown in a few country-specific studies, including Bangladesh (Mashreky and others 2010), Belize (Perez-Nunez and others 2010), China (Zhou and others 2003), Uganda (Benmaamar, Dunkerley, and Ellis 2002), and Vietnam (Nguyen and others 2013; Nguyen and others 2015).

Using the human capital approach, researchers in Vietnam estimated that each RTI cost about 6 months of average salary during hospitalization (US$420 [in 2012 US$]), and the average costs during recovery (12 months after hospital discharge) were equivalent to an entire year of income (US$919 [in 2012 US$]) (Nguyen and others 2013, Nguyen and others 2015). Similarly, the total economic costs of injury including direct and indirect costs in Belize represented 0.9 percent of the GDP in 2007 (Perez-Nunez and others 2010). In addition, researchers using the willingness-to-pay approach estimated that each motorist fatality cost $0.55 million (in 2012 US$) in Malaysia (Mohd Faudzi, Mohamad, and Ghani 2011), and the value of a Sudanese pedestrian ranged between US$0.02 million to US$0.10 million (Mofadal, Kanitpong, and Jiwattanakulpaisarn 2015). Although these studies clearly demonstrate the adverse impact of RTIs on economic and social development, more studies and improved health information systems in LMICs are needed to document and understand the full extent and nature of this burden.

### Societal Burden

Despite the progress made in understanding the epidemiology and economic burden of RTIs, understanding of the long-term societal impact of RTIs remains inadequate. Evidence of the significant societal impact of RTIs is limited and mostly available only for HICs. For example, the European Commission estimates that more than 30,000 people were killed and more than 120,000 were permanently disabled by RTIs in 2011; as a result, nearly 150,000 families struggled with the consequent devastation (European Commission 2014). A similar study in the United Kingdom estimated that about 1.1 percent of the total population (more than 130,000 individuals) in the whole of England and Wales had lost a close family member in a fatal RTI since 1971, subjecting many of them to mental health and other consequences (Sullivan and others 2009).

In LMICs, because of the scarcity of good medical care, rehabilitation services, and financial protection mechanisms, individuals often rely heavily on their social networks for support. In these settings, injuries often have far-reaching implications that need to be understood to better address the burden. Studies examining the social impact of RTIs in LMICs are almost nonexistent (Peden and others 2004). However, those that do exist show that road traffic crashes and resultant deaths or disabilities can take a heavy toll on families and friends of injured persons, many of whom experience adverse financial, physical, social, and psychological stresses. For example, families and friends of injured persons reallocate work or change work patterns to provide care. Often, debts are incurred because of the expensive rehabilitation services and reduced income (Mock, Arreola-Risa, and Quansah 2003). Children in these households can be pressured to leave school or can suffer from decreased supervision (Mock, Arreola-Risa, and Quansah 2003).

## RISK FACTORS FOR ROAD TRAFFIC INJURIES

The Haddon matrix revolutionized the understanding of the multifactorial nature of the causes and risk factors of RTIs, and it has made a substantial contribution to the reduction of RTIs (Haddon 1968, 1973). The matrix

**Table 3.2** Risk Factors of Road Traffic Injuries: The Haddon Matrix

| Phase | Host (human) | Agent (vehicles and equipment) | Environment | |
|---|---|---|---|---|
| | | | Physical | Socioeconomic |
| Precrash | Speeding | Insufficient lighting | Flaws in road design (for example, lack of lane separation) | Lack of comprehensive traffic safety law |
| | Driving while impaired (for example, alcohol-impaired driving) | Compromised braking | Flaws in road layout (for example, lack of separation of vehicles and vulnerable road users) | Inadequate licensing system for drivers |
| | Inexperienced and young drivers | Inadequate maintenance | Improper speed limits | Economic pressure (for example, social deprivation) |
| | Distracted driving | | Lack of pedestrian facilities | |
| | Poor road user eyesight | | | |
| | Substance use | | Lack of alternative modes of traveling | |
| | | | Insufficient visibility | |
| Crash | Failure to use restraints (for example, seatbelt, child seat) | Lack of occupant restraints | Non-forgiving roadside (for example, lack of crash barriers) | |
| | Failure to wear a helmet | Compromised braking Insufficient crash-protective design | Poorly designed and maintained roads | |
| Postcrash | No first-aid skills | Fire risk | Inadequate rescue facilities | Inadequately trained EMS[a] and rehabilitation personnel |
| | Lack of access to medical personnel | Leakage of hazardous materials | Congestion | Inadequate prehospital care |

a. Emergency Medical Services.

provided a framework to integrate the traditional epidemiological triangle of host, vector, and environment with a temporal perspective in terms of precrash, crash, and postcrash phases (table 3.2) (Haddon 1973). This approach facilitates the analysis of potential interventions covering the spectrum from primary prevention to rehabilitation. The matrix has been broadly applied in both HICs and LMICs to assist with a systematic understanding of the epidemiology and risk factors, and to facilitate the ability to prioritize the most appropriate preventive and curative measures (Brice and others 2011; Chorba 1991; Short, Mushquash, and Bedard 2013).

## Precrash Risk Factors

Risk factors at the precrash phase include those that predispose individuals to be involved in a crash. At the individual level, these include speeding, driving while impaired, driving while distracted, being inexperienced or young, and using substances; at the vehicle level, these include compromised braking and inadequate lighting and maintenance; and at the environmental level, these include both physical and socioeconomic factors (Herbert and others 2011).

## Crash Risk Factors

Risk factors at the crash phase mainly affect the outcomes in terms of injury severity and fatality. Risk factors at the individual level include failure to use seatbelts, helmets, and child restraints. Vehicles without occupant restraints and crash-protective design or with compromised braking lead to a higher risk of injury death and more severe disability. At the environmental level, poorly designed and maintained roads, low visibility, and lack of crash-protective roadside objects also put road users in danger. Although failure to use seatbelts, helmets, or child restraints significantly increases risk of RTIs and deaths among vehicle occupants, many LMICs have no mandatory requirements; even if they do, compliance and law enforcement often are limited (Peden and others 2004).

## Postcrash Risk Factors

While preventing road traffic crashes is always desirable, a comprehensive road safety strategy is incomplete without a focus on improving postcrash care for injured persons to reduce fatalities and improve outcomes. Many LMICs lack appropriate and adequate postcrash care, contributing to the high burden of deaths and disability resulting from RTIs (Khorasani-Zavareh and others 2009; Miranda and others 2013; Paravar and others 2013; Solagberu and others 2014).

In 2007, global efforts to improve postcrash care, including trauma and emergency care services, gained major momentum when a World Health Assembly adopted a resolution that called on governments and the WHO to increase their efforts to improve care for victims of injuries and other medical emergencies (WHO 2011). It also called on the WHO to raise awareness about affordable ways in which trauma and emergency care services can be strengthened, especially through universally applicable means, such as improvements in organization and planning (WHO 2011). Other studies from LMICs have highlighted a similar need and opportunities to improve care for injured patients (Hyder and Razzak 2013). Documented case studies have shown that improvements can be made even in the poorest and most difficult settings (Mock and others 2010). For example, the simple administration of tranexamic acid to actively bleeding patients in the acute care phase could prevent thousands of premature deaths (Ker and others 2012). Therefore, implementing interventions based on the assessment of risk factors, together with good postcrash care practices, has the potential to save and improve the lives of RTI victims and move closer to the goal of the Decade of Action for road safety (United Nations Road Safety Collaboration 2010).

## INTERVENTIONS

Most road traffic deaths and serious injuries are preventable, because crash risk is largely predictable; therefore, many proven or promising countermeasures can be implemented. RTIs respond well to targeted interventions that prevent the occurrence of the injury, minimize the severity of the injury sustained, and mitigate the sequelae.

Although no blueprint for road safety exists, a broad consensus exists on several principles for interventions:

- Reducing risk exposure by stabilizing motorization levels, providing alternative modes of travel, and improving land-use planning practices
- Reducing risk factors directly related to crash causation, such as speeding, drinking and driving, using unsafe vehicles on unsafe roads (with inadequate safety features for the traffic mix), and failing to enforce road safety laws effectively
- Reducing severity of injuries by mandating and enforcing the use of seat belts, child restraints, and helmets, as well as by improving road infrastructure and vehicle design to protect all road users

- Improving postcrash outcomes, from appropriate and life-saving measures at the scene of the crash through rehabilitation services.

In addition to these fundamental principles, political will and commitment are essential to reducing the burden of RTIs.

The Decade of Action for Road Safety 2011–2020 adopts a systems approach to addressing the burden of RTIs, and proposes five pillars: road safety management, safer roads and mobility, safer vehicles, safer road users, and postcrash care (United Nations Road Safety Collaboration 2010).

### Safer Road Users

Effective legislation that establishes safety codes and punishes unsafe behavior is the first and foremost intervention needed to reduce RTIs. Currently, 91 out of 180 countries have national laws that address the key risk factors, including speeding; driving under the influence; and failing to use motorcycle helmets, seat belts, and child restraints. Since 2011, 17 countries have amended their laws on one or more key risk factors for RTIs to bring them in line with best practice (WHO 2015a). However, little progress has been made globally in extending the coverage of national laws to include all key risk factors (WHO 2015a).

Encouraging a culture of safe road behavior guided by legislation requires not only a high level of enforcement but also a high public perception of enforcement (WHO 2013a). A large body of research (although few studies were conducted in LMICs) shows that:

- Establishing and enforcing speed limits according to designated functions of the roads can reduce RTIs by up to 34 percent (WHO 2013a).
- Setting legislative limits on blood alcohol concentrations at 0.05 grams per deciliter (g/dl) and conducting random breath tests can significantly reduce alcohol-related RTIs (Elvik and others 2009; Shults and others 2001). Despite global progress in strengthening legislation that penalizes alcohol-impaired driving, LMICs are less likely than HICs to adopt the practices (WHO 2013a).
- Introducing and enforcing the use of motorcycle helmets can reduce the risk of death by 40 percent and the risk of serious head injuries by more than 70 percent, yet LMICs are less likely to adopt the practices (Liu and others 2008).
- Introducing and enforcing the use of seatbelts can reduce the risk of fatal injuries by up to 50 percent for front seat occupants and up to 75 percent for rear seat

occupants (Zhu and others 2007). Although most countries have mandatory seatbelt laws, the legislation often does not extend to rear seat occupants (WHO 2013a).

- Mandating the use of child restraints can reduce the likelihood of a fatal crash for children by up to 80 percent (Zaza and others 2001). However, such laws do not always exist in LMICs. For example, only 1 out of 10 South-East Asian countries has a law requiring child restraints (WHO 2015a).

Effective enforcement of traffic laws in low-resource settings could provide economic benefits. Research shows that observance of traffic codes (Bishai and Hyder 2006) and the use of motorcycle helmets (Bishai and Hyder 2006) and seatbelts (Chisholm and others 2012) can be very cost-effective in preventing RTIs in LMICs. While a paucity of good evidence in LMICs of the effectiveness of education exists (as indicated by a systematic review of 15 randomized controlled trials on the effectiveness of safety education programs), some have testified to the synergistic effects of approaches that combine education with legislation and enforcement (Duperrex, Bunn, and Roberts 2002; Sedlák, Grivna, and Cihalova 2006).

## Safer Vehicles

More than 1.8 billion vehicles are registered globally, and more than half of them are in LMICs (WHO 2015a). The increasing demand for mobility has led to rapid motorization (especially in LMICs), creating challenges for safer transport. Strategies focusing on safer vehicles have expanded, from protecting those inside of vehicles to protecting those outside of vehicles. As automakers have refined advanced technology designed to prevent or mitigate crashes, they have introduced it into passenger vehicle models. While limited data on the effectiveness of safety technologies exists, some (such as crash avoidance systems) showed the potential to mitigate RTIs (Jermakian 2011; WHO 2013a). A study in France shows that while public safety measures (such as speed cameras) contributed to a greater than 75 percent reduction in road crash fatalities, enhanced vehicle safety technologies directly saved 27,365 car occupants and 1,083 pedestrian from fatal crashes between 2000 and 2010 (Page, Hermitte, and Cuny 2011). Furthermore, a literature review on road safety interventions shows that electronic stability control systems were associated with a 2–41 percent reduction in RTIs (Novoa, Pérez, and Borrell 2009). The study also noted that the most successful interventions are those that reduce or eliminate the hazard of RTIs and do not rely on changes in road users' behavior (Novoa, Pérez, and Borrell 2009).

Safer vehicles in LMICs are scarce, however, because of costs and inadequate government safety regulations on the automotive industry (IIHS 2013). For example, the Latin New Car Assessment Program (NCAP) evaluated car models in the Latin America market and found that those earning the lowest rating in safety equipment (one out of five stars) were among the top selling cars (IIHS 2013). Furthermore, while frontal airbags for the driver and front passenger have been standard equipment on vehicles in the United States since 1999, they typically were optional equipment on car models in LMICs (IIHS 2013).

In addition to four-wheeled vehicles, the surge of motorized two-wheelers (motorcycles and electric bikes, or e-bikes) in LMICs is even more concerning, especially in South-East Asia and Africa. For example, in Malaysia and Thailand, these vehicles were adopted at a ratio of three persons per vehicle and four persons per vehicle, respectively, in 2011 (Sekine 2014). Both countries had significantly higher fatality rates in motorcycles crashes: 62 percent in Malaysia and 73 percent in Thailand (WHO 2015a).

Looking to address the safety of vehicles in LMICs, the Global NCAP offers a stakeholder movement (as part of the UN's Decade of Action for Road Safety) to encourage adoption and enforcement of harmonized motor vehicle standards in LMICs to promote safer vehicles (NCAP 2011).

## Safer Infrastructure

Poorly designed road networks that lack sufficient safety measures significantly increase RTIs. Results of the International Road Assessment Program in LMICs show that about half of the roads assessed in these countries are rated in the highest risk category, largely because 84 percent of the roads assessed where pedestrians are present have no footpaths (WHO 2013a). This contributes in part to the high proportion (60 percent) of all road traffic deaths in these countries among vulnerable road users (WHO 2013a).

A growing number of countries have amended their national transport policies to encourage alternative modes of transport, such as walking and cycling, or to increase investment in public transport systems to deal with increased motorization and RTIs (WHO 2013a). However, these approaches often have lacked the appropriate strategies for heterogeneous traffic environments or the required resources to ensure the safety of vulnerable road users; these deficits have the potential to counteract the intended effect of the interventions (WHO 2013a). For example, separating vulnerable road users (pedestrians, motorcyclists, and cyclists) from larger and faster vehicles while promoting programs such as city cycling has been shown to reduce injuries and fatalities (Herrstedt 1998; Radin, Mackay, and Hills 2000; Vieira Gomes and Cardoso 2012; Wittink 2001). However, only 91 countries have policies that physically separate vulnerable road users from other road users (WHO 2015a). Other safety features with proven effectiveness include adequate lighting (Radin, Mackay, and Hills 1996, 2000); adequate lane markings or signage (Ward and others 1989); appropriate pedestrian crossings (Dalby 1981); and roadside barriers (Bambach, Mitchell, and Grzebieta 2013), among others (Duduta and others 2011; Fuentes and Hernandez 2013; Mock, Arreola-Risa, and Quansah 2003).

Traffic calming measures (such as the use of speed bumps or rumble strips) are effective in reducing RTIs (Changchen and others 2010; Lines and Machata 2000; Novoa, Pérez, and Borrell 2009). Those and other measures that limit vehicle speed in areas with high concentrations of vulnerable road users were found to reduce the risk of vehicle crashes with pedestrians by 67 percent (WHO 2013a). However, only 47 countries representing 950 million people have set effective urban speed limits; of those, only 27 countries rate their enforcement of the speed laws as good (WHO 2015a).

## Proven and Promising Interventions

The *World Report on Road Traffic Injury Prevention* remains the seminal document discussing proven and promising interventions for road traffic injury prevention (Peden and others 2004). Randomized controlled trials (RCTs) are the gold standard for assessing effectiveness of interventions; however, given the resources that such trials require and the ethical issues of randomizing life-saving interventions, RCTs are rarely used to evaluate road safety interventions.

Consequently, proven interventions rely heavily on case-control or before-and-after studies, but even these are largely concentrated in HICs. Road safety approaches in LMICs in recent years have focused on adapting strategies that worked in HICs and achieved good results. As table 3.3 shows, some interventions focus on reducing or eliminating exposure to risk factors among vulnerable road users, such as promoting alternative modes of transport (Duduta and others 2011), constructing exclusive lanes for motorcyclists (Radin, Mackay, and Hills 2000), increasing visibility of pedestrians and cyclists (Radin, Mackay, and Hills 1996, 2000), and supervising children walking to school (Muchaka and Behrens 2012; Muda and Ali 2006).

**Table 3.3** Examples of Proven and Promising Road Safety Interventions Implemented in LMICs

| Interventions proven in HICs | Implementation and evaluation in LMICs | | |
|---|---|---|---|
| | Country | Study design | Results |
| Providing and encouraging use of alternative forms of mass transportation | Guadalajara, Mexico | Before-and-after study of the impact of Macrobus on crashes | 46 percent reduction in crashes after Macrobus was implemented (Duduta and others 2011) |
| Increasing the visibility of pedestrians and cyclists | Seremban and Shah Alam, Malaysia | Time series study of the use of daytime running lights for motorcycles | 29 percent reduction in visibility-related motorcycle crashes (Radin, Mackay, and Hills 1996, 2000) |
| Supervising children walking to school | Kuala Teregganu, Malaysia | Case–control study assessing the risk of injury to children walking or cycling to school who were supervised by parents | Risk of injury was reduced by 57 percent among supervised children (Muda and Ali 2006) |
| Separating different types of road users | Selagor, Malaysia | Video observational study of crashes and outcomes after introduction of an exclusive motorcycle lane | 39 percent reduction in motorcycle crashes, and 600 percent decrease in fatalities (Radin, Mackay, and Hills 2000) |
| Reducing average speeds through traffic calming measures | China | Before-and-after study of simple engineering measures (such as speed humps, raised intersections, and crosswalks) on speed and casualties | Average speed dropped by 9 percent in three of four intervention sites; overall number of casualties dropped by 60 percent (Changchen and others 2010) |
| Setting and enforcing speed limits appropriate to the function of roads | Londrina, Brazil | Time series study on enforcement of speed control, seat belt use, new traffic code, and improved prehospital care | Reduction in mortality to 27.2 per 100,000 population after one year of implementing a new traffic code (De Andrade and others 2008) |

*table continues next page*

**Table 3.3** Examples of Proven and Promising Road Safety Interventions Implemented in LMICs (continued)

| Interventions proven in HICs | Implementation and evaluation in LMICs | | |
|---|---|---|---|
| | Country | Study design | Results |
| Setting and enforcing blood alcohol concentration limits | Kampala, Uganda | Time series study on enforcement of alcohol-impaired driving and speed laws | 17 percent reduction in traffic fatalities after intervention (Bishai and others 2008) |
| | Villa Clara, Cuba | Time series study on enforcement of alcohol-impaired driving during weekends | 29.9 percent reduction in traffic crashes, 70.8 percent reduction in deaths, and 58.7 percent reduction in injuries, compared with previous year (2002) (Garcell and others 2008) |
| Setting and enforcing the use of seat belts for all motor vehicle occupants | Iran, Islamic Rep. | Before-and-after study of seat belt and helmet enforcement and social marketing | Death rates reduced from 38.2 per 100,000 population in 2004 to 31.8 in 2007 (p < 0.001); death rate per 10,000 vehicles reduced from 24.2 to 13.4. (Soori and others 2009) |
| | Guangzhou, China | Before-and-after study of enhanced enforcement and social marketing on seat-belt wearing | 12 percent increase in prevalence of seat belt use (p = 0.001) (Stevenson and others 2008) |
| Setting and enforcing motorcycle helmet use | Cali, Colombia | Time series analysis of fatalities following implementation of mandatory helmet law, reflective vests, restrictions on when motorcycles can be used, and compulsory driving training | 52 percent reduction in motorcyclist deaths (Espitia-Hardeman and others 2008) |
| | Thailand | Before-and-after survey using trauma registry data following implementation of helmet law | Helmet use increased 5-fold, injuries decreased by 41 percent, and deaths decreased by 20.8 percent (Ichikawa, Chadbunchachai, and Marui 2003) |
| | Vietnam | Time series observational study in three provinces following introduction of mandatory motorcycle helmet law | 16 percent reduction in injuries, and 18 percent reduction in deaths (Passmore, Tu, and others 2010) |
| | Malaysia | Time series study of motorcycle-related crashes, injuries, and fatalities following implementation of a Motorcycle Safety Program using annual police statistics | 25 percent reduction in motorcycle-related crashes, 27 percent reduction in motorcycle-related casualties, and 35 percent reduction in motorcycle fatalities (Law and others 2005) |
| Encouraging helmet use among child bicycle riders | Czech Republic | Case–control study of helmet enforcement, education, and reward campaign at schools | 100 percent increase in helmet use, and 75 percent reduction in head injury admission rates (Sedlák, Grivna, and Cihalova 2006) |

*Note:* LMICs = low- and middle-income countries.

Other interventions focus on addressing the five major behavioral risk factors of RTIs by setting blood alcohol concentration limits (Bishai and others 2008; Garcell and others 2008), setting or reducing speed limits (Changchen and others 2010; De Andrade and others 2008), and enforcing the use of seatbelts for drivers and passengers and helmets for motorcyclists and bicyclists (Espitia-Hardeman and others 2008; Ichikawa, Chadbunchachai, and Marui 2003; Law and others 2005; Passmore, Nguyen, and others 2010; Passmore, Tu, and others 2010; Sedlák, Grivna, and Cihalova 2006; Soori and others 2009; Stevenson and others 2008).

Four additional types of interventions that have proven applicability in HICs but that have yet to be eval-uated in LMICs (or the results of studies yet to be pub-lished in the peer-reviewed literature) are as follows:

- Setting and enforcing lower blood alcohol limits for novice drivers
- Setting and enforcing the usage of appropriate child restraints
- Reducing speed limits around areas with high pedes-trian densities, such as schools and hospitals
- Implementing graduated driver licensing systems for new drivers.

However, challenges exist when adapting interven-tions to the LMIC context. The "effectiveness" realized often is subject to a variety of factors, including the law-making process and long-standing values, norms, and behaviors. Moreover, when trying to identify and quantify the interventions in LMICs, research and implementation capacity (as well as access to funding and costs) play important roles in the effectiveness element (Perel and others 2007).

## Economic Analysis of Interventions

Data on the economic benefits of these interventions, especially in LMICs, are limited. Although some data are available in HICs (such as the net economic benefits of these interventions), the starkly different costs associated with property losses, disability, and medical care make simply translating the conclusions from HICs to LMICs difficult. A recent systematic review of studies on costs, cost-effectiveness, and economic benefits of interventions for RTIs and other types of unintentional injuries in LMICs found that, of the 30 economic evaluations published before February 2013, only two studies analyzed the costs of road safety interventions or devices (Wesson and others 2013). The costs reported below have been updated to 2012 US$ for easier comparison.

Bishai and others (2003) estimated that the budgetary expenditure on road safety at all levels of government in Uganda and Pakistan is US$0.12 and US$0.11 per capita, respectively. Hendrie and others (2004) examined availability, urban price, and affordability of child and family safety devices across 18 economically diverse countries and found that child safety seats and bicycle helmets were more expensive in lower-income countries than higher-income countries. For example, a bicycle helmet cost 10 hours of factory work in lower-income countries, while the cost in higher-income countries was equivalent to less than one hour of work. The study also noted that booster seats were usually not available in lower-income countries, and the average price of one was US$277 based on limited data from eight LMICs in the study sample.

The systematic review (Wesson and others 2013) also includes six cost-effectiveness analyses exploring costs associated with RTI interventions. When comparing across interventions that report costs in terms of years of life saved (YLSs) or DALYs averted, the authors applied the WHO standards of the Choosing Interventions that Are Cost-Effective (WHO-CHOICE) project. WHO-CHOICE considers an intervention "very cost-effective" if it generates a healthy life year for less than the GDP per capita; "cost-effective" if it produces a healthy life year for less than three times the GDP per capita; and

"non-cost-effective" if it produces a healthy life year for more than three times the GDP per capita (Tan-Torres Edejer and others 2003). The authors found four cost-effectiveness studies, which have been updated to US$ 2012:

- Bishai and Hyder (2006) modeled the cost-effectiveness of four potential interventions to increase enforcement of traffic codes (including media coverage, speed bumps, bicycle helmet legislation, and motorcycle helmet legislation) in several LMICs, using previous research findings on effective interventions in LMICs. The results indicated that the average costs per DALY averted (discounted at 3 percent) are US$12 for installing speed bumps at high-risk junctions where 25 percent of RTIs occurred, US$84 for providing traffic enforcement, and US$615 for setting and enforcing motorcycle helmet use, all of which were very cost-effective.
- Chisholm and others (2012) studied the global public health responses to RTIs by estimating the population costs and effects of five enforcement strategies—speed cameras, alcohol-impaired driving and breath testing campaigns, seatbelt use, helmets for motorcyclists, and helmets for bicyclists—on reducing the RTI burden in South-East Asia and Sub-Saharan Africa. In addition to confirming the previous studies, the results suggested that simultaneous enforcement of multiple road safety laws could lead to the most health gains at the least expense.
- Ditsuwan and others (2013) focused on RTIs related to alcohol-impaired driving in Thailand and associated interventions. From a health sector perspective, they found that, when compared with doing nothing and considering only intervention costs (average costs per DALY averted), selective breath testing (US$555), random breath testing (US$611), mass media campaign (US$440), selective breath testing with mass media campaign (US$542), and random breath testing with mass media campaign (US$576) were all very cost-effective. They also estimated that implementing all the interventions together would potentially reduce the burden of alcohol-related RTIs by 24 percent in Thailand.
- Bishai and others (2008) modeled the costs and potential effectiveness of enhanced traffic safety patrols in the capital of Uganda from the perspective of the police department. The evaluation concluded that traffic enforcement could be very cost-effective (US$32 per YLS) in low-income countries, even from a government perspective.

Although limited, these studies demonstrate that road safety interventions are among the most cost-effective interventions. In environments of limited resources and competing priorities, such studies have resonated with policy makers. More economic evaluations of road safety interventions need be conducted in LMICs to advance this important agenda.

## IMPLEMENTATION OF PREVENTION AND CONTROL PROGRAMS

### Safe Systems Approach

Road traffic crashes and their outcomes depend on complex interactions, which makes a systems approach to addressing road safety desirable. The safe systems approach recognizes that multiple sectors need to work in harmony to minimize the occurrence of these crashes and their impacts (SafetyNet 2009). This approach has taken center stage and is being adapted in many settings globally (Elvik and others 2009; Gururaj 2011; WHO 2009). Among the key principles of this approach are recognizing human error in transport systems; appreciating human physical vulnerability and fallibility; promoting accountability of systems and shared responsibilities; integrating interventions; developing intersectoral approaches; highlighting ethical values; and promoting societal values for economic development, human health, and individual choices (WHO 2013a). Some well-known and successful examples of such an approach include the Swedish Vision Zero (Swedish Road Safety 2013), the Sustainable Safety Model of the Netherlands (SWOV 2006), and the Safe Systems approach of Australia (Australian Transport Council 2011).

### Road Safety Policies and Integrated Approaches

To work effectively, the safe systems concept needs to be part of an integrated policy framework and a national road safety plan that define goals and objectives based on burden of RTIs at population level. Some components of the integrated strategic approach for road safety include the following:

- Developing a sound road safety management system
- Building institutional capabilities and mechanisms for interaction
- Developing sustainable policies
- Strengthening human and financial resources and capabilities
- Providing advocacy approaches

- Developing epidemiologically sound and robust information systems on road crashes, injuries, and fatalities
- Promoting intersectoral approaches
- Developing a suitable choice of evidence-based scientific interventions in conjunction with integrated monitoring and evaluation (Schopper, Lormand, and Waxweiler 2006).

The safe systems approach builds on the unique strength of each sector—ministries, other governmental agencies, private organizations, and NGOs—to integrate road safety into different policies systematically, both vertically within each sector and horizontally across sectors. The European Commission, for example, advocates that road safety policies need to utilize other related policy avenues to identify areas of integration, thereby creating opportunities for useful synergies that are in line with the safe systems approach (Elvik and others 2009; International Transport Forum 2008). The United Nations Road Safety Collaboration (UNRSC) is a great example of bringing together different sectors and stakeholders at the global level to advocate for comprehensive multisectoral approaches to addressing the burden of RTIs (United Nations Road Safety Collaboration 2010). Another great example is the Bloomberg Philanthropies Global Road Safety Program (box 3.1), a large-scale initiative that brings together a multisectoral consortium at the global and national levels to implement promising interventions to reduce the burden of RTIs in LMICs (Hyder and others 2012; Peden 2010).

The health sector is well-positioned to play a leading role in developing and integrating road safety into its mainstream agenda. Reducing occurrence of RTIs not only improves population health but also likely has far-reaching health benefits by addressing the key risk factors for road safety (Schopper, Lormand, and Waxweiler 2006). For example, limiting alcohol-impaired driving will help control noncommunicable diseases, as well as improve the social welfare of the population (Global Road Safety Partnership 2007; Gururaj and others 2011). Similarly, health professionals can use their close involvement in the delivery of trauma care and rehabilitation services to advocate road safety practices, such as use of motorcycle helmets, seat belts, and child restraints. In short, the health sector needs to expand its traditional caregiving role and be involved in areas that are relevant to promoting road safety, such as data collection, advocacy, policy development, and capacity building (WHO 2013a).

## Box 3.1

## Case Study: Improving Seatbelt Use in the Russian Federation

**Background:** The Russian Federation is an upper-middle-income country with one of the highest road traffic injuries (RTIs) mortality rates (18.9 per 100,000 population in 2013 in the European Region (WHO 2015a). Every year, nearly 30,000 people are killed from RTIs, and an additional 260,000 are injured or permanently disabled on Russian roads (Department of the Federal Road Safety Inspectorate of the Russian Ministry of Interior [http://www.gibdd.ru/stat/]; Institute for Health Metrics and Evaluation 2013).

**Intervention:** The Bloomberg Philanthropies Global Road Safety Program (the Global Road Safety Program) in Russia aims to support the government's implementation of its national objectives in preventing deaths and serious injury on the country's roads. The program focuses on increasing the use of seatbelts and child restraints, as well as speed management, through three key activities: legislation, enhanced police enforcement, and social marketing campaigns.

**Key Stakeholders and Setting:** The program is administered by the Department of Road Safety within the Russian Ministry of Interior and jointly implemented by other governmental departments at the national and regional levels in two intervention sites: Ivanovskaya and Lipetskaya Oblast.

**Results:** Prevalence of seatbelt and child restraint use was monitored using observation studies. Results from these studies show a steady increase in seatbelt use rates in the two sites over time. As figure B3.1.1 shows, the overall prevalence of seatbelt use increased from 47.5 percent to 88.8 percent among all occupants in Ivanovskaya Oblast. Similar trends were observed in Lipetskaya Oblast, where overall seatbelt use increased from 52.4 percent to 73.5 percent over the same period. Although lower than seatbelt use, child restraint use also has increased over this period in both intervention regions.

The preliminary results of observational studies show promising signs that seatbelt use is moving in the right direction in both Oblasts since the implementation of the measures.

**Figure B3.1.1** Seatbelt Use in Ivanovskaya, Russia, following Implementation of a Seatbelt Program

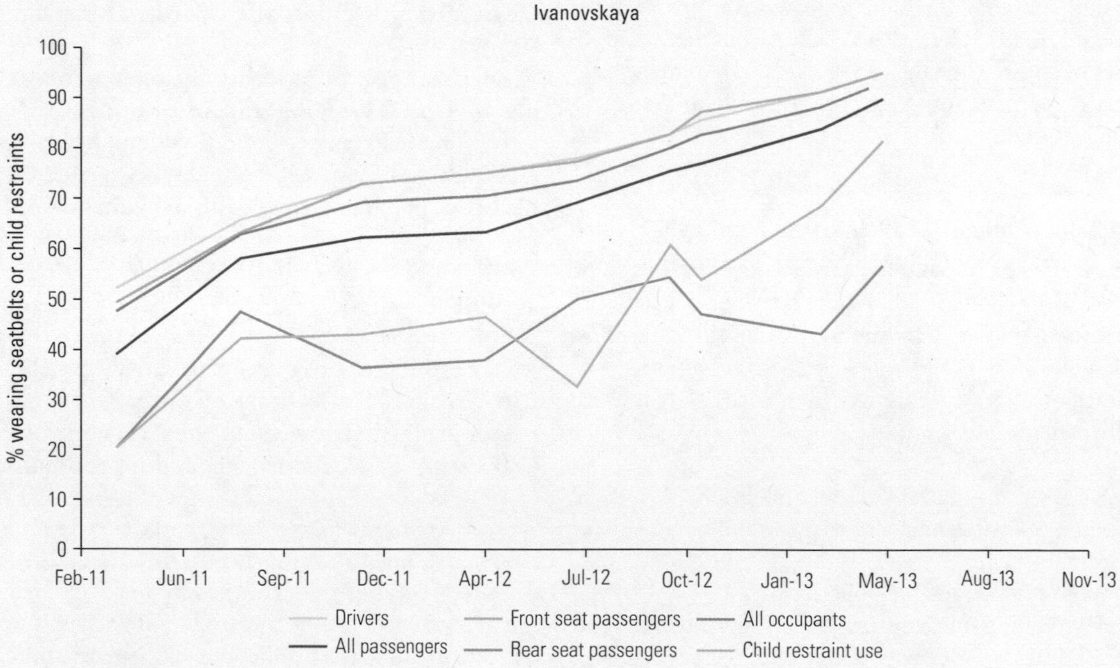

*Source:* Slyunkina and others 2013.

## OPERATIONALIZING ACTION FOR ROAD SAFETY

The information presented throughout this chapter can be crystallized into actionable items that can be undertaken by countries or organizations to enhance road safety. As described in previous sections of the chapter, countries around the world have diverse landscapes for road safety, with different financial and infrastructural contexts, policy and legislative environments, as well as human resource capacities. As such, a *one-size fits all* list of "must-dos" for road safety may not be practical, but the principles of injury prevention and evidence base of road safety must guide all actions. Accordingly, we highlight five key areas of focus: resource mobilization; policy and legislative environment; intervention implementation; data systems; and capacity development.

### Resource Mobilization

Despite the increasing burden of deaths and disabilities from RTIs, generating financial and political support for road safety has not been without its challenges. The health sector, for example, often pays relatively little attention to RTIs as a significant health issue, which has contributed to the limited support from government health sectors and health funders generally. This calls for a multifaceted approach that could involve the following areas:

- Forming intersectoral partnerships
- Targeting high-risk individuals and groups
- Promoting effective interventions
- Developing a clinical research agenda.

#### Forming Intersectoral Partnerships

While the health sector primarily deals with treating and caring for RTIs, effective solutions to road safety require a multisectoral approach. In order to contribute to the evidence base in this area and ultimately to reductions in the incidence and burden of RTIs, health professionals ought to work with nonhealth sector colleagues. Given their expertise and experience in dealing with RTIs, health professionals, for example, could make significant contributions to the design of preventive interventions, or provide input to product manufacturers working to improve the effectiveness of safety devices. This would enable them to leverage financial and political support for their activities from nonhealth sector funders. Countries or cities could promote these linkages by supporting intersectoral working groups, providing seed funding for multidisciplinary research, or both.

#### Targeting High-Risk Individuals and Groups

Continuing to document and highlight the significance of the health and economic burdens of RTIs on individuals and their families is a major part of a profile-raising strategy. Highlighting the burden in high-risk populations (such as adolescents and young people) might well prove to be a more effective strategy than a population-wide approach, given the overwhelming burden of RTIs in these age groups. Additionally, highlighting the greater impact of these injuries on poor people might provide an impetus for some governments and some funders to take action.

#### Promoting Effective Interventions

Continuing to identify and promote cost-effective, evidence-based strategies for the prevention of RTIs could form an important component of a profile-raising strategy. In particular, promoting the implementation and evaluation of the initiatives that have produced sustained reductions in RTI-related crashes or those that are proven cost-effective and feasible among low socioeconomic groups might be particularly effective.

#### Developing a Clinical Research Agenda

Partnering with clinicians involved in the acute and postacute care for the victims might form another strand of the approach to fostering intersectoral engagements on this issue. Our knowledge about the longer-term physical, psychological, and economic impacts is still scant, as is our knowledge about the impact of RTIs on health care systems. Consequently, developing a research agenda in partnership with clinicians to access this information might provide a useful stimulus to mobilize resources and action.

### Policy and Legislative Environment

The WHO has published *Strengthening Road Safety Legislation*, a manual that outlines the strategies and resources that might be used to facilitate implementation and enforcement of such legislation (WHO 2013c). The manual presents some enabling factors for countries to adopt and implement legislation, including the following:

- Recent trends in injuries and fatalities
- Social norms and values
- Financial, human, and other resources.

The manual outlines a framework to support governments and those working with governments to facilitate the implementation of legislation. The framework includes conducting an institutional assessment to identify local, regional, and national bodies responsible for making and enforcing legislation; reviewing and assessing the gaps in national laws and regulations; and improving their comprehensiveness based on evidence. The manual also outlines an advocacy process to facilitate the legislative and regulatory changes.

In addition to a focus on behavioral risk factors, policies and legislation to prevent RTIs need to focus on issues such as safe road infrastructure, protection of vulnerable road users, land use, and safer vehicles. Furthermore, research examining factors that influence policy change around the prevention of RTIs is much needed. Such research, especially in LMICs, ought to include intervention studies to test what approaches have the greatest success in bringing about legislation, as well as studies that show which approaches might be the most cost-effective. Unfortunately, funding for such implementation or policy research is woefully inadequate, and a significant challenge remains in undertaking such research and developing a strong, policy-oriented evidence base.

## Intervention Implementation

As evidenced from the findings in the most recent *Global Status Report on Road Safety*, those countries without adequate laws were almost exclusively LMICs (WHO 2015a), and the implementation challenge for road safety interventions is greatest in these countries. An implementation research agenda may help in overcoming this challenge.

In the case of legislation implementation, undertaking research to gain a systematic understanding of why relevant legislation has not been implemented might provide a useful starting point to determining what sort of additional research might be needed to facilitate change.

Some governments, even when evidence of efficacy is strong, require the evidence of effectiveness within their specific jurisdictions. However, to provide such evidence, legislative action must be implemented first, which usually is difficult. In such cases, the most useful approach would be to undertake small scale efforts or even simulation exercises that could show governments the potential reductions in disease burden and the potential cost-savings of introducing specific legislations or interventions.

The identification of evidence to support the efficacy and effectiveness of non-legislative interventions must also be a continuing endeavor.

## Data Systems

Accurately and regularly collecting comprehensive data on RTIs is vital to monitoring a country's progress in addressing road safety. Such information can be instrumental in guiding a country's health system in planning for and addressing the burden. In addition to mortality and morbidity estimates, reliable information and data on modifiable risk factors, costs associated with RTIs, and age- and gender-specific RTI data at both the national and local levels could inform researchers and policy makers about cost-effective interventions, as well as provide implications of the future health and economic burden—which could be a powerful advocacy tool for action.

Current efforts in HICs such as the EU project JAMIE (2011–2014, Joint Action for Injury Monitoring in Europe) have enabled participating member states to have a relatively limited but useful set of injury data collected from emergency departments. This project has significantly improved comparable injury surveillance systems across EU Member States (Bauer and others 2014; Rogmans 2012).

In LMICs, however, the absence or limited availability of strong and robust injury information systems presents a significant challenge to obtaining consistent and quality data on injuries. These measurement limitations render demonstrating the magnitude of the injury problem or even tracking a nation's progress in addressing it difficult. Establishing simple yet robust data systems in LMICs would facilitate the flow of continuous, reliable, and systematic information on key variables to all stakeholders (Chandran, Hyder, and Peek-Asa 2010; Hofman and others 2005; Kruk and others 2010; Lett, Kobusingye, and Sethi 2002; Mock and others 2004; Razzak, Sasser, and Kellermann 2005). Integrating systems for collecting key information on risk factors and outcomes into new and existing programs to address RTIs in LMICs therefore is essential to begin closing this gap (Bachani, Koradia, and others 2012; Bachani and others 2013; Hyder and others 2013; Slyunkina and others 2013).

## Capacity Development

A recurring theme in the preceding sections is the scarcity of appropriately skilled human resources in LMICs to address the burden of RTIs effectively. This scarcity is evidenced by the relatively few studies on the burden (health, economic, and social) of RTIs and effectiveness of interventions for RTIs originating from LMICs in the peer-reviewed literature (Wesson and others 2013). Clearly, the level of investment in research and development on RTIs in LMICs must increase. This investment will be critical for generating local evidence and for promoting injury on the global public health agenda. Key areas for such capacity include epidemiological research to describe the existing burden, causes, and distribution of RTIs, as well as intervention research.

**Table 3.4** Example of Intersectoral Contributions across the Five Domains to Increase the Use of Seatbelts and Child Restraints

| | Health | Police | Finance/donors | NGOs | Academia |
|---|---|---|---|---|---|
| Resource mobilization for increasing seatbelt/child restraint use | Leadership; Stakeholder engagement | — | Funding | Advocacy | Generation of evidence/data |
| Seatbelt/child restraint policy and legislation | Review of laws | Implement law | Leverage networks/ influence | Review of laws | Policy analysis |
| Intervention implementation | Technical assistance | Enforcement | Funding | Creating awareness; implementation | Monitoring |
| Data systems | Indicators defined | Evidence for enforcement | — | Technical or logistical support | Evaluation; technical support |
| Capacity development | Technical training | — | Funding | — | Training |

*Note:* — = not available; NGO = nongovernmental organization.

Any technical assistance delivered to countries for road safety must include a capacity development component, with the ultimate goal of improving local capacity to conduct injury research, plan services needed, and reduce the burden of injuries. The Global Road Safety Partnership, an organization that works with LMICs to promote the Decade of Action for Road Safety, is a good example (United Nations Road Safety Collaboration 2010).

More accessible training and mentoring programs for road safety also are needed. Although many road safety training programs exist globally, not all are accessible to interested individuals from LMICs, mainly because of the training programs' locations or associated costs or both. A few (such as the Teach-VIP and Mentor-VIP developed by the WHO) make training materials and mentorship for LMIC researchers available at no cost (Hyder, Meddings, and Bachani 2009; Meddings 2010, 2015; Meddings and others 2005). Another online training program for prevention and control offered by the Johns Hopkins International Injury Research Unit takes advantage of the increasing internet connectivity in LMICs to provide free formal classroom-type instruction on key topics, ranging from understanding the burden of RTIs to selecting and implementing interventions and evaluating them (JHU-IIRU 2013). The reach and effectiveness of these new approaches have not yet been determined; however, they are a step in the right direction, and more such efforts are needed to improve road safety globally.

An example of an action agenda for increasing seatbelt use using the five elements described is provided in table 3.4.

## CONCLUSIONS

RTIs continue to contribute to a significant amount of the health, social, and economic burden to society, and global interest in slowing or even halting this trend has been renewed. By implementating interventions and legislation targeted to behavioral factors, vehicle and equipment factors, and infrastructure, as well as the availability of adequate postcrash care, addressing this burden is possible, especially in LMICs. However, more research is needed to better understand the specific needs in LMICs, as well as policy and legislation frameworks that may be appropriate for such settings. Systems must be established that will yield the data necessary to inform these activities; adequately trained human resources also are needed both to generate new research and design and to implement the appropriate policies and programs.

## ACKNOWLEDGMENTS

The authors would like to express their gratitude to Xiaoge Julia Zhang and Jeffrey C. Lunnen for the editorial support they provided in the preparation of this chapter.

## NOTES

WHO Member States are grouped into six geographical regions: African, the Americas, South-East Asia, Europe, Eastern Mediterranean, and Western Pacific.

World Bank Income Classifications as of July 2014 are as follows, based on estimates of gross national income (GNI) per capita for 2013:

- Low-income countries (LICs) = US$1,045 or less
- Middle-income countries (MICs) are subdivided:
  a) lower-middle-income = US$1,046 to US$4,125
  b) upper-middle-income (UMICs) = US$4,126 to US$12,745
- High-income countries (HICs) = US$12,746 or more.

1. *The Global Status Report on Road Safety 2015* by the World Health Organization aims to describe the burden of road

traffic injuries and implement effective interventions in all Member States using a standardized methodology, and it aims to assess changes since the first and second *Global Status Reports* in 2009 and 2013. The data presented in the report were collected from 180 countries and areas, covering 6.97 billion people (97.3 percent of the world's population). Data collection in each country was coordinated by a National Data Collector and driven by a number of individual respondents from different sectors within a country, each of whom completed a self-administered questionnaire with information on key variables. This group was then required to come to a consensus on the data that best represented their country, which is presented in the report. Response rates by region covered were between 95 percent of the population in the European region to 99.6 percent in the Western Pacific region. Data collection was carried out in 2014; accordingly, while data on legislation and policies were related to 2014, data on fatalities were related to 2013 (WHO 2015a).

## REFERENCES

Australian Transport Council. 2011. *National Road Safety Strategy 2011–2020*. Canberra, Australia. https://www.infrastructure.gov.au/roads/safety/national_road_safety_strategy/files/NRSS_2011_2020_15Aug11.pdf.

Bachani, A. M., E. Galiwango, D. Kadobera, J. A. Bentley, D. Bishai, and others. 2014. "A New Screening Instrument for Disability in Low-Income and Middle-Income Settings: Application at the Iganga-Mayuge Demographic Surveillance System (IM-DSS), Uganda." *BMJ Open* 4 (12): e005795. doi:10.1136/bmjopen-2014-005795. PubMed PMID: 25526793; PubMed Central PMCID: PMC4275668.

Bachani, A. M., E. Galiwango, D. Kadobera, J. A. Bentley, D. Bishai, and others. 2015. "Characterizing Disability at the Iganga-Mayuge Demographic Surveillance System (IM-DSS), Uganda." *Disability and Rehabilitation*: 1–9. [Epub ahead of print] PubMed PMID: 26457663.

Bachani, A. M., Y. W. Hung, S. Mogere, D. Akungah, J. Nyamari, and others. 2013. "Prevalence, Knowledge, Attitude and Practice of Speeding in Two Districts in Kenya: Thika and Naivasha." *Injury* 44 (Suppl 4): S24–30. doi:10.1016/S0020-1383(13)70209-2. PubMed PMID: 24377774.

Bachani, A. M., P. Koradia, H. K. Herbert, S. Mogere, D. Akungah, and others. 2012. "Road Traffic Injuries in Kenya: The Health Burden and Risk Factors in Two Districts." *Traffic Injury Prevention* 13 (Suppl 1): 24–30. doi:10.1080/15389588.2011.633136. PubMed PMID: 22414125.

Bachani, A. M., X. J. Zhang, K.A. Allen, and A.A. Hyder. 2014. Injuries and Violence in the Eastern Mediterranean Region: A Review of the Health, Economic and Social Burden." *Eastern Mediterranean Health Journal* 20 (10): 643–52. Review. PubMed PMID: 25356696.

Bambach, M. R., R. J. Mitchell, and R. H. Grzebieta. 2013. "The Protective Effect of Roadside Barriers for Motorcyclists." *Traffic Injury Prevention* 14 (7): 756–65.

Bauer, R., M. Steiner, R. Kisser, S. M. Macey, and D. Thayer. 2014. "Accidents and Injuries in the EU. Results of the EuroSafe Reports." *Bundesgesundheitsblatt Gesundheitsforschung Gesundheitsschutz* 57 (6): 673–80.

Benmaamar, M., C. Dunkerley, and S. D. Ellis. 2002. "Urban Transport Services in Sub-Saharan Africa: Recommendations for Reforms in Uganda." Presentation at the 81st Annual Meeting of the Transportation Research Board, Washington, DC, January 2002. Transport Research Laboratory, Crowthorne, United Kingdom.

Bishai, D., B. Asiimwe, S. Abbas, A. A. Hyder, and W. Bazeyo. 2008. "Cost-Effectiveness of Traffic Enforcement: Case Study from Uganda." *Injury Prevention* 14 (4): 223–27.

Bishai, D., and A. Bachani. 2012. "Chapter 19: Injury Costing Frameworks." In *Injury Research: Theories, Methods, and Approaches*, edited by G. Li and S. P. Baker, 371–79. New York, NY: Springer Science + Business Media, LLC.

Bishai, D., and A. A. Hyder. 2006. "Modeling the Cost Effectiveness of Injury Interventions in Lower and Middle Income Countries: Opportunities and Challenges." *Cost Effectiveness and Resource Allocation* 4 (2).

Bishai, D., A. A. Hyder, A. Ghaffar, R. H. Morrow, and O. Kobusingye. 2003. "Rates of Public Investment for Road Safety in Developing Countries: Case Studies of Uganda and Pakistan." *Health Policy and Planning* 18: 232–35.

Blincoe, L., T. R. Miller, E. Zaloshnja, and A. B. Lawrence. 2015. "The Economic and Societal Impact of Motor Vehicle Crashes, 2010 (Revised)." Technical Report DOT HS-812 013. Washington, DC: National Center for Statistics and Analysis, National Highway Traffic Safety Administration.

Brice, J. H., J. R. Studnek, B. L. Bigham, C. Martin-Gill, C. B. Custalow, and others. 2011. "EMS Provider and Patient Safety during Response and Transport: Proceedings of an Ambulance Safety Conference." *Prehospital Emergency Care* 16 (1): 3–19.

Chandran, A., A. A. Hyder, and C. Peek-Asa. 2010. "The Global Burden of Unintentional Injuries and an Agenda for Progress." *Epidemiologic Reviews* 32 (1): 110–20.

Changchen L., Z. Gaowuiang, Z. Jianjun, and Z. Hao. 2010. "First Engineering Practice of Traffic Calming in Zhaitang Town in China." *Proceedings of the 2010 International Conference on Optoelectronics and Image Processing* (volume 1), 565–68. Washington, DC: Institute of Electrical and Electronic Engineering (IEEE). Computer Society.

Chisholm, D., H. Naci, A. A. Hyder, N. T. Tran, and M. Peden. 2012. "Cost Effectiveness of Strategies to Combat Road Traffic Injuries in Sub-Saharan Africa and South East Asia: Mathematical Modelling Study." *BMJ* 344: e612. doi:10.1136/bmj.e612.

Chorba, T. L. 1991. "Assessing Technologies for Preventing Injuries in Motor Vehicle Crashes." *International Journal of Technology Assessment in Health Care* 7 (3): 296–314.

Connelly, L. B., and R. Supangan. 2006. "The Economic Costs of Road Traffic Crashes: Australia, States and Territories." *Accident and Analysis Prevention* 38 (6): 1087–93.

Dalby, E. 1981. "Applications of Low-Cost Road Accident Countermeasures According to an Area-Wide Strategy." *Traffic Engineering and Control* 22: 567–74.

De Andrade, S. M., D. A. Soares, T. Matsuo, C. L. Barrancos Liberatti, and M. L. Hiromi Iwakura. 2008. "Road Injury-Related Mortality in a Medium-Sized Brazilian City after

Some Preventive Interventions." *Traffic Injury Prevention* 9 (5): 450–55.

Department of the Federal Road Safety Inspectorate of the Russian Ministry of Interior. http://www.gibdd.ru/stat/.

Ditsuwan, V., J. Lennert Veerman, M. Bertram, and T. Vos. 2013. "Cost-Effectiveness of Interventions for Reducing Road Traffic Injuries Related to Driving under the Influence of Alcohol." *Value in Health* 16 (1): 23–30.

Duduta, N., C. Adriazola, C. Wass, D. Hidalgo, and L. A. Lindau. 2011. *Traffic Safety on Bus Corridors: Pilot Version—Road Test*. Washington, DC: EMBARQ.

Duperrex, O., F. Bunn, and I. Roberts. 2002. "Safety Education of Pedestrians for Injury Prevention: A Systematic Review of Randomised Controlled Trials." *British Medical Journal* 324 (7346): 1129.

Elvik, R. 2000. "How Much Do Road Accidents Cost the National Economy?" *Accident Analysis and Prevention* 32: 849–51.

Elvik, R., T. Vaa, A. Hoye., and M. Sorensen, eds. 2009. *The Handbook of Road Safety Measures*. UK: Emerald Group Publishing Limited.

Espitia-Hardeman, V., L. Vélez, F. Muñoz, M. I. Gutiérrez-Martínez, R. Espinosa-Vallín, and others. 2008. "Impact of Interventions Directed toward Motorcyclist Death Prevention in Cali, Colombia: 1993–2001." *Salud Pública de México* 50 (Suppl 1): S69–77.

European Commission. 2014. *Statistics—Accidents Data*. Brussels, Belgium. http://ec.europa.eu/transport/road _safety/specialist/statistics/index_en.htm.

Fuentes, C. M., and V. Hernandez. 2013. "Spatial Environmental Risk Factors for Pedestrian Injury Collisions in Ciudad Juarez, Mexico (2008–2009): Implications for Urban Planning." *International Journal of Injury Control and Safety Promotion* 20 (2): 169–78. doi:10.1080/17457300.2012.724690.

Garcell, H. G., T. S. Enríquez, F. G. Garcia, C. M. Quesada, R. P. Sandoval, and others. 2008. "Impact of a Drink-Driving Detection Program to Prevent Traffic Accidents [Villa Clara Province, Cuba]. Impacto de un programa de detección de conductores bajo los efectos del alcohol en la prevención de accidentes de tráfico (provincia de Villa Clara [Cuba])." 22 (4): 344–47.

Garcia-Altes, A., J. M. Suelves, and E. Barberia. 2013. "Cost Savings Associated with 10 Years of Road Safety Policies in Catalonia, Spain." *Bulletin of the World Health Organization* 91 (1): 28–35.

Global Road Safety Partnership. 2007. *Drinking and Driving: A Road Safety Manual for Decision-Makers and Practitioners*. Geneva: Global Road Safety Partnership. Global New Car Assessment Program, http://www.globalncap.org.

Gururaj, G. 2011. "Road Safety in India: A Framework for Action." Publication 83, National Institute of Mental Health and Neurosciences, Bangalore.

Gururaj, G., P. Murthy, G. N. Rao, and V. Benegal. 2011. "Alcohol Related Harm: Implications for Public Health and Policy in India." Publication 73, National Institute of Mental Health and Neurosciences, Bangalore, India. http://www.nimhans.kar.nic.in/cam/CAM/Alcohol_report _NIMHANS.pdf.

Haddon, W., Jr. 1968. "The Changing Approach to the Epidemiology, Prevention, and Amelioration of Trauma: The Transition to Approaches Etiologically Rather Than Descriptively Based." *American Journal of Public Health and the Nation's Health* 58 (0002-9572): 8.

———. 1973. "Energy Damage and the Ten Countermeasure Strategies." *Journal of Trauma* 13: 321–31.

Hendrie, D., T. R. Miller, M. Orlando, R. S. Spicer, C. Taft, and others. 2004. "Child and Family Safety Device Affordability by Country Income Level: An 18 Country Comparison." *Injury Prevention* 10: 338–43.

Herbert, H. K., A. A. Hyder, A. Butchart, and R. Norton. 2011. "Global Health: Injuries and Violence." *Infectious Disease Clinics of North America* 25 (3): 653–68.

Herrstedt, L. 1998. "Planning and Safety of Bicycles in Urban Areas." In *Proceedings of the Traffic Safety on Two Continents Conference*, 43–58. Lisbon, September 22–24, 1997. Linköping: Swedish National Road and Transport Research Institute.

Hofman, K., A. Primack, G. Keusch, and S. Hrynkow. 2005. "Addressing the Growing Burden of Trauma and Injury in Low- and Middle-Income Countries." *American Journal of Public Health* 95 (1): 13–17.

Hyder, A. A., K. A. Allen, G. Di Pietro, C. A. Adriazola, R. Sobel, and others. 2012. Addressing the Implementation Gap in Global Road Safety: Exploring Features of an Effective Response and Introducing a 10-Country Program. *American Journal of Public Health* 102 (6): 1061–67. doi:10.2105 /AJPH.2011.300563. Epub 2012 Apr 19. PubMed PMID: 22515864; PubMed Central PMCID: PMC3483956.

Hyder, A. A., K. A. Allen, D. H. Peters, A. Chandran, and D. Bishai. 2013. Large-Scale Road Safety Programmes in Low- and Middle-Income Countries: An Opportunity to Generate Evidence." *Global Public Health* 8 (5): 504–18. doi:10.1080/17441692.2013.769613. Epub 2013 Feb 27. PubMed PMID: 23445357.

Hyder, A. A., and D. Bishai. 2012. "Road Safety in 10 Countries: A Global Opportunity." *Traffic Injury Prevention* 13 (Suppl 1): 1–2. doi:10.1080/15389588.2011.650023. PubMed PMID: 22414120.

Hyder, A. A., A. Ghaffar, and T. I. Masood. 2000. "Motor Vehicle Crashes in Pakistan: The Emerging Epidemic." *Injury Prevention* 6 (3): 199–202. Review. PubMed PMID: 11003185; PubMed Central PMCID: PMC1730645.

Hyder, A. A., M. Labinjo, and S. S. Muzaffar. 2006. A New Challenge to Child and Adolescent Survival in Urban Africa: An Increasing Burden of Road Traffic Injuries." *Traffic Injury Prevention* 7 (4): 381–88. Review. PubMed PMID: 17114096.

Hyder, A. A., D. Meddings, and A. M. Bachani. 2009. "MENTOR-VIP: Piloting a Global Mentoring Program for Injury and Violence Prevention." *Academic Medicine* 84 (6): 793–96. doi:10.1097/ACM.0b013e3181a407b8. Review. PubMed PMID: 19474562.

Hyder, A. A., S. S. Muzaffar, and A. M. Bachani. 2008. Road Traffic Injuries in Urban Africa and Asia: A Policy Gap in Child and Adolescent Health. *Public Health* 122 (10): 1104–10. doi:10.1016/j.puhe.2007.12.014. Epub 2008 Jul 1. PubMed PMID: 18597800.

Hyder, A. A., and M. Peden. 2003. "Inequality and Road-Traffic Injuries: Call for Action." *The Lancet* 362 (9401): 2034–35. PubMed PMID: 14697797.

Hyder, A. A., and J. A. Razzak. 2013. The Challenges of Injuries and Trauma in Pakistan: An Opportunity for Concerted Action." *Public Health* 127 (8): 699–703. doi:10.1016/j .puhe.2012.12.020. Epub 2013 Mar 13. Review. PubMed PMID: 23489711; PubMed Central PMCID: PMC4313547.

Ichikawa, M., W. Chadbunchachai, and E. Marui. 2003. "Effect of the Helmet Act for Motorcyclists in Thailand." *Accident Analysis and Prevention* 35 (2): 183–89.

Institute for Health Metrics and Evaluation (IHME). 2013. "Global Burden of Disease Data." http://www.healthdata .org/gbd/data.

Insurance Institute for Highway Safety (IIHS). 2013. "Safety Gains Aren't Global: Some Regions Lag U.S., Europe, Australia in Protecting People in Crashes." Status Report. 48 (5). http:// www.iihs.org/iihs/sr/statusreport/article/48/5/1.

International Transport Forum. 2008. "Towards Zero: Ambitious Road Safety Targets and the Safe System Approach." Organisation for Economic Co-operation and Development. Paris. http://www.internationaltransportforum.org/Pub /pdf/08TowardsZeroE.pdf.

Jacobs, G., A. Aeron-Thomas, and A. Astrop. 2000. *Estimating Global Road Fatalities.* Report 445. Crowthorne, United Kingdom: Transport Research Laboratory.

Jermakian, J. S. 2011. "Crash Avoidance Potential of Four Passenger Vehicle Technologies." *Accident Analysis Prevention* 43 (3): 732–40.

JHU-IIRU (Johns Hopkins International Injury Research Unit). 2013. *Courses in Injury Prevention.* http://www .jhsph.edu/research/centers-and-institutes/johns -hopkins-international-injury-research-unit/training/.

Ker, K., J. Kiriya, P. Perel, P. Edwards, H. Shakur, and others. 2012. "Avoidable Mortality from Giving Tranexamic Acid to Bleeding Trauma Patients: An Estimation Based on WHO Mortality Data, A Systematic Literature Review and Data from the CRASH-2 Trial." *BMC Emergency Medicine* 12: 3 (Published online).

Khorasani-Zavareh, D., B. J. Haglund, R. Mohammadi, M. Naghavi, and L. Laflamme. 2009. "Traffic Injury Deaths in West Azarbaijan Province of Iran: A Cross-Sectional Interview-Based Study on Victims' Characteristics and Pre-Hospital Care." *International Journal of Injury Control and Safety Promotion* 16 (3): 119–26.

Kruk, M. E., A. Wladis, N. Mbembati, S. K. Ndao-Brumblay, R. Y. Hsia, and others. 2010. "Human Resource and Funding Constraints for Essential Surgery in District Hospitals in Africa: A Retrospective Cross-Sectional Survey." *PLoS Medicine* 7 (3): 1–11.

Kudryavtsev A. V., O. Nilssen, J. Lund, A. M. Grjibovski, and B. Ytterstad. 2013. "Road Traffic Crashes with Fatal and Non-Fatal Injuries in Arkhangelsk, Russia in 2005–2010." *International Journal of Injury Control and Safety Promotion* 20 (4): 349–57. doi:10.1080/17457300.2012.745576. Epub 2012 Dec 7. PubMed PMID: 23216194.

Law, T. H., R. S. Umar, S. Zulkaurnain, and S. Kulanthayan. 2005. Impact of the Effect of Economic Crisis and the Targeted Motorcycle Safety Programme on Motorcycle-Related Accidents, Injuries and Fatalities in Malaysia. *International Journal of Injury Control and Safety Promotion* 12 (1): 9–21.

Lett, R., O. Kobusingye, and D. Sethi. 2002. "A Unified Framework for Injury Control: The Public Health Approach and Haddon's Matrix Combined." *Injury Control and Safety Promotion* 9 (3): 199–205.

Lim, S. J., W. J. Chung, and W. H. Cho. 2011. "Economic Burden of Injuries in South Korea." *Injury Prevention* 17 (5): 291–96.

Lin, T., N. Li, W. Du, X. Song, and X. Zheng. 2013. "Road Traffic Disability in China: Prevalence and Socio-Demographic Disparities." *Journal of Public Health (Oxford)* 35 (4): 541–7. doi:10.1093/pubmed/fdt003. Epub 2013 Feb 5. PubMed PMID: 23386326.

Lines, C., and K. Machata. 2000. "Changing Streets, Protecting People: Making Roads Safer for All." In *Proceedings of Best in Europe 2000 Road Safety Conference,* Brussels, September 12.

Liu, B. C., R. Ivers, R. Norton, S. Boufous, S. Blows, and S. K. Lo. 2008. "Helmets for Preventing Injury in Motorcycle Riders." Cochrane Database of Systematic Reviews 1: CD004333.

Lozano, R., M. Naghavi, K. Foreman, S. Lim, K. Shibuya, and others. 2012. "Global and Regional Mortality from 235 Causes of Death for 20 Age Groups in 1990 and 2010: A Systematic Analysis for the Global Burden of Disease Study 2010." *The Lancet* 380 (9859): 2095–128.

Madans, J. H., and M. Loeb. 2013. "Methods to Improve International Comparability of Census and Survey Measures of Disability." *Disability and Rehabilitation* 5 (13): 1070–73. doi:10.3109/09638288.2012.720353. Epub 2012 Oct 1. PubMed PMID: 23020151.

Madans, J. H., M. E. Loeb, and B. M. Altman. 2011. Measuring Disability and Monitoring the UN Convention on the Rights of Persons with Disabilities: The Work of the Washington Group on Disability Statistics. *BioMed Central Public Health* 11 (Suppl 4): S4. doi:10.1186/1471-2458-11-S4-S4. PubMed PMID: 21624190; PubMed Central PMCID: PMC3104217.

Mashreky, S. R., A. Rahman, T. F. Khan, M. Faruque, L. Svanstrom, and others. 2010. "Hospital Burden of Road Traffic Injury: Major Concern in Primary and Secondary Level Hospitals in Bangladesh." *Public Health* 124 (4): 185–89.

Meddings, D. R. 2010. "WHO Launches TEACH-VIP E-Learning." *Injury Prevention* 16 (2): 143. doi:10.1136 /ip.2010.026468. PubMed PMID: 20363825.

———. 2015. "MENTOR-VIP and Broader Capacity Building for Injury and Violence Prevention." *Injury Prevention* 2: 142. doi:10.1136/injuryprev-2015-041585. PubMed PMID: 25805772.

Meddings, D. R., L. M. Knox, M. Maddaleno, A. Concha-Eastman, and J. S. Hoffman. 2005. "World Health Organization's TEACH-VIP: Contributing to Capacity Building for Youth Violence Prevention." *American Journal of Preventive Medicine* 5 (Suppl 2): 259–65. PubMed PMID: 16376728.

Miranda, J. J., E. Rosales-Mayor, D. A. Quistberg, A. Paca-Palao, C. Gianella, and others. 2013. "Patient Perspectives on the

Promptness and Quality of Care of Road Traffic Incident Victims in Peru: A Cross-Sectional, Active Surveillance Study." *F1000Res* 2: 167.

Mock, C. N., C. Arreola-Risa, and R. Quansah. 2003. "Strengthening Care for Injured Persons in Less Developed Countries: A Case Study of Ghana and Mexico." *Injury Control and Safety Promotion* 10 (1–2): 45–51.

Mock, C. N., C. Juillard, M. Joshipura, and J. Goosen, eds. 2010. *Strengthening Care for the Injured: Success Stories and Lessons Learned from Around the World.* Geneva: World Health Organization.

Mock, C. N., R. Quansah, R. Krishnan, C. Arreola-Risa, and F. Rivara. 2004. "Strengthening the Prevention and Care of Injuries Worldwide." *The Lancet* 363 (9427): 2172–79.

Mofadal, A. I., K. Kanitpong, and P. Jiwattanakulpaisarn. 2015. "Analysis of Pedestrian Accident Costs in Sudan Using the Willingness-to-Pay Method." *Accident Analysis and Prevention* 78: 201–11. doi:10.1016/j.aap.2015.02.022. Epub 2015 Mar 17.

Mohd Faudzi, M. Y., N. A. Mohamad, and N. Ghani. 2011. "Malaysian Value of Fatal and Non Fatal Injury Due to Road Accident: The Willingness to Pay Using Conjoint Analysis Study." *Eastern Asia Society for Transportation Studies* 8.

Muchaka, P., and R. Behrens. 2012. "Evaluation of a 'Walking Bus' Demonstration Project in Cape Town: Qualitative Findings, Implications and Recommendations." Paper presented to the 31st Southern African Transport Conference, Pretoria, July 9–12.

Muda, F., and O. Ali. 2006. "Road Traffic Accidents among Primary School Children Who Cycle or Walk to School in Kuala Terengganu District, 1996." *Journal Kesihatan Masyarakat* 12 (1): 1.

NCAP (National Car Assessment Programs). 2011. "Vehicle Safety Is Global." Global NCAP.

Nguyen, H., R. Q. Ivers, S. Jan, A. L. Martiniuk, L. Segal, and others. 2015. Cost and Impoverishment 1 Year after Hospitalisation Due to Injuries: A Cohort Study in Thai Binh, Vietnam. *Injury Prevention.*

Nguyen, H., R. Q. Ivers, S. Jan, A. L. Martiniuk, Q. Li, and others. 2013. The Economic Burden of Road Traffic Injuries: Evidence from a Provincial General Hospital in Vietnam." *Injury Prevention* 19 (2): 79–84.

Novoa, A. M., K. Pérez, and C. Borrell. 2009. "Evidence-Based Effectiveness of Road Safety Interventions: A Literature Review." *Gaceta Sanitaria* 23 (6): 553–e1.

O'Dea, D., and J. Wren. 2010. *New Zealand Estimates of the Total Social and Economic Cost of "All Injuries" and the Six Priority Areas Respectively, at June 2008 Prices: Technical Report Prepared for NZIPS Evaluation.* Wellington, New Zealand: Accident Compensation Corporation.

Odero, W., M. Khayesi, and P. M. Heda. 2003. Road Traffic Injuries in Kenya: Magnitude, Causes, and Status of Intervention. *Injury Control and Safety Promotion* 10 (1–2), 53–61.

Page, Y., T. Hermitte, and S. Cuny. 2011. How Safe is Vehicle Safety? The Contribution of Vehicle Technologies to the Reduction in Road Casualties in France from 2000 to 2010. *Annals of Advances in Automotive Medicine* 55: 101–12.

Paravar, M., M. Hosseinpour, S. Salehi, M. Mohammadzadeh, A. Shojaee, and others 2013. "Pre-Hospital Trauma Care in Road Traffic Accidents in Kashan, Iran." *Archives of Trauma Research* 1 (4): 166–71.

Passmore, J., L. H. Nguyen, N. Phuong Nguyen, and J. M. Olivé. 2010. "The Formulation and Implementation of a National Helmet Law: A Case Study from Viet Nam." *Bulletin of World Health Organization* 88 (10): 783–87.

Passmore, J., N. T. H. Tu, M. A. Luong, N. D. Chinh, and N. P. Nam. 2010. "Impact of Mandatory Motorcycle Helmet Wearing Legislation on Head Injuries in Viet Nam: Results of a Preliminary Analysis." *Traffic Injury Prevention* 11 (2): 202–06.

Peden, M. 2010. Road Safety in 10 Countries. *Injury Prevention* 16 (6): 433. doi:10.1136/ip.2010.030155. Epub 2010 Nov 11. PubMed PMID: 21071768.

Peden, M., R. Scurfield, D. Sleet, D. Mohan, A. A. Hyder, and others. 2004. *World Report on Road Traffic Injury Prevention.* Geneva: World Health Organization.

Perel, P., K. Ker, R. Ivers, and K. Blackhall. 2007. "Road Safety in Low- and Middle-Income Countries: A Neglected Research Area." *Injury Prevention* 13 (4): 227.

Perez-Nunez, R., M. Hijar-Medina, I. Heredia-Pi, S. Jones, and E. M. Silveira Rodrigues. 2010. "Economic Impact of Fatal and Nonfatal Road Traffic Injuries in Belize in 2007." *Revista Panamericana de Salud Pública* 28 (5): 326–36.

Radin, U. R. S., G. M. Mackay, and B. L. Hills. 1996. "Modelling of Conspicuity-Related Motorcycle Accidents in Seremban and Shah Alam, Malaysia." *Accident Analysis and Prevention* 28 (3): 325–32.

Radin, U. R. S., G. M. Mackay, and B. L. Hills. 2000. "Multivariate Analysis of Motorcycle Accidents and the Effect of Exclusive Motorcycle Lanes in Malaysia." *Journal of Crash Prevention and Injury Control* 2: 11–17.

Razzak, J. A., S. M. Sasser, and A. L. Kellermann. 2005. "Injury Prevention and Other International Public Health Initiatives." *Emergency Medicine Clinics of North America* 23 (1): 85–98.

Rogmans, W. H. 2012. "Joint Action on Monitoring Injuries in Europe (JAMIE)." *Archives of Public Health* 70 (1): 19.

SafetyNet. 2009. *Road Safety Management. European Road Safety Observatory.* Brussels, Belgium: European Commission. http://ec.europa.eu/transport/road_safety /specialist/knowledge/pdf/road_safety_management.pdf.

Schopper, D., J. D. Lormand, and R. Waxweiler, eds. 2006. *Developing Policies to Prevent Injuries and Violence: Guidelines for Policy-Makers and Planners.* Geneva: World Health Organization.

Sedlák, M., M. Grivna, and J. Cihalova. 2006. "On Bike in Helmet Only: Results of a Three-Year Community Campaign Promoting Bicycle Helmets for Children." Book of Abstracts, 1st European Conference on Injury Prevention and Safety Promotion, Vienna, Austria, June 25–27.

Sekine, T. 2014. "Utilization of Probe Powered Two-Wheeler Vehicles to Realize a Safe Mobile Society." *IATSS Research* 38 (1): 58–70.

Short, M. M., C. J. Mushquash, and M. Bedard. 2013. "Motor Vehicle Crashes among Canadian Aboriginal People:

A Review of the Literature." *Canadian Journal of Rural Medicine* 18 (3): 86–98.

Shults, R. A., R. W. Elder, D. A. Sleet, J. L. Nichols, M. O. Alao, and others. 2001. "Reviews of Evidence Regarding Interventions to Reduce Alcohol-Impaired Driving." *American Journal of Preventive Medicine* 21 (Suppl 4): 66–88.

Slyunkina, S. E., V. E. Kliavin, E. A. Gritsenko, A. B. Petruhin, F. Zambon, and others. 2013. "Activities of the Bloomberg Philanthropies Global Road Safety Program (formerly RS10) in Russia: Promising Results from a Sub-National Project." *Injury* 44 (Suppl 4): S64–69.

Solagberu, B. A., R. I. Osuoji, N. A. Ibrahim, M. A. Oludara, R. A. Balogun, and others. 2014. "Child Pedestrian Injury and Fatality in a Developing Country." *Pediatric Surgery International* 30 (6): 625–32.

Soori, H., M. Royanian, A. R. Zali, and A. Movahedinejad. 2009. "Road Traffic Injuries in Iran: The Role of Interventions Implemented by Traffic Police." *Traffic Injury Prevention* 10 (4): 375–78.

Stevenson, M., J. Yu, D. Hendrie, L. P. Li, R. Ivers, and others. 2008. "Reducing the Burden of Road Traffic Injury: Translating High-Income Country Interventions to Middle-Income and Low-Income Countries." *Injury Prevention* 14 (5): 284–89.

Sullivan, R., P. Edwards, A. Sloggett, and C. E. Marshall. 2009. Families Bereaved by Road Traffic Crashes: Linkage of Mortality Records with 1971–2001 Censuses. *Injury Prevention* 15 (6): 364–68.

Swedish Road Safety. 2013. "Vision Zero: A Safe Road Traffic Concept." http://www.swedishroadsafety.se/vision-zero.html.

SWOV Institute for Road Safety Research. 2006. *Advancing Sustainable Safety: National Road Safety Outlook for 2005–2020*, edited by F. Wegman and L. Aarts. The Netherlands: SWOV Institute for Road Safety Research. http://www.sustainablesafety.nl.

Tan-Torres Edejer, T., R. Baltussen, T. Adam, R. Hutubessy, A. Acharya, and others, eds. 2003. "Making Choices in Health: WHO Guide to Cost-Effectiveness Analysis." Geneva, World Health Organization.

United Nations Road Safety Collaboration. 2010. *Global Plan for the Decade of Action for Road Safety 2011–2020*. http://www.who.int/roadsafety/decade_of_action/plan/en/.

Vieira Gomes, S., and J. L. Cardoso. 2012. "Safety Effects of Low-Cost Engineering Measures: An Observational Study in a Portuguese Multilane Road." *Accident Analysis and Prevention* 48: 346–52.

Ward, H., J. Norrie, R. E. Allsop, and A. P. Sang. 1989. *Urban Safety Project: The Bristol Scheme.* Contractor Report 192. Crowthorne, Berkshire, U.K: Transport and Road Research Laboratory.

Wesson, H. K., N. Boikhutso, A. M. Bachani, K. J. Hofman, and A. A. Hyder. 2013. "The Cost of Injury and Trauma Care in Low- and Middle-Income Countries: A Review of Economic Evidence." *Health Policy and Planning* 29 (6): 795–808.

Wittink, R. 2001. "Promotion of Mobility and Safety of Vulnerable Road Users: Final Report of the European Research Project PROMISING (Promotion of Measures for Vulnerable Road Users)." D-2001-3. Leidschendam, Netherlands: SWOV Institute for Road Safety Research. http://www.swov.nl/rapport/d-2001-03.pdf.

WHO (World Health Organization). 2007. "Youth and Road Safety." WHO, Geneva.

———. 2009. *European Status Report on Road Safety Towards Safer Roads and Healthier Transport Choices.* Geneva: WHO.

———. 2011. *66th World Health Assembly Adopts Resolution Calling for Better Health Care for People with Disabilities.* WHO news archive. http://www.who.int/disabilities/media/news/2013/28_05/en/index.html.

———. 2013a. *Global Status Report on Road Safety 2013: Supporting a Decade of Action.* Geneva: WHO.

———. 2013b. *Fact Sheet on Road Safety.* WHO, Geneva.

———. 2013c. *Strengthening Road Safety Legislation: A Practice and Resource Manual for Countries.* Geneva: WHO.

———. 2014. *Global Health Estimates 2014.* Geneva, WHO. http://www.who.int/healthinfo/global_burden_disease/en/.

———. 2015a. *Global Status Report on Road Safety 2015.* Geneva: WHO.

———. 2015b. *Fact Sheet on Road Safety.* WHO, Geneva.

Zaza, S., D. A. Sleet, R. S. Thompson, D. M. Sosin, and J. C. Bolen. 2001. "Reviews of Evidence Regarding Interventions to Increase Use of Child Safety Seats." *American College of Preventive Medicine* 21 (Suppl 4): 31–47.

Zhou, Y., T. D. Baker, K. Rao, and G. Li. 2003. "Productivity Loses from Injury in China." *Injury Prevention* 9: 124–27.

Zhu, M., P. Cummings, H. Chu, and L. J. Cook. 2007. "Association of Rear Seat Safety Belt Use with Death in a Traffic Crash: A Matched Cohort Study." *Injury Prevention* 13 (3): 183–85.

# Chapter 4

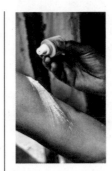

# Nontransport Unintentional Injuries

Robyn Norton, Rajeev B. Ahuja, Connie Hoe, Adnan A. Hyder,
Rebecca Ivers, Lisa Keay, David Mackie, David Meddings,
and Fazlur Rahman

## INTRODUCTION

Injuries are most commonly categorized as unintentional or intentional, based on the injured party's presumed intent (Norton and Kobusingye 2013). Unintentional injuries comprise both transport and nontransport injuries. This chapter examines in detail the leading causes of nontransport unintentional injuries, namely falls, drowning, burns, and poisoning.

The chapter also briefly discusses the burden of injuries resulting from the other two main categories of nontransport unintentional injuries, namely exposure to forces of nature and all other unintentional injuries combined. All other unintentional injuries combined constitute approximately 38 percent of nontransport unintentional injuries. However, because the numbers of deaths for each cause-specific injury within this group are comparatively small, and because the nature of, risk factors for, and interventions for each cause are unique, this chapter does not include a detailed examination of risk factors or interventions for this group as a whole, nor for any individual cause-specific injury.

Individuals in low- and middle-income countries (LMICs) sustain a higher proportion of deaths and disability-adjusted life years (DALYs) from nontransport unintentional injuries compared with those in high-income countries (HICs). The mortality rates for almost all of these injuries are higher in LMICs than in HICs. The best available evidence suggests that the numbers of deaths from most nontransport unintentional injuries are decreasing globally, with the exception of deaths from falls and possibly from burns, which are increasing.

This chapter places injuries in a global context but documents the burden and known risk factors for nontransport unintentional injuries in LMICs. It also provides an overview of the best available evidence about interventions and policies that are shown to effectively reduce such injuries in those countries. The key focus of the chapter is preventive strategies, although the importance of acute care and rehabilitation is clear, as discussed elsewhere in this volume. Where data are available, the costs and economic benefits of these interventions are outlined.

A consistent theme for every category of cause-specific, nontransport unintentional injury is the dearth of reliable evidence from LMICs on risk factors, interventions, and cost-effective approaches to prevention. This theme reflects the limited availability of human and other resources that would enable researchers to access such information, and it also reflects the low priority key stakeholders place on addressing the burden of such injuries.

The final section makes recommendations about what policy makers need to do to continue the trend of declines in the burden of death and disability from nontransport unintentional injuries; to achieve similar declines for falls; and to reduce the disparities in injury rates between HICs and LMICs.

Corresponding author: Robyn Norton, Principal Director, The George Institute for Global Health; Professor of Global Health, University of Oxford, Oxford, United Kingdom; Professor of Public Health, University of Sydney, Sydney, Australia; rnorton@georgeinstitute.org.

This chapter follows the World Health Organization (WHO) classification of regions: Africa, the Americas, South-East Asia, Europe, the Eastern Mediterranean, and the Western Pacific.

## BURDEN OF NONTRANSPORT UNINTENTIONAL INJURIES

Recent estimates of the global burden of death and disability resulting from nontransport unintentional injuries are available from the Global Burden of Disease study for 2013 (Haagsma and others 2015) and from the Global Health Estimates provided through WHO for 2012 (WHO 2014).

Global Health Estimates data suggest that, collectively, nontransport unintentional injuries account for more than 6,700 deaths a day and 2.4 million deaths annually (WHO 2014)—almost twice the number of deaths from transport injuries and twice the number of deaths from intentional injuries. The total is comparable to the number of deaths from HIV/AIDS and tuberculosis combined. Nontransport unintentional injuries also account for more than 148 million DALYs annually— almost twice the number from transport injuries and from intentional injuries (WHO 2014).

### Falls

Falls are the leading cause of nontransport unintentional injury deaths, accounting for almost 700,000 deaths a year (figure 4.1). In contrast to most other nontransport

unintentional injuries, deaths from falls have increased since 2000, in large part as a consequence of the increasing numbers of older people, who are at greatest risk. Falls are the leading cause of DALYs; between 2000 and 2012, the numbers of DALYs from falls increased by 19.2 percent (figure 4.2).

Men account for a slightly higher proportion of deaths from falls (54 percent) than women, with approximately 50 percent of all fall-related deaths occurring in individuals ages 70 years and older. The rates of death from falls in that age group (96.6 per 100,000 population) are strikingly higher than in all other age groups (table 4.1). Although the death rates in LMICs are comparable to those in HICs, they are highest in the LMICs of South-East Asia (16 per 100,000 population) (table 4.2).

### Drowning

Drowning is the second most common cause of death and DALYs from nontransport unintentional injuries. Drowning accounts for approximately 15 percent of both deaths and DALYs, with approximately 372,000 individuals dying each year as a consequence (figures 4.1 and 4.2). Over the past two decades, deaths and DALYs from drowning have decreased by approximately 20 percent and 30 percent, respectively, although those figures may be underestimates, given the known data limitations in LMICs (WHO 2012).

Almost all drowning deaths occur in LMICs (95 percent), and rates of drowning are substantially higher in almost all LMICs compared with HICs (table 4.2). Death rates from drowning are about twice as

**Figure 4.1** Nontransport Unintentional Injury Deaths, by Cause, 2000 and 2012

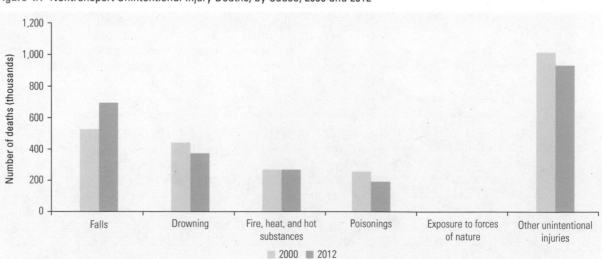

Source: WHO 2014.
Note: The WHO data suggest that negligible numbers of deaths resulted from forces of nature in low- and middle-income countries.

**Figure 4.2** Nontransport Unintentional Injury Disability-Adjusted Life Years, by Cause, 2000 and 2012

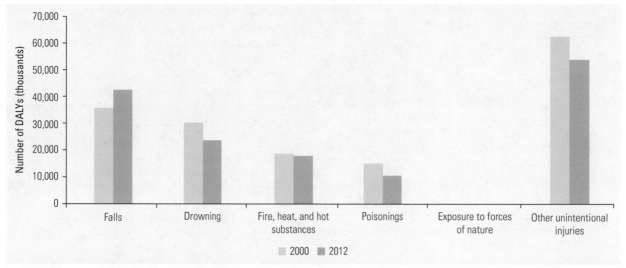

Source: WHO 2014.
Note: The WHO data suggest that negligible numbers of deaths resulted from forces of nature in low- and middle-income countries.

**Table 4.1** Nontransport Unintentional Injury Deaths, by Proportion of Males and Age Group, 2012
*Deaths per 100,000 population*

| Cause-specific injury category | Male (percent) | Age group (years) | | | | | |
|---|---|---|---|---|---|---|---|
| | | <5 | 5–14 | 15–29 | 30–49 | 50–69 | 70+ |
| Falls | 54 | 5.0 | 2.5 | 2.5 | 4.0 | 13.5 | 96.6 |
| Drowning | 67 | 10.1 | 6.1 | 4.2 | 3.2 | 4.9 | 10.9 |
| Burns | 53 | 9.6 | 3.4 | 2.7 | 2.3 | 3.1 | 9.7 |
| Poisoning | 61 | 3.6 | 1.0 | 2.1 | 2.7 | 3.9 | 6.4 |
| Forces of nature | 60 | 0.0 | 0.0 | 0.0 | 0.0 | 0.1 | 0.1 |
| Other | 63 | 17.8 | 6.3 | 8.1 | 9.3 | 16.9 | 61.1 |

Source: WHO 2014.

**Table 4.2** Nontransport Unintentional Injury Deaths, by Income and Region, 2012
*Deaths per 100,000 population*

| Cause-specific injury category | Income and region | | | | | | |
|---|---|---|---|---|---|---|---|
| | High-income countries | Low- and middle-income countries | | | | | |
| | | Africa | Americas | South-East Asia | Europe | Eastern Mediterranean | Western Pacific |
| Falls | 9 | 10 | 5 | 16 | 5 | 4 | 8 |
| Drowning | 3 | 8 | 3 | 7 | 4 | 5 | 4 |
| Burns | 2 | 14 | 1 | 4 | 3 | 4 | 1 |
| Poisoning | 2 | 4 | 1 | 3 | 2 | 4 | 3 |
| Forces of nature | 0 | 0 | 0 | 0 | 0 | 0 | 0 |
| Other | 14 | 20 | 10 | 14 | 14 | 16 | 8 |

Source: WHO 2014.
Note: The WHO data suggest that negligible numbers of deaths resulted from forces of nature in low- and middle-income countries.

high for men and boys than for women and girls (table 4.3). Death rates are highest for those younger than age five years, for both genders, followed by those ages 50 years and older.

## Burns

Burns are the third most common cause of death and DALYs from nontransport unintentional injuries, accounting for approximately 15 percent of deaths and 14 percent of DALYs. Between 250,000 and 350,000 individuals die each year as a consequence of burns (figures 4.1 and 4.2). Unlike most other unintentional injuries, rates of burn deaths for women and girls are comparable to those for men and boys (47 percent versus 53 percent, as shown in table 4.1). Rates of death from burns are highest in those younger than age five years and those ages 70 years and older. However, as with drowning, almost all deaths occur in LMICs (97 percent); rates of death are highest in LMICs in Africa, followed by South-East Asia, Europe, and the Eastern Mediterranean (table 4.2). The rates in Africa, for example, are 14 per 100,000 population, compared with 2 per 100,000 in HICs.

Although these figures clearly identify a significant burden of death and disability, almost all LMICs lack comprehensive data on burns. The International Society for Burn Injuries (ISBI), WHO, the U.S. Centers for Disease Control and Prevention (CDC), and the Global Alliance for Clean Cookstoves (GACC) have launched initiatives to develop minimal datasets and software platforms for better surveillance of burn incidence in domestic settings.

**Table 4.3** Drowning Deaths, by Gender, Age Group, and Country Type, 2012

*Deaths per 100,000 population*

| Gender | Age group (years) | Global | LMICs |
|--------|-------------------|--------|-------|
| Males | 0–4 | 11.5 | 12.6 |
| | 5–14 | 7.9 | 8.7 |
| | 15–49 | 5.5 | 5.9 |
| | 50+ | 8.1 | 8.9 |
| | Total | 7.0 | 7.6 |
| Females | 0–4 | 8.6 | 9.6 |
| | 5–14 | 4.3 | 4.8 |
| | 15–49 | 1.8 | 2.0 |
| | 50+ | 4.8 | 5.9 |
| | Total | 3.5 | 4.0 |

*Source:* WHO 2014.

## Poisoning

Poisoning constitutes approximately 8 percent of nontransport unintentional injury deaths and 7 percent of DALYs, resulting in an estimated 193,000 deaths and almost 11 million DALYs annually (figures 4.1 and 4.2).

Of poisoning victims, 61 percent are men and boys; the highest rates are in those under age five years and over age 50 years (table 4.1). The rates of poisoning deaths in most LMICs are higher than those in HICs, with the rates being twice as high in the LMIC regions of Africa and the Eastern Mediterranean (table 4.2).

## Forces of Nature

Deaths and DALYs caused by forces of nature include those arising from exposure to excessive natural heat or cold, earthquakes, and floods. These can vary significantly by year. For 2012, WHO data suggest that forces of nature accounted for only around 2,000 deaths. However, the numbers of deaths and DALYs have increased in recent years.

WHO data also suggest that men are at greater risk than women and that forces of nature primarily impact older adults (table 4.1).

## All Other Nontransport Unintentional Injuries

All other causes combined account for approximately 38 percent of deaths from nontransport unintentional injuries and a similar proportion for DALYs (figures 4.1 and 4.2). WHO Global Health Estimates give little additional detail on these. However, the Global Burden of Disease report breaks out several subgroups, the largest of which are exposure to mechanical forces, adverse effects of medical treatment, and animal contact (Lozano and others 2012).

As with most deaths from unintentional injuries, men and boys account for a disproportionate number of all other causes (63 percent) (table 4.1). The rates of death are highest in those ages 70 years and older, and among deaths occurring in LMICs, the rates are highest in Africa (table 4.2).

## RISK FACTORS FOR INJURIES

### Falls

**Falls in Older People**

The high burden of fall-related deaths in older people is due in part to the physical, sensory, and cognitive changes associated with aging, in combination with environments that are not adapted for this population (Lord and others 2007). Risk factors in LMICs are largely similar to those in HICs: age, female gender, previous falls, mobility problems, declining vision, medication use, unsafe environments, and chronic health problems (Kalula and others 2011; Ranaweera and others 2013).

However, the nature of the environmental risks differs in LMICs, with more falls resulting from factors relating to street and house design, transport, violence, and rural locations (Dandona and others 2010; Jagnoor and others 2014; Jitapunkul, Yuktananandana, and Parkpian 2001; Kalula and others 2011; Ranaweera and others 2013). Often, access to water is limited only to locations outside of the home (Hestekin and others 2013). The risk factors for fall-related injuries, including osteoporotic fractures, may differ across settings because of variations in diet and in load-bearing exercise (Lau and others 2001).

### Falls in People of Working Age

Research to examine risk factors for falls in people of working age in HICs is scarce, but studies of falls in the home may have some relevance. Those have highlighted the role of alcohol (Kool and others 2008) as well as structural or environmental hazards (Kool and others 2010). Falls in people of working age in LMICs are reported more commonly for men and are reported as occupational injuries, including those on farms (Dandona and others 2010; Gururaj, Sateesh, and Rayan 2008).

### Falls in Children

The risk factors for falls for children in HICs include male gender, younger age, and low socioeconomic status. Fall-related injuries are commonly sustained on playgrounds; on bunk beds and equipment, such as baby change tables or baby walkers (Khambalia and others 2006); or from windows (Harris, Rochette, and Smith 2011). The risk factors in LMICs are similar, with falls reported from ladders or stairs, or beds or other furniture (Hyder and others 2009). More falls occur in boys and in rural locations (Jiang and others 2010).

## Drowning

The International Life Saving Federation World Drowning Report (International Life Saving Federation 2007) divides drowning risk factors into two groups: human factors and environmental factors.

### Human Factors

Sociodemographic factors, socioeconomic conditions, behavioral factors, and medical conditions have all been postulated or shown to be risk factors for drowning. Higher rates among men and boys purportedly result from their increased exposure to water and riskier behaviors (Peden and McGee 2003). Children under age

five years have the highest drowning mortality rates worldwide. Deaths in this age group frequently occur as a result of children's inherent vulnerability—the inability to keep their airway clear of water—combined with a lapse in adult supervision. Individuals with lower education levels are at increased risk of drowning; across all regions and countries, lower socioeconomic groups are more vulnerable to drowning than higher socioeconomic groups (Giashuddin and others 2009).

The absence of, or a lapse in, adult supervision has been shown to be an important, potentially modifiable risk factor for drowning incidents in children (Bierens 2006; Chalmers, McNoe, and Stephenson 2004; International Life Saving Federation 2007; WHO 2006; Yang and others 2007), and individuals with few swimming skills or those who have not received swimming lessons have been shown to be at increased risk (Yang and others 2007). Alcohol consumption is one of the most frequently reported contributory factors associated with adolescent and adult drowning (WHO 2006). Some medical conditions such as epilepsy, which are often poorly controlled in LMICs, also place individuals at increased risk (Bell and others 2008).

### Environmental Factors

Children who live near open water sources are particularly at risk (Peden and McGee 2003). People who work on or near water, travel on water, or use surface water or open wells for household water are all likely to face increased risk of unintentional immersion in a water hazard. Similarly, those who live in settings susceptible to flash floods, river flooding, storm surges, or tsunamis are at increased risk of drowning.

## Burns

The etiological factors responsible for the majority of burn injuries in LMICs are very different from those in HICs. In the United States, for example, 69 percent of burns happen at home, with factors such as alcohol, smoking, and high bathing temperatures dominating (American Burn Association 2012). Almost 50 percent of burn deaths have been attributed to the combination of alcohol and smoking.

In LMICs a large proportion of burn injuries is sustained in the kitchen or cooking area and is related to the nature of the cooking appliances, the source of heat, and the heating of liquids (Hyder and others 2009; Mashreky and others 2010). Several studies have implicated kerosene stoves in a large percentage of burn injuries (Ahuja and Bhattacharya 2002; Ahuja, Bhattacharya, and Rai 2009; Ahuja, Dash, and Shrivastava 2011; Mabrouk, El Badawy, and Sherif 2000). As the source of heating moves up the energy ladder from biomass products to kerosene to liquefied petroleum gas (LPG) to electricity, the fuel becomes safer, cleaner, and more expensive. Cooking appliances that use LPG appear to be safer and less polluting than those fueled by kerosene, but they still pose serious risks if not properly used and maintained (Ahuja, Dash, and Shrivastava 2011).

In India, most domestic burns are sustained by women ages 16–35 years; almost 70 percent of these injuries are due to the traditional practice of cooking at floor level or over an open fire, compounded by wearing loose-fitting clothing made from non-flame-retardant fabric (Sanghavi, Bhalla, and Das 2009).

Burns from incidents involving traditional home-made bottle lamps or commercial wick lamps are a cause of major morbidity and mortality in Bangladesh, India, Mozambique, Nepal, and Sri Lanka. In a study in Sri Lanka, 41 percent of the burns in patients admitted with unintentional flame burns resulted from homemade kerosene bottle lamps tipping over (Laloë 2002). A case-control study of childhood burn injuries in 2008 in rural Bangladesh revealed that households using traditional kerosene lamps (*kupi bati*) had a greater than threefold risk of childhood burns relative to households not using such lamps (Mashreky and others 2010).

## Poisoning

Although some studies have been conducted in LMICs to examine victims of all ages admitted to hospitals for unintentional poisoning (Akbaba and others 2007; Peiris-John and others 2013; Sawalha and others 2010), much of the available literature on unintentional poisoning in these countries focuses on young children. Findings from these studies show that, consistent with overall trends, boys tend to be at higher risk than girls (Balan and Lingam 2012; Lifshitz and Gavrilov 2000; Soori 2001). Paraffin and kerosene, other types of chemical products, medicines, and drugs are the most common agents in unintentional child poisoning cases (Balan and Lingam 2012; Balme and others 2012; Kohli and others 2008; Lifshitz and Gavrilov 2000; Ozdemir and others 2012; Zia and others 2012).

Case-control studies in LMICs have also highlighted the importance of risk factors such as unsafe storage of chemicals or medicines (Ahmed, Fatmi, and Siddiqui 2011; Chatsantiprapa, Chokkanapitak, and Pinpradit 2001; Ramos and others 2010; Soori 2001); history of previous poisoning (Ahmed, Fatmi, and Siddiqui 2011; Soori 2001); distraction or lack of adult supervision (Ramos and others 2010; Soori 2001); hyperactive child behavior; low socioeconomic status; and low maternal educational status (Ahmed, Fatmi, and Siddiqui 2011).

## INTERVENTIONS, EFFECTIVENESS, AND COVERAGE

Evidence for the effectiveness of interventions and policies associated with nontransport unintentional injuries, and especially interventions that are effective in LMICs, is extremely limited. Few randomized controlled trials have been undertaken; some before-and-after studies are available, but much information derives from observational studies. This section outlines the best available evidence and highlights those interventions that show the greatest likelihood of being effective in LMICs (table 4.4).

## Falls

### Falls in Older People
Substantial progress has been made in the development of effective fall prevention programs for older people in HICs. The incidence of falls in older people living in the community has been reduced by either group and home-based exercise programs, usually containing some balance and strength-training exercises, or by Tai Chi programs (Gillespie and others 2012). Successful multifactorial interventions include home safety modifications, cataract surgery, withdrawal of psychotropic medication, and insertion of a pacemaker for those with carotid sinus hypersensitivity (Gillespie and others 2012). The effectiveness of fall prevention programs for older people in acute and subacute hospital settings, though promising, especially in high-risk groups, is limited and requires further investigation (Cameron and others 2012).

Although a substantial body of work is emerging on the burden and risk factors for falls in older people in LMICs, little or no evidence exists about the effectiveness of fall prevention programs in these settings (Kalula and others 2011). Although many of the interventions shown to be effective in HICs might be effective in LMICs, implementing them can be difficult. Competing health care demands that are perceived to be more urgent, combined with a lack of trained health care professionals, create challenges for implementing or translating evidence-based policy for fall prevention in LMICs. Further, the lack of systematic care for older people places much of the burden on family members. Without substantial investment in prevention programs, elder-care facilities, acute-care hospital services, and rehabilitation, the burden on families will increase.

### Falls in People of Working Age
Fall prevention for those of working age in LMICs requires a systematic approach, with a focus on industrial and construction safety standards. Little work has

**Table 4.4** Interventions for Cause-Specific Injuries, with Promising or Good Evidence, in HICs and LMICs

| Cause-specific injury | Age group | HICs | LMICs |
|---|---|---|---|
| Falls | Older people | Group and home-based exercise programs, containing balance and strength-training exercises, or Tai Chi (Gillespie and others 2012) | — |
| | | Multifactorial interventions, including home safety modifications (Gillespie and others 2012) | — |
| | | Targeted interventions involving cataract surgery, withdrawal from psychotropic medication, and pacemaker insertion (Gillespie and others 2012) | — |
| | Working age | Company-oriented safety campaigns and drug-free workplace programs (van der Molen and others 2012) | — |
| | Children | Home safety interventions providing free, low-cost, or subsidized safety equipment (Kendrick and others 2012) | — |
| Drowning | Children | Legislation and enforcement of swimming pool fencing (Stevenson and others 2003; Thompson and Rivara 2000) | Parental or other adult supervision and swimming lessons (Rahman 2010; Rahman and others 2009; Rahman and others 2012) |
| | | Provision of swimming lessons (Brenner, Saluja, and Smith 2003; Brenner and others 2009) | — |
| | | Legislation and enforcement of PDF use for recreational boaters (Bugeja and others 2014) | — |
| Burns | All ages | Installation and maintenance of smoke detectors (Mock and others 2011; Norton and others 2006) | Improvements in stove design (Mock and others 2011) |
| | | Education, legislation, and enforcement to regulate the temperature of household taps (Norton and others 2006) | — |
| Poisoning | Children | Home safety education, with the provision of safety equipment (Kendrick and others 2013) | Community-based educational interventions (Schwebel and others 2009) |
| | | | Child-resistant containers (Krug and others 1994) |

*Note:* — = not available; HICs = high-income countries; LMICs = low- and middle-income countries.

been done to evaluate the effectiveness of programs to reduce falls at building sites or in industrial settings, either in high- or low-income environments. Low-quality evidence suggests that company-oriented safety interventions–such as multifaceted safety campaigns and drug-free workplace programs—can reduce non-fatal injuries among construction workers (van der Molen and others 2012). Further improvements in construction safety standards and regulations are likely to reduce fall-related injuries, but these will require the development and implementation of appropriate policies, as well as education and enforcement.

**Falls in Children**

In HICs, home safety interventions for the prevention of falls in children have been shown to increase the use of stair gates and to reduce the use of baby walkers, although no evidence suggests that such programs increase the possession of window locks, screens, or windows with limited openings (Kendrick and others 2008; Kendrick and others 2012). Interventions that provide free, low-cost, or subsidized safety equipment appear to be more effective in improving safety practices than interventions that do not do so (Kendrick and others 2012). However, little research has been conducted on adapting known effective interventions to LMICs (Kendrick and others 2008).

Although many important challenges face efforts to prevent falls for both young and older people in rural settings, the increasing and rapid urbanization of LMICs will present additional challenges. The development of high-rise apartments is likely to increase the risk of falls from windows and stairways, particularly in poorly lit buildings. Urban slums and squatter camps pose particular risks (Rizvi and others 2006). Urban planning and architectural design can play a major role in mitigating the risks of falls, as can regulation of sidewalks to provide a safe walking environment free of roadside stalls.

## Drowning

### Evidence for Drowning Prevention

The scientific literature on drowning prevention studies published since the late 1990s identifies a number of possible and promising options for drowning prevention. In HICs, much of the evidence relates to the prevention of drowning in recreational settings. Evidence from observational studies suggests that legislation and enforcement of swimming pool fencing are likely to significantly reduce drowning, especially among children (Stevenson and others 2003; Thompson and Rivara 2000). Also, a growing body of evidence shows the contribution of alcohol consumption to recreational drowning in young people and adults, so legislation and enforcement to control alcohol use, especially in relation to aquatic activities, are likely to have an important effect (Diplock and Jamrozic 2006).

Some evidence indicates that providing swimming lessons may reduce drowning risks (Brenner, Saluja and Smith 2003; Brenner and others 2009; Rahman and others 2012). Increased knowledge of water safety, both for children and adults, also may decrease the risk of drowning. However, little evidence shows that water safety knowledge alone leads to improved safety (Kendrick and others 2007; Moran 2006; Solomon and others 2013). By comparison, increasingly strong evidence supports legislation requiring and enforcing the use of personal flotation devices (PFDs) by recreational boaters as an effective intervention strategy (Bugeja and others 2014).

In LMICs, evidence has shown that both increased parental or other adult supervision of and swimming lessons for children reduce child drownings (Rahman 2010; Rahman others 2009; Rahman and others 2012). The Prevention of Child Injury through Social Intervention and Education (PRECISE) was implemented in Bangladesh between 2006 and 2010 and covered more than 750,000 people in rural villages in three separate subdistrict intervention areas. The research design involved a comparison between very large cohorts of children participating in the interventions with nonparticipating children who were matched for age, gender, and location of residence. For children ages one to five years, a village *crèche* (child care) program called Anchal was established to provide a safe haven where mothers could drop off their children for four hours a day while they tended to domestic work. Children ages four years and older received training in a program called SwimSafe, which taught water safety, safe rescue, and survival swimming in the village pond, which had been converted into a safe training site. Both program components appeared to reduce the incidence of drowning in the intervention villages (Rahman 2010; Rahman and others 2009; Rahman and others 2012).

The *World Report on Child Injury Prevention* summarized the evidence on key strategies to prevent drowning among children. It suggested that four interventions should be considered as effective: removing or covering water hazards, requiring isolation fencing around swimming pools, wearing PFDs, and ensuring immediate resuscitation (Peden and others 2008). The report suggested that although other strategies are promising, including ensuring the presence of lifeguards in swimming areas and raising targeted awareness about drowning, for the remainder, the evidence is insufficient, ineffective, or potentially harmful.

### Prevention Challenges in LMICs

A 2012 report prepared on behalf of the Working Group on Child Drowning in LMICs has highlighted the challenges in addressing drowning prevention, especially among children (Linnan and others 2012):

- Most LMICs are predominantly rural.
- Water and other environmental hazards are ubiquitous around the home and throughout the community.
- Building codes and zoning ordinances are lacking or unenforced.
- Universal primary education is a goal, not a reality, resulting in high levels of illiteracy across large segments of the population.
- Parents often have many children and must rely on older children to supervise younger ones.
- Essential social services are lacking, such as emergency medical and rescue services that extend lifesaving services outside hospitals or other safety infrastructure.
- Sufficient financial resources are lacking.
- Adequate human resources for drowning prevention are lacking.

In contrast, the report suggests, HICs have built a culture of water safety on these foundations, using the wealth of financial and social capital that they possess. Introducing drowning prevention and the creation of a culture of water safety was a natural progression in the process of developing strong public health and public safety institutions connected to effective civil governance and enforcement structures.

Although, in theory, the principles underlying drowning prevention are the same among all population groups, whether in LMICs or HICs, they require thoughtful and extensive adaptation, given the different societal contexts and norms (Hyder and others 2008). It may not be possible to adapt the drowning prevention strategies for HICs in low-resource settings. The report by Linnan and others (2012) highlights, in particular, that of the four interventions deemed to have sufficient evidence for effectiveness in the *World Report on Child Injury Prevention*, three—fencing around swimming pools, legislating the use of PFDs, and ensuring immediate resuscitation—are likely to be unfeasible or unsustainable in LMICs.

## Burns

In HICs, prevention efforts have focused on education and on the installation and maintenance of smoke detectors for the prevention of fire-related burns. To reduce the incidence of scald-related burns, efforts have included legislation and enforcement to regulate the temperature of household taps (Mock and others 2011; Norton and others 2006). In LMICs, strategies have primarily focused on the prevention of fire-related burns.

### Education and Increasing Awareness in Communities
Education alone is unlikely to lead to behavioral changes. However, in many LMICs, especially in areas with high levels of literacy, educating the public on safe practices may be an important strategy in improving awareness levels. This education may lead to increased pressure on authorities to pass appropriate prevention legislation and to provide the necessary impetus for resources to address the problem.

### Improvements in Stove Design
Between 1992 and 1994, a household randomized trial, RESPIRE (randomized exposure study of pollution indoors and respiratory effects), was implemented in rural highland Guatemala to determine the effects of having an improved wood stove with a chimney (*plancha*) on the health of young children younger than 18 months, compared with continued use of open fires (Smith and others 2011). Prior to the intervention, the burn incidence rate among young children was 42.1 per 1,000 per year. Six months postintervention the rates were 18.1 and 35.2 per 1,000 children per year among the intervention and control groups, respectively. In addition, the plancha group had fewer serious burns (Mock and others 2011).

Another intervention with tremendous potential to prevent burn injuries is the use of a safer and cleaner kerosene stove design that is competitively priced. The Global Alliance for Clean Cookstoves is investing significant resources in research and design improvements for kerosene stoves (http://www.cleancookstoves.org).

### Platform Cooking
Floor-level cooking has been implicated in increasing the incidence of burn injuries, whether on a woodstove, a kerosene stove, or an open three-stone fire. Cooking on a platform immediately distances children from fires and from toppling cooking vessels. Platform cooking also renders irrelevant, to an extent, the type of clothing worn by women while cooking. Loose-fitting clothes are much less likely to get caught in the fire if the stove is on a platform. However, there is no published literature outlining the development and implementation of platform design, nor evaluation of their effectiveness.

## Poisoning

The traditional three "E" approach to preventing injuries—education, engineering, and enforcement—can be used as a framework to select intervention strategies for preventing unintentional poisonings in LMICs. Because these three Es generally refer to two broad concepts, behavior and environment, the focus is first on strategies to change the behavior of individuals and communities and then on strategies to alter the environment.

### Behavioral Strategies for the Prevention of Poisoning
Many experts have highlighted the need to target behavioral change to prevent accidental poisoning. Suggested interventions include safe storage of poisons, that is, where they are stored as well as the types of containers used (Ahmed, Fatmi, and Siddiqui 2011; Kohli and others 2008; Schwebel and Swart 2009). Ozdemir and others (2012), for example, recommended storing poisons in high places or locked cupboards after finding that 70 percent of responsible agents were easily accessible to child victims.

Unfortunately, the few studies that have assessed the effectiveness of behavioral approaches to addressing unintentional poisoning, such as paraffin- and kerosene-related injuries in LMICs, have mixed results (Schwebel and Swart 2009). One strategy, known as community-based educational interventions, has shown promise in South Africa. In 2008, Swart and others evaluated the effectiveness of a paraprofessional home visitation program to prevent child injuries. Intervention households received four visits from home visitors recruited from the community. During these visits, the trained home visitors gave caregivers safety information, as well as devices to improve safety. Although statistically insignificant, the findings showed a decline in risks associated with poisoning, as well as other injuries (Swart and others 2008).

Complementing this work, Schwebel and others (2009) examined the effectiveness of a trainer-to-trainer model, in which experts from the Paraffin Safety

Association of Southern Africa trained local community members to distribute educational materials to an intervention community in South Africa. The educational materials were based on the theory of health behavioral change. The findings showed that the intervention was effective at significantly changing the level of kerosene safety knowledge in the intervention community. The researchers found slight behavioral changes related to kerosene safety as well as to perceptions of risk (Schwebel and others 2009).

Results from these two studies are consistent with findings from HICs. A meta-analysis conducted in 2013, for example, showed that home safety education used in interventions that included the provision of safety equipment were effective at increasing safety practices for preventing injury, including poisoning (Kendrick and others 2013).

### Environmental Strategies for the Prevention of Poisoning

Some of the identified risk factors point to the need to target broader environmental risk factors, such as by enacting and enforcing poisoning prevention legislation. Krug and others (1994), for example, demonstrated in a controlled before-and-after study in South Africa that the incidence rate of paraffin ingestion decreased by 47 percent when child-resistant containers were widely distributed (Krug and others 1994). However, government policies mandating the use of such child-resistant containers do not exist in many LMICs (Balan and Lingam 2012). In Turkey, only a limited number of medications are sold with child safety caps (Ozdemir and others 2012); in Pakistan, a call for child-resistant packaging legislation has been made (Ahmed, Fatmi, and Siddiqui 2011).

Other types of legislation, such as laws that mandate standards for wick stoves in South Africa, are lacking in many LMICs (Schwebel and Swart 2009). Suggested interventions include ensuring that labels possess all the necessary safety information and are in languages that people can understand. Nonyelum and others (2010), for example, showed that safety warnings on pharmaceutical and consumer products still need improvement in Nigeria. Their study revealed that only 70 percent of the 600 products examined had adequate warning labels. Moreover, despite English being Nigeria's official language, 5 percent of products had only non-English labels.

## COSTS AND COST-EFFECTIVENESS OF INTERVENTIONS

Not surprisingly, given the dearth of evidence on effective interventions for the prevention of nontransport unintentional injuries in LMICs, the published data on the costs and cost-effectiveness of interventions are limited. This section presents information on the costs incurred by such injuries, where data are available, and on potential cost-effective interventions for LMICs, supplemented by the best available information from HICs (table 4.5). All costs presented in this section have been converted to 2012 U.S. dollars.

### Falls

The costs of falls are well documented in HICs, but few data are available on the costs of falls in LMICs. However, the costs are likely to be substantial. Falls and road traffic injuries accounted for the largest out-of-pocket health care costs for those hospitalized for injuries in Vietnam. Of road traffic victims, 26 percent experience catastrophic expenditure as a result of their injuries (Nguyen and others 2013).

There are no published data showing the cost-effectiveness of fall prevention programs in LMICs. However, growing evidence suggests that some community-based fall prevention programs among older people in HICs can be cost-effective. Data from Australia on older adults living in the community show that the most cost-effective intervention is the practice of Tai Chi; the cost per quality-adjusted life year (QALY) is US$49,119; the incremental cost per fall avoided is US$3,484 (Church and others 2011). And although evidence for effectiveness is still emerging, the data suggest that cataract surgery is potentially extremely cost-effective (the cost per QALY is US$3,818; the incremental cost per fall avoided is US$275. For those taking psychotropic medications, medication withdrawal is also highly cost-effective (with the cost per QALY of $22,711, and the incremental cost per fall avoided of US$1,251 (Church and others 2011).

The evidence on cost-effective interventions in residential care settings in Australia is still emerging. The data suggest that medication review and the use of hip protectors among medium- and high-risk groups are highly cost-effective strategies. The former is more effective and less costly than no intervention; the cost per QALY of the latter is US$2,002, and the incremental cost per fall avoided is US$114 (Church and others 2011). Among all individuals living in residential settings, vitamin D supplementation has the potential to be extremely cost-effective at a cost of US$7,970 per QALY, and an incremental cost per fall avoided of US$444.

### Drowning

Cost and cost-effectiveness data for interventions to prevent drowning in LMICs are scarce, given the paucity of

**Table 4.5** Promising and Cost-Effective Interventions for Cause-Specific Injuries for HICs and LMICs, US$ 2012

| Cause-specific injury | HICs | LMICs |
|---|---|---|
| Falls | Tai Chi: cost per QALY—$49,119; incremental cost per fall avoided—$3,484 (Church and others 2011) | — |
| | Cataract surgery: cost per QALY—$3818; incremental cost per fall avoided—$275 (Church and others 2011) | — |
| | Psychotropic medication withdrawal: cost per QALY—$22,711; incremental cost per fall avoided—$1,251 (Church and others 2011) | — |
| | In residential settings, medication review: more effective and less costly than no intervention (Church and others 2011) | — |
| | In residential settings, use of hip protectors: cost per QALY—$2,002; incremental cost per fall avoided—$114 (Church and others 2011) | — |
| | In residential settings, vitamin D supplementation: cost per QALY—$7,970; incremental cost per fall avoided—$444 (Church and others 2011) | — |
| Drowning | Fencing of residential swimming pools in homes with children younger than age 18 years: cost per QALY—$35,212 to $43,663 (Segui-Gomez 2001) | Supervision of children: $256 per DALY averted and $8,703 per death averted (Rahman and others 2012) |
| | Purchase of personal flotation devices for boats: cost per QALY—$5,634 (Segui-Gomez 2001) | Swimming training for children ages four years and older: $27 per DALY averted and $949 per death averted (Rahman and others 2012) |
| Poisoning | | Distribution of child-resistant containers: $127 per DALY averted; $3,329 per death averted (Norton and others 2006) |

*Note:* — = not available; DALY = disability-adjusted life year; HICs = high-income countries; LMICs = low- and middle-income countries; QALY = quality-adjusted life year.

information on effective interventions in these settings. However, data have been published on the cost-effectiveness of the PRECISE study in Bangladesh (Rahman and others 2012). Cost-effectiveness was calculated using the WHO-CHOICE guidelines (CHOosing Interventions that are Cost Effective), by determining the numbers of DALYs and deaths averted and the costs associated with both (http://www.who.int/choice/interventions/en/?)

The cost-effectiveness of Anchal—the component of the intervention that involved supervision of children ages one to five years in a community crèche—in reducing mortality was US$256 per DALY averted and US$8,703 per death averted. The cost-effectiveness of SwimSafe—the component of the intervention that involved children ages four years and older receiving swimming training—was US$27 per DALY averted and US$949 per death averted. Overall, the cost-effectiveness of PRECISE was US$114 per DALY averted and US$3,970 per death averted.

By comparison, earlier research focusing on interventions in HICs has shown that the cost-effectiveness of fencing around residential pools in homes with children younger than age 18 years ranged from US$35,212 to US$43,663 per QALY gained, depending on whether the fenced pools belonged to homes with children of different age subgroups and whether an incremental installation was considered (Segui-Gomez 2001).

Modeling of the cost-effectiveness of PFDs resulted in figures of US$5,634 per QALY gained. Sensitivity analyses were also conducted, suggesting that installing fencing around in-ground pools in homes with children younger than age 18 years and purchasing PFDs for recreational boats resulted in cost-effectiveness figures well below those of many interventions implemented in the clinical and public health realms.

## Burns

Many burn injuries lead to prolonged hospital stays. In addition to acute burn care, patients often require a protracted period of rehabilitation. Only recently has the cost of providing reasonable burn care in LMICs been reported. Ahuja and Goswami (2013) calculated the cost per patient (all medications and consumables, dressing material, investigations, blood products, dietary costs, and salaries of all personnel) in a third-level teaching hospital in northern India to be US$1,102.

Although the cost of burn care is relatively easy to calculate and reflects the cost of survival from a major injury, albeit with disability, the cost-effectiveness of prevention programs is not easy to calculate. National or regional statistics need to be available to measure the effectiveness of prevention interventions. Interventions need to be combined with educational campaigns to institute safe behavioral practices, and studies evaluating all costs against all benefits with regard to burn injuries are not available. Also, to establish the cost-effectiveness of any action for preventing burns, one needs to factor in the elimination of the high cost of burn care and the prevention of disability, in addition to the decrease in burn incidence.

## Poisoning

Limited data exist on the cost of unintentional poisonings in LMICs. A study in Pakistan revealed that the costs of treatment to patients were considerable; approximately 37 percent had to pay out of pocket. However, only 9 percent of the patients were able to obtain government support to cover the treatment cost (Zia and others 2012).

A detailed analysis of the cost-effectiveness of providing child-resistant containers in 2006 showed that, as a means of preventing paraffin poisoning among children in South Africa, the intervention had a cost-effectiveness ratio of $3,329 per death averted (Norton and others 2006). The impact of this intervention was calculated to be 263 DALYs averted, and cost-effectiveness was estimated to be US$127 per DALY at a 3 percent discount rate.

## CONCLUSIONS

### Burden of Unintentional Injuries

Recent global estimates provide a strong foundation for understanding the burden of death and disability associated with nontransport unintentional injuries. Falls, which are the most important cause of death and disability, are likely to become even more important as populations in LMICs continue to age. Drowning and burns are important contributors to the burden and predominantly affect LMICs, especially younger children. Poisonings constitute the next leading contributor to the unintentional injury burden and affect both HICs and LMICs, and particularly adults ages 70 years and older. With the exception of burn injuries, and to a lesser extent falls, men and boys account for a much higher proportion of all injuries than women and girls. However, the reliability and validity of data from LMICs remain uncertain, and improved data collection in these countries needs to be prioritized.

### Risk Factors, Interventions, and Cost-Effectiveness

#### Falls

Despite evidence of a rising burden of falls in older people in LMICs worldwide, few evidence-based prevention programs have been implemented in these countries. Governments have failed to recognize the costs of this burden, resulting in inadequate policy development and investment in prevention programs or prevention research.

Although HICs have an increasingly strong evidence base for effective and cost-effective programs to prevent falls in older people, policymakers in these countries need to better understand how such programs may be put into practice, both at the community level and in residential care settings. Further, significant work needs to be undertaken by health care providers to adapt fall prevention programs from HICs to LMICs, where risk factors may vary. Such programs will likely have to be substantially modified for LMIC environments.

Consequently, more research is needed to enhance understanding of the likely contextual factors and unique contributors to falls among older people in LMICs. Such factors include the influence of diet, physical activity, environment, and transportation, and the role of health services. Fall prevention programs that target the physical environment, inside and outside the home, may significantly affect the success of such programs in older people in those countries.

Falls are also a significant cause of death and injury in children and working-age adults in HICs and LMICs. Although HIC studies suggest that environmental factors, including urban and street design as well as building design, contribute significantly to falls in these population groups, the evidence base is weak. Nevertheless, fall prevention programs involving environmental modification may have more of an impact in LMICs, particularly in countries with rapid urbanization or areas with high levels of poverty. Similarly, focusing on building design and safety standards for construction sites and workplaces is likely to reduce falls for people of working age. Increasing regulation of consumer products by governments, as well as community education on the appropriate use of such products, will be relevant as the use of these products increases in LMICs.

#### Drowning

The need to address the burden of drowning in LMICs is a neglected health issue in many countries, with very few researchers focused on identifying effective interventions or on examining differences in risk factors between HICs and LMICs. The development of successful drowning prevention strategies in LMICs faces a number of obstacles:

- The absence of and need by researchers to better identify risk factors for drowning, not only among young children, but also among other age groups
- The absence of and need by researchers to identify effective intervention strategies, especially for older age groups
- The need by governments and other stakeholders to scale up effective drowning interventions into national, regional, and global programs
- Capacity building for implementing drowning prevention at all levels of program development
- The need to stimulate and sustain investment in drowning prevention interventions and activities
- Incorporation of research into program design and implementation.

## Burns

Major causes of burn injuries in LMICs include poverty and hazardous work environments, including in the home. Therefore, progress on burn prevention can be expected with countries' socioeconomic growth and government enforcement of regulations. In HICs, the introduction of smoke detectors and flame-retardant sleepwear, along with enforced safety practices in the workplace, have led to significant reductions in fire injuries. These efforts will be less effective in LMICs until the infrastructure improves.

In the meantime, policymakers and health providers need to develop a better understanding of (1) risk factors for burn injuries in LMICs, (2) the economic impact of burn injuries on survivors, and (3) the effectiveness and cost-effectiveness of burn prevention programs. Sufficient data are available from HICs to support the claim that burn injuries can be successfully prevented using education, engineering changes, enforcement of legislative protections, and environmental modifications (Peck, Molnar, and Swart 2009).

In addition to focusing on prevention strategies, health care organizations should encourage providers to be involved in specialized burn treatment at a local level. Moreover, encouraging participation with global initiatives, such as the Global Alliance for Clean Cookstoves, can further the success of local initiatives.

## Poisoning

Most of the available studies on risk factors associated with unintentional poisoning in LMICs focus on young children, despite the fact that older adults are at highest risk. Data on the cost of unintentional poisoning are limited, so the true economic burden of this public health problem is unknown. Few researchers have investigated the effectiveness of interventions in these settings; even fewer have studied their cost-effectiveness. More studies are urgently needed. Cost studies, as well as benefit-cost analysis of successful behavioral programs, for example, can be vitally important. Findings could encourage donors and governments to invest in preventive measures in LMICs.

## Summary Conclusions

Nontransport unintentional injuries are comparable to transport injuries in terms of the burden of death and disability, but they have not received the same attention from government agencies or researchers. Recognition of the need to prevent falls and fall-related injuries among older people is likely to grow in LMICs as governments in these countries begin to address the growing numbers of older people and the potential cost-effectiveness of prevention strategies. However, given the observed declines in the burden of other unintentional injuries, it seems less likely that government initiatives will drive a strengthened evidence base or facilitate prevention initiatives for these injuries. Consequently, global support from the United Nations, WHO, academia, nongovernmental organizations, and commercial enterprises, in tandem with the injury control community and health practitioners, will be important to move the unintentional injury agenda forward.

## NOTE

World Bank Income Classifications as of July 2014 are as follows, based on estimates of gross national income (GNI) per capita for 2013:

- Low-income countries (LICs) = US$1,045 or less
- Middle-income countries (MICs) are subdivided:
  a) lower-middle-income = US$1,046 to US$4,125
  b) upper-middle-income (UMICs) = US$4,126 to US$12,745
- High-income countries (HICs) = US$12,746 or more.

## REFERENCES

Ahmed, B., Z. Fatmi, and A. R. Siddiqui. 2011. "Population Attributable Risk of Unintentional Childhood Poisoning in Karachi Pakistan." *PLoS One* 6 (10): e26881.

Ahuja, R. B., and S. Bhattacharya. 2002. "An Analysis of 11,196 Burn Admissions and Evaluation of Conservative Management Techniques." *Burns* 28 (6): 555–61.

Ahuja, R. B., S. Bhattacharya, and A. Rai. 2009. "Changing Trends of an Endemic Trauma." *Burns* 35 (5): 650–56.

Ahuja R. B., J. K. Dash, and P. Shrivastava. 2011. "A Comparative Analysis of Liquefied Petroleum Gas (LPG) and Kerosene Related Burns." *Burns* 37 (8): 1403–10.

Ahuja, R. B., and P. Goswami. 2013. "Cost of Providing Inpatient Burn Care in a Tertiary Teaching Hospital of North India." *Burns* 39 (4): 558–64.

Akbaba, M., E. Nazlican, H. Demirhindi, Z. Sütoluk, and Y. Gökel. 2007. "Etiological and Demographical Characteristics of Acute Adult Poisoning in Adana, Turkey." *Human and Experimental Toxicology* 26 (5): 401–6.

American Burn Association. 2012. National Burn Repository. Chicago, IL: American Burn Association.

Balan, B., and L. Lingam. 2012. "Unintentional Injuries among Children in Resource Poor Settings: Where Do the Fingers Point?" *Archives of Disease in Childhood* 97 (1): 35–38.

Balme, K. H., J. C. Roberts, M. Glasstone, L. Curling, and M. D. Mann. 2012. "The Changing Trends of Childhood Poisoning at a Tertiary Children's Hospital in South Africa." *South African Medical Journal* 102 (3): 142–46.

Bell, G. S., A. Gaitatzis, C. L. Bell, A. L. Johnson, and J. W. Sander. 2008. "Drowning in People with Epilepsy: How Great Is the Risk?" *Neurology* 71: 578–82.

Bierens, J. J. L. M. 2006. *Handbook on Drowning: Prevention, Rescue, Treatment.* Berlin: Springer-Verlag.

Brenner, R. A., G. Saluja, and G. S. Smith. 2003. "Swimming Lessons, Swimming Ability, and the Risk of Drowning." *Injury Control and Safety Promotion* 10 (4): 211–16.

Brenner, R. A., G. S. Taneja, D. L. Haynie, A. C. Trumble, C. Qian, and others. 2009. "Association between Swimming Lessons and Drowning in Childhood: A Case-Control Study." *Archives of Pediatrics and Adolescent Medicine* 163 (3): 203–10.

Bugeja, L., E. Cassell, L. R. Brodie, and S. J. Walter. 2014. "Effectiveness of the 2005 Compulsory Personal Flotation Device (PFD) Wearing Regulation in Reducing Drowning Deaths among Recreational Boaters in Australia." *Injury Prevention* 20 (6): 387–92. doi:10.1136/injuryprevention-2014-041169.

Cameron, I. D., L. D. Gillespie, M. C. Robertson, G. R. Murray, K. D. Hill, and others. 2012. "Interventions for Preventing Falls in Older People in Care Facilities and Hospitals." *Cochrane Database of Systematic Reviews* 12: CD005465.

Chalmers, D., B. McNoe, and S. Stephenson. 2004. *Drowning, Near-Drowning and Other Water-Related Injury: Literature Review and Analysis of National Injury Data. A Report to the Accident Compensation Corporation.* Dunedin: Injury Prevention Research Centre.

Chatsantiprapa, K., J. Chokkanapitak, and N. Pinpradit. 2001. "Host and Environment Factors for Exposure to Poisons: A Case-Control Study of Preschool Children in Thailand." *Injury Prevention* 7 (3): 214–17.

Church, J., S. Goodall, R. Norman, and M. Haas. 2011. *An Economic Evaluation of Community and Residential Aged Care Falls Prevention Strategies in NSW.* Sydney: NSW Ministry of Health.

Dandona, R., G. A. Kumar, R. Ivers, R. Joshi, B. Neal, and others. 2010. "Characteristics of Non-Fatal Fall Injuries in Rural India." *Injury Prevention* 16 (3): 166–71.

Diplock, S., and K. Jamrozic. 2006. "Legislative and Regulatory Measures for Preventing Alcohol-Related Drownings and Near-Drownings." *Australian and New Zealand Journal of Public Health* 30 (4): 314–17.

Giashuddin, S. M., A. Rahman, F. Rahman, S. R. Mashreky, S. M. Chowdhury, and others. 2009. "Socioeconomic Inequality in Child Injury in Bangladesh—Implication for Developing Countries." *International Journal for Equity in Health* 8: 7.

Gillespie, L. D., M. C. Robertson, W. J. Gillespie, C. Sherrington, S. Gates, and others. 2012. "Interventions for Preventing Falls in Older People Living in the Community." *Cochrane Database of Systematic Reviews* 9: CD007146.

Gururaj, G., V. Sateesh, and A. Rayan. 2008. *Bengaluru Injury/Road Traffic Injury Surveillance Programme: A Feasibility Study.* Bengaluru: National Institute of Mental Health and Neuro Sciences.

Haagsma, J. A., N. Graetz, I. Bolliger, M. Naghavi, H. Higashi, and others. 2015. "The Global Burden of Injury: Incidence, Mortality, Disability-Adjusted Life Years and Time Trends from the *Global Burden of Disease Study 2013.*" *Injury Prevention.* 0: 1–15. E-published 3 December 2015. doi:10.1136/injuryprev-2015-041616.

Harris, V. A., L. M. Rochette, and G. A. Smith. 2011. "Pediatric Injuries Attributable to Falls from Windows in the United States in 1990–2008." *Pediatrics* 128 (3): 455–62.

Hestekin, H., T. O'Driscoll, J. S. Williams, P. Kowal, K. Peltzer, and others. 2013. "Measuring Prevalence and Risk Factors for Fall-Related Injury in Older Adults in Low- and Middle-Income Countries: Results from the WHO Study on Global AGEing and Adult Health (SAGE)." SAGE Working Paper 6, World Health Organization, Geneva. http://cdrwww.who.int/healthinfo/sage/SAGEWorkingPaper6_Wave1Falls.pdf.

Hyder, A. A., N. N. Borse, L. Blum, R. Khan, S. El Arifeen, and others. 2008. "Childhood Drowning in Low- and Middle-Income Countries: Urgent Need for Intervention Trials." *Journal of Paediatrics and Child Health* 44 (4): 221–27.

Hyder, A. A., D. E. Sugerman, P. Puvanachandra, J. Razzak, H. El-Sayed, and others. 2009. "Global Childhood Unintentional Injury Surveillance in Four Cities in Developing Countries: A Pilot Study." *Bulletin of the World Health Organization* 87 (5): 345–52.

International Life Saving Federation. 2007. *World Drowning Report.* Gemeenteplein, Belgium: International Life Saving Association.

Jagnoor, J., L. Keay, N. Jaswal, M. Kaur, and R. Ivers. 2014. "A Qualitative Study on the Perceptions of Preventing Falls as a Health Priority among Older People in Northern India." *Injury Prevention* 20 (1): 29–34.

Jiang, X., Y. Zhang, Y. Wang, B. Wang, Y. Xu, and others. 2010. "An Analysis of 6215 Hospitalized Unintentional Injuries among Children Aged 0–14 in Northwest China." *Accident Analysis and Prevention* 42 (1): 320–26.

Jitapunkul, S., P. Yuktananandana, and V. Parkpian. 2001. "Risk Factors of Hip Fracture among Thai Female Patients." *Journal of the Medical Association of Thailand* 84 (11): 1576–81.

Kalula, S. Z., V. Scott, A. Dowd, and K. Brodrick. 2011. "Falls and Fall Prevention Programmes in Developing Countries: Environmental Scan for the Adaptation of the Canadian Falls Prevention Curriculum for Developing Countries." *Journal of Safety Research* 42 (6): 461–72.

Kendrick, D., C. Coupland, C. Mulvaney, J. Simpson, S. J. Smith, and others. 2007. "Home Safety Education and Provision of Safety Equipment for Injury Prevention." *Cochrane Database of Systematic Reviews* 1: CD005014.

Kendrick, D., M. C. Watson, C. A. Mulvaney, S. J. Smith, A. J. Sutton, and others. 2008. "Preventing Childhood Falls at Home: Meta-Analysis and Meta-Regression." *American Journal of Preventive Medicine* 35 (4): 370–79.

Kendrick, D., B. Young, A. J. Mason-Jones, N. Ilyas, F. A. Achana, and others. 2012. "Home Safety Education and Provision of Safety Equipment for Injury Prevention." *Cochrane Database Systematic Reviews* 9: CD005014.

———. 2013. "Home Safety Education and Provision of Safety Equipment for Injury Prevention (Review)." *Evidence-Based Child Health* 8 (3): 761–939.

Khambalia, A., P. Joshi, M. Brussoni, P. Raina, B. Morrongiello, and others. 2006. "Risk Factors for Unintentional Injuries Due to Falls in Children Aged 0–6 Years: A Systematic Review." *Injury Prevention* 12 (6): 378–81.

Kohli, U., V. S. Kuttiat, R. Lodha, and S. K. Kabra. 2008. "Profile of Childhood Poisoning at a Tertiary Care Centre in North India." *Indian Journal of Pediatrics* 75: 791–94.

Kool, B., S. Ameratunga, M. Lee, E. Robinson, S. Crengle, and others. 2010. "Prevalence of Risk and Protective Factors for Falls in the Home Environment in a Population-Based Survey of Young and Middle-Aged Adult New Zealanders." *Australian and New Zealand Journal of Public Health* 34 (1): 63–66.

Kool, B., S. Ameratunga, E. Robinson, S. Crengle, and R. Jackson. 2008. "The Contribution of Alcohol to Falls at Home among Working-Aged Adults." *Alcohol* 42 (5): 383–88.

Krug, A., J. B. Ellis, I. T. Hay, N. F. Mokgabudi, and J. Robertson. 1994. "The Impact of Child-Resistant Containers on the Incidence of Paraffin (Kerosene) Ingestion in Children." *South African Medical Journal* 84 (11): 730–34.

Laloë, V. 2002. "Epidemiology and Mortality of Burns in a General Hospital of Eastern Sri Lanka." *Burns* 28 (8): 778–81.

Lau, E. M., P. Suriwongpaisal, J. K. Lee, S. Das De, M. R. Festin, and others. 2001. "Risk Factors for Hip Fracture in Asian Men and Women: The Asian Osteoporosis Study." *Journal of Bone and Mineral Research* 16 (3): 572–80.

Lifshitz, M., and V. Gavrilov. 2000. "Acute Poisoning in Children." *The Israel Medical Association Journal* 2 (7): 504–6.

Linnan, M., A. Rahman, J. Scarr, T. Reinten-Reynolds, H. Linnan, and others. 2012. "Child Drowning: Evidence for a Newly Recognized Cause of Child Mortality in Low and Middle Income Countries in Asia." Working Paper 2012-07, Special Series on Child Injury 2, UNICEF Office of Research, Florence.

Lord, S. R., C. Sherrington, H. B. Menz, and J. C. T. Close. 2007. *Falls in Older People: Risk Factors and Strategies for Prevention*. 2nd ed. Cambridge, U.K.: Cambridge University Press.

Lozano, R., M. Naghavi, K. Foreman, S. Lim. K. Shibuya, V. Aboyans, and others. 2012. "Global and Regional Mortality from 235 Causes of Death for 20 Age Groups in 1990 and 2010: A Systematic Analysis for the Global Burden of Disease Study 2010." *The Lancet* 380 (9859): 2095–128.

Mabrouk, A., A. El Badawy, and M. Sherif. 2000. "Kerosene Stove as a Cause of Burns Admitted to the Ain Shams Burn Unit." *Burns* 26 (5): 474–77.

Mashreky, S. R., A. Rahman, T. F. Khan, L. Svanström, and F. Rahman. 2010. "Determinants of Childhood Burns in Rural Bangladesh: A Nested Case-Control Study." *Health Policy* 96 (3): 226–30.

Mock, C., M. Peck, C. Juillard, D. Meddings, A. Gielen, and others. 2011. *Burn Prevention: Success Stories and Lessons Learned*. Geneva: World Health Organization.

Moran, K. 2006. "Water Safety Knowledge, Attitudes and Behaviours of Asian Youth in New Zealand." In *Proceedings of the Second International Asian Health and Wellbeing Conference*, November 13–14, edited by S. Tse, M. Hoque, K. Rasanathan, M. Chatterji, R. Wee, and others. Auckland, New Zealand: University of New Zealand.

Nguyen, H., R. Ivers, S. Jan, A. Martiniuk, and C. Pham. 2013. "Catastrophic Household Costs Due to Injury in Vietnam." *Injury* 44 (5): 684–90.

Nonyelum, S. C., N. Nkem, C. N. Ofeyinwa, and O. E. Orisakwe. 2010. "Safety Warnings and First Aid Instructions on Consumer and Pharmaceutical Products in Nigeria: Has There Been an Improvement?" *Journal of the Pakistan Medical Association* 60 (10): 801–4.

Norton, R., A. A. Hyder, D. Bishai, and M. Peden. 2006. "Unintentional Injuries." In *Disease Control Priorities in Developing Countries*, second edition, edited by D. T. Jamison, J. G. Breman, A. R. Measham, G. Alleyne, M. Claeson, D. B. Evans, P. Jha, A. Mills, and P. Musgrove. Washington, DC: Oxford University Press and World Bank.

Norton, R., and O. Kobusingye. 2013. "Injuries." *New England Journal of Medicine* 368 (18): 1723–30.

Ozdemir, R., B. Bayrakci, Ö. Tekşam, B. Yalçın, and G. Kale. 2012. "Thirty-Three-Year Experience on Childhood Poisoning." *Turkish Journal of Pediatrics* 54 (3): 251–59.

Peck, M., J. Molnar, and D. Swart. 2009. "A Global Plan for Burn Prevention and Care." *Bulletin of the World Health Organization* 87 (10): 802–03.

Peden, M., K. Oyegbite, J. Ozanne-Smith, A. A. Hyder, C. Branche, and others, eds. 2008. *World Report on Child Injury Prevention*. Geneva: World Health Organization.

Peden, M. M, and K. McGee. 2003. "The Epidemiology of Drowning Worldwide." *Injury Control and Safety Promotion* 10 (4): 195–99.

Peiris-John, R., B. Kafoa, I. Wainiqolo, R. K. Reddy, E. McCaig, and others. 2013. "Population-Based Characteristics of Fatal and Hospital Admissions for Poisoning in Fiji: TRIP Project-11." *Injury Prevention* 19 (5): 355–57.

Rahman, A. 2010. "A Community Based Child Drowning Prevention Programme in Bangladesh: A Model for Low Income Countries." Doctoral thesis, Public Health Science Department, Karolinska Institutet, Solna, Sweden.

Rahman, A., S. R. Mashreky, S. M. Chowdhury, M. S. Giashuddin, I. J. Uhaa, and others. 2009. "Analysis of the Childhood Fatal Drowning Situation in Bangladesh: Exploring Prevention Measures for Low-Income Countries." *Injury Prevention* 15: 75–79.

Rahman, F., S. Bose, M. Linnan, A. Rahman, S. Mashreky, and others. 2012. "Cost-Effectiveness of an Injury and Drowning Prevention Program in Bangladesh." *Pediatrics* 130 (6): e1621–28.

Ramos, C. L., H. M. Barros, A. T. Stein, and J. S. Costa. 2010. "Risk Factors Contributing to Childhood Poisoning." *Jornal de Pediatria* 86 (5): 435–40.

Ranaweera, A. D., P. Fonseka, A. PattiyaArachchi, and S. H. Siribaddana. 2013. "Incidence and Risk Factors of Falls among the Elderly in the District of Colombo." *Ceylon Medical Journal* 58: 100–106.

Rizvi, N., S. Luby, S. I. Azam, and F. Rabbani. 2006. "Distribution and Circumstances of Injuries in Squatter Settlements of Karachi, Pakistan." *Accident Analysis and Prevention* 38 (3): 526–31.

Sanghavi, P., K. Bhalla, and V. Das. 2009. "Fire-Related Deaths in India in 2001: A Retrospective Analysis of Data." *The Lancet* 373 (9671): 1282–88.

Sawalha, A. F., W. M. Sweileh, M. T. Tufaha, and D. Y. Al-Jabi. 2010. "Analysis of the Pattern of Acute Poisoning in Patients Admitted to a Governmental Hospital in Palestine." *Basic and Clinical Pharmacology and Toxicology* 107 (5): 914–18.

Schwebel, D. C., and D. Swart. 2009. "Preventing Paraffin-Related Injury." *Journal of Injury and Violence Research* 1 (1): 3–5.

Schwebel, D. C., D. Swart, J. Simpson, P. Hobe, and S. K. Hui. 2009. "An Intervention to Reduce Kerosene-Related Burns and Poisonings in Low-Income South African Communities." *Health Psychology* 28 (4): 493–500.

Segui-Gomez, M. 2001. "Cost Effectiveness of Interventions to Prevent Drowning and Near-Drowning." Abstract at 129th Annual Meeting of the American Public Health Association, October 23. https://apha.confex.com/apha/129am/techprogram/paper_23731.htm.

Smith, K. R., J. P. McCracken, M. W. Weber, A. Hubbard, A. Jenny, and others. 2011. "Effect of Reduction in Household Air Pollution on Childhood Pneumonia in Guatemala (RESPIRE): A Randomised Controlled Trial." *The Lancet* 378 (9804): 1717–26.

Solomon, R., M. J. Giganti, A. Weiner, and M. Akpinar-Elci. 2013. "Water Safety Education among Primary School Children in Grenada." *International Journal of Injury Control and Safety Promotion* 20 (3): 266–70.

Soori, H. 2001. "Developmental Risk Factors for Unintentional Childhood Poisoning." *Saudi Medical Journal* 22 (3): 227–30.

Stevenson, M. R., M. Rimajova, D. Edgecombe, and K. Vickery. 2003. "Childhood Drowning: Barriers Surrounding Private Swimming Pools." *Pediatrics* 3 (2): e115–19.

Swart, L., A. van Niekerk, M. Seedat, and E. Jordaan. 2008. "Paraprofessional Home Visitation Program to Prevent Childhood Unintentional Injuries in Low-Income Communities: A Cluster Randomized Controlled Trial." *Injury Prevention* 14 (3): 164–69.

Thompson, D. C., and F. P. Rivara. 2000. "Pool Fencing for Preventing Drowning in Children." *Cochrane Database of Systematic Reviews* 2: CD001047.

van der Molen, H. F., M. M. Lehtola, J. Lappalainen, P. L. Hoonakker, H. Hsiao, and others. 2012. "Interventions to Prevent Injuries in Construction Workers." *Cochrane Database of Systematic Reviews* 12: CD006251.

WHO (World Health Organization). 2006. *Guidelines for Safe Recreational Water Environments*. Vol. 2: *Swimming Pools and Similar Environments*. Geneva: WHO.

———. 2012. "Drowning." Fact Sheet, WHO, Geneva. http://www.who.int/mediacentre/factsheets/fs347/en/index.html.

———. 2014. "Global Health Estimates." http://www.who.int/healthinfo/global_burden_disease/en/.

Yang, L., Q. Q. Nong, C. L. Li, Q. M. Feng, and S. K. Lo. 2007. "Risk Factors for Childhood Drowning in Rural Regions of a Developing Country: A Case-Control Study." *Injury Prevention* 13 (3): 178–82.

Zia, N., U. R. Khan, J. A. Razzak, P. Puvanachandra, and A. A. Hyder. 2012. "Understanding Unintentional Childhood Home Injuries: Pilot Surveillance Data from Karachi, Pakistan." *BMC Research Notes* 5: 37.

# Chapter 5

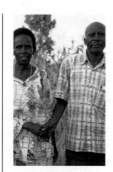

# Interpersonal Violence: Global Impact and Paths to Prevention

James A. Mercy, Susan D. Hillis, Alexander Butchart,
Mark A. Bellis, Catherine L. Ward, Xiangming Fang,
and Mark L. Rosenberg

## INTRODUCTION

Interpersonal violence is a pervasive public health, human rights, and development challenge (Rosenberg and others 2006). Its effects reverberate through families, communities, and nations and across generations. It is a leading cause of death among adolescents and young adults in most parts of the world. Exposure to interpersonal violence increases individuals' lifelong vulnerability to a broad range of emotional, behavioral, and physical health problems. Interpersonal violence directly affects health care expenditures worldwide; indirectly, it affects national and local economies—stunting development, increasing inequality, and eroding human capital (WHO 2008).

Attention to interpersonal violence as a global issue has expanded dramatically since the World Health Assembly identified violence as a public health priority in 1996. Reports by the United Nations (UN) have contributed greatly to increased awareness (Krug and others 2002; Pinheiro 2006; UN 2006). These and other efforts culminated in specific targets for eliminating interpersonal violence in the UN's post-2015 Action Agenda for Sustainable Development (UN 2015).

## NATURE AND BURDEN OF INTERPERSONAL VIOLENCE

Globally, the three primary forms of violence are interpersonal violence; self-directed violence, including suicide; and collective violence, including war, terrorism, and state-perpetrated violence in the form of genocide or torture (Dahlberg and Krug 2002). This chapter focuses on interpersonal violence.

### Definitions of Interpersonal Violence

The World Health Organization (WHO) defines *violence* as follows: "The intentional use of physical force or power, threatened or actual, against oneself, another person, or against a group or community that either results in or has a high likelihood of resulting in injury, death, psychological harm, mal-development, or deprivation" (Dahlberg and Krug 2002, 5). This definition encompasses interpersonal, self-directed, and collective violence.

Interpersonal violence involves the intentional use of physical force or power against other persons by an individual or small group of individuals. Interpersonal violence may be physical, sexual, or psychological (also called emotional violence), and it may involve

Corresponding author: James A. Mercy, U.S. Centers for Disease Control and Prevention, Atlanta, Georgia, United States; jam2@cdc.gov.

deprivation and neglect. Acts of interpersonal violence can be further divided into family or partner violence and community violence.

- *Family* or *partner violence* refers to violence within the family or between intimate partners. It includes child maltreatment, dating and intimate partner violence (IPV), and elder maltreatment.
- *Community violence* occurs among individuals who are not related by family ties but who may know each other. It includes youth violence, bullying, assault, rape or sexual assault by acquaintances or strangers, and violence that occurs in institutional settings such as schools, workplaces, and prisons.

## The Burden of Interpersonal Violence

Information on the magnitude, nature, and consequences of interpersonal violence is critical for program and policy development.

### Deaths Resulting from Interpersonal Violence

WHO's Global Health Estimates (GHE) indicate that approximately 1.4 million people died in 2011 as a result of all three major forms of violence (table 5.1). Of those deaths, 35.3 percent, or 504,587, were due to interpersonal violence. GBD estimates find that 83 percent of all violence-related deaths occur in low- and middle-income countries (LMICs), and 91.4 percent of deaths due to interpersonal violence occur in LMICs. In 2011, the estimated rate of deaths due to interpersonal violence or homicide in LMICs was 8.0 per 100,000 people, compared with 3.3 per 100,000 in high-income countries (HICs).

Rates and patterns of violent death varied by region (figure 5.1). Homicide rates were highest in LMICs in Latin America and the Caribbean and in Sub-Saharan Africa, and lowest in East Asia and the Pacific and in some countries in northern Africa. In 2010, homicide was the leading cause of years of life lost in tropical and central Latin America, the fourth leading cause in southern Sub-Saharan Africa, and the eighth leading cause in the Caribbean and Eastern Europe (Lozano and others 2012). Poorer countries, especially those with large gaps between the rich and the poor, tend to have higher rates of homicide than wealthier countries (Butchart and Engstrom 2002).

Homicide rates differed markedly by age and gender (table 5.2). For infants and young children ages 0–4 years, the rates for male and female homicide victims are 2.9 and 3.2 per 100,000, respectively; this is the only age range in which the female rate exceeds the male rate. For the 15- to 29-year-old age group, rates for males were nearly five times those for females; for the remaining older age groups, rates for males were around two to four times those for females. Homicide rates for females doubled between the ages of 5–14 and 15–29 years and then decreased; however, the rates increased again in women ages 70 years and above. Rates for males increased almost tenfold for

**Table 5.1** Estimated Violence-Related Deaths, by Type and Income Level, 2011

| Category | Number | Rate per 100,000 people[a] | Proportion of total (percent) |
|---|---|---|---|
| **Suicide** | 803,900 | 11.4 | 56.3 |
| LMICs | 606,698 | 10.5 | 75.5 |
| HICs | 197,201 | 15.2 | 24.5 |
| **Interpersonal** | 504,587 | 7.1 | 35.3 |
| LMICs | 461,429 | 8.0 | 91.4 |
| HICs | 43,158 | 3.3 | 8.6 |
| **Conflict related** | 119,463 | 1.7 | 8.4 |
| LMICs | 117,131 | 2.0 | 98.0 |
| HICs | 2,332 | 0.2 | 2.0 |
| **All types of violence** | 1,427,949 | 20.2 | 100.0 |
| LMICs | 1,185,259 | 20.5 | 83.0 |
| HICs | 242,691 | 18.8 | 17.0 |

*Source:* WHO 2014.
*Note:* HIC = high-income country; LMIC = low- and middle-income country.
a. Age standardized.

**Figure 5.1** Homicide, Suicide, and Conflict-Related Fatality Rates, by Region, 2011

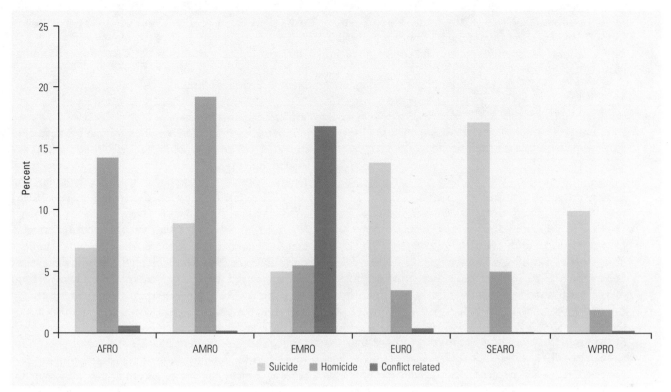

*Source:* WHO 2014.
*Note:* AFRO = African Regional Office; AMRO = Americas Regional Office; EMRO = Eastern Mediterranean Regional Office; EURO = European Regional Office; SEARO = South-East Asia Regional Office; WPRO = Western Pacific Regional Office.

**Table 5.2** Estimated Global Homicide and Suicide Rates, by Age and Gender, 2012

| Age | Homicides[a] | | Suicides[a] | |
|---|---|---|---|---|
| | **Males** | **Females** | **Males** | **Females** |
| 0–4 years | 2.9 | 3.2 | 0.0 | 0.0 |
| 5–14 years | 2.0 | 1.6 | 1.2 | 1.2 |
| 15–29 years | 19.4 | 3.7 | 15.6 | 11.3 |
| 30–49 years | 15.4 | 2.8 | 17.6 | 7.8 |
| 50–59 years | 9.6 | 2.0 | 21.7 | 9.3 |
| 60–69 years | 6.8 | 2.2 | 24.6 | 13.1 |
| 70+ years | 6.4 | 3.5 | 43.2 | 20.8 |
| Total | 11.4 | 2.8 | 14.5 | 8.2 |

*Source:* WHO 2014.
a. Per 100,000 people.

males 15 to 29, declined slightly for those 30 to 49, and then decreased with age. Overall, homicides resulted in the deaths of slightly more than 4 males for every 1 female. Recent estimates indicate that, globally, about one in seven homicides, and more than one in three homicides of females, are perpetrated by an intimate partner (Stöckl and others 2013).

Firearms are associated with a substantial number of homicides around the world. In 2010, an estimated 196,200 firearm homicides were committed in nonconflict situations (Lozano and others 2012). Firearm suicides are also an important problem in many countries, such as in the United States, where more than 60 percent of all firearm deaths are suicides. The number of suicides committed with firearms globally is unknown.

### Nonfatal Interpersonal Violence

In recent years, multiple reports using household survey data have characterized the prevalence of interpersonal violence.

### Violence against Children and Youth

Results from the United Nations Children's Fund (UNICEF) Multiple Indicator Cluster Surveys and Demographic and Health Surveys (DHS) in 33 countries found that an average of 76 percent of children ages 2 to 14 years had experienced some form of violent physical or psychological discipline during the previous month (UNICEF 2010). Surveys of violence against children in five countries (Haiti, Kenya, Swaziland, Tanzania, and Zimbabwe) found that the prevalence of sexual violence against girls was 26 percent to 38 percent, and against boys it was 9 percent to 21 percent (CDC, INURED, and the Comité de Coordination, 2014; Reza and others 2009; UNICEF, CDC, and KNBS 2012; UNICEF, CDC, and Muhimbili University 2012; ZIMSTAT, UNICEF, and CCORE 2012). The prevalence of physical violence against girls was 61 percent to 74 percent, and against boys it was 57 percent to 76 percent. The prevalence of emotional violence against girls was 24 percent to 35 percent, and against boys it was 27 percent to 39 percent. Regardless of the type of violence, perpetrators are largely known to the victim, and violence tends to occur in homes.

In meta-analyses of studies worldwide, 11 percent to 22 percent of girls and 4 percent to 19 percent of boys have experienced child sexual abuse, 14 percent to 55 percent have experienced child physical abuse, 12 percent to 22 percent have experienced physical neglect, and 13 percent to 25 percent have experienced emotional neglect (Stoltenborgh and others 2011; Stoltenborgh and others 2013a; Stoltenborgh, Bakermans-Kranenburg, and van Ijzendoorn 2013b). The hidden nature of child sexual and physical abuse is poignant. When compared with official reports, self-reported prevalence of child sexual abuse was more than 30 times the official rate (Stoltenborgh and others 2011); self-reported prevalence of physical abuse was more than 75 times the official rate (Stoltenborgh and others 2013a).

In youth ages 10 to 24 years, interpersonal violence was the fifth leading cause of disability-adjusted life years (DALYs) in 2004, accounting for 3.5 percent of all DALYs in this age group (Gore and others 2011). Unfortunately, few studies in LMICs examine the nonfatal consequences of youth violence. This research gap urgently requires filling.

### Violence against Women

The prevalence of violence against women has been documented by Demographic and Health Surveys conducted in Sub-Saharan African countries (Cameroon, Kenya, Malawi, Rwanda, Uganda, Zambia, and Zimbabwe) and by Reproductive Health Surveys (RHS) conducted in Central and South American countries (Ecuador, El Salvador, Guatemala, Jamaica, Nicaragua, and Paraguay). In Sub-Saharan Africa, the DHS findings show that the prevalence of physical violence against women ranged from 30 percent in Malawi to 60 percent in Uganda, with most perpetrators being intimate partners; the prevalence of sexual and emotional violence by intimate partners was also high (Borwankar, Diallo, and Sommerfelt 2008). For Central and South America, RHS findings show prevalence of physical violence against women ranging from 17 percent in Jamaica to 31 percent in Ecuador (Bott and others 2012). Global and regional estimates of violence against women demonstrate that 35 percent of women worldwide have experienced physical or sexual violence (or both), and most of that violence was perpetrated by intimate partners (WHO 2013).

### Violence against Elderly People

Elder maltreatment has been examined using population-based surveys and records from adult protective services. In surveys, 6.0 percent of older people reported significant abuse in the past month, and 5.6 percent of couples reported physical violence in their relationship in the past year (Cooper, Selwood, and Livingston 2008). In studies involving vulnerable elders in nursing or care homes, nearly 25 percent reported significant levels of psychological abuse. Rates of abuse reported to adult protective services are generally very low (1 percent to 2 percent).

### Consequences of Interpersonal Violence

The consequences of experiencing interpersonal violence are pervasive and enduring. Evidence confirms that exposure to violence increases the risks of injuries, infectious diseases, mental health problems, reproductive health problems, and noncommunicable diseases (NCDs).

## Cause of Physical or Psychological Injury

Although *injury* historically has been defined as an individual's experience of physical damage, the definition has been expanded to include damage that is psychological, with the potential to lead to maldevelopment or deprivation (Norton and Kobusingye 2013). Whether they are physical or psychological, violence-associated injuries commonly go unrecognized and range from self-limiting to severe. Physical injuries include lacerations, bruises, wounds, fractures, broken teeth, ocular damage, burns, internal injuries, and head injuries. Such injuries, especially those associated with highly lethal means such as firearms, may lead to disability, including brain damage, amputations, or paralysis (Buchanan 2013).

## Link to Infectious Diseases

The association between sexual and physical violence and infectious diseases, particularly sexually transmitted infections (STIs) and human immunodeficiency virus/acquired immune deficiency syndrome (HIV/AIDS) is well supported. Evidence across multiple studies demonstrates that these associations are strong, largely consistent, graded, and biologically plausible (Andersson, Cockcroft, and Shea 2008; Machtinger, Wilson, and others 2012). Emerging evidence suggests that violence may be associated with the transmission and progression of infections, increases in antiretroviral failure, high-risk behaviors, and an independently elevated risk of HIV/AIDS-associated death (Machtinger, Haberer, and others 2012). The importance of gender-based violence as a driver of HIV/AIDS in women is so prominent that multilateral donors such as UN Women view elimination of violence against women and children as a key strategy for advancing prevention (IOM 2013).

## Increased Risk of Reproductive Problems

Multiple studies document the reproductive consequences of exposure to child maltreatment and IPV. These forms of violence are associated with unintended pregnancy and teen pregnancy, and they influence victims' associated risk behaviors, such as multiple partners and early initiation of sexual activity (Hillis and others 2004). The intergenerational effects of exposure to childhood violence may be extreme. For example, violence against girls increases the future risk of adverse pregnancy outcomes, such as fetal death (Hillis and others 2004). In addition, mortality for young children is significantly higher when their mothers are victims of IPV (Silverman and others 2011). A review of studies from 17 LMICs shows that IPV leads to an increased prevalence of pregnancy-associated mental health disorders, such as postpartum depression, which impair a mother's ability to provide a safe, stable, and nurturing environment for her children (Fisher and others 2012).

## Increased Risk of Mental Health Problems

Globally, studies from high-, middle-, and low-income countries document that violent experiences lead to various mental health consequences. The WHO World Mental Health Survey findings from 21 countries demonstrate that violence during childhood is associated with mood, anxiety, behavior, and substance disorders, as well as suicidal behavior, during adulthood (Kessler and others 2010). Furthermore, studies involving 21,000 women from Asia, Sub-Saharan Africa, and Latin America and the Caribbean confirm strong associations between various forms of violence—including experiencing and witnessing IPV, nonpartner physical violence, and childhood sexual abuse—and suicides (Devries and others 2011).

## Increased Risk of Future Violence

Exposure to violence during childhood increases the risk of experiencing or perpetrating violence later in life. Experiencing child maltreatment and witnessing partner abuse have consistently been shown to increase the risk of becoming either a perpetrator or a victim of sexual violence and IPV as an adult (Capaldi and others 2012; Tharp and others 2012). This intergenerational effect of childhood violence increases the risk that men will become perpetrators and that women will become victims. An assessment of Reproductive Health Surveys in six countries in the Americas found that the proportion of women reporting IPV was more than twice as high for those who experienced sexual or physical abuse in childhood as for those who did not (Bott and others 2012).

## Increased Risk to Special Populations

Although most reports addressing interpersonal violence focus on the general population, some recent studies have addressed infectious, reproductive, and mental health consequences of violence for children outside of family care, including street children, trafficked children, those affected by crises and armed conflict, and those living in institutions such as orphanages. For street children, studies from LMICs report HIV/AIDS seroprevalences of 40 percent and higher among those who experienced childhood violence, in contrast to general population prevalences of 1 percent (Kissin and others 2007; Robbins and others 2010). Associations between violence and elevated risks of HIV/AIDS and STIs, pregnancy, psychiatric pathology, depression, anxiety, posttraumatic stress disorder, and suicide have been reported among victims of sex trafficking and armed conflict, as well as among those in orphanages (Reed and others 2012; Silverman and others 2009; Zapata and others 2011, 2013).

### Increased Risk of NCDs

Violence during childhood is also associated with non-communicable diseases (NCDs) that often only become evident decades later. Exposure to childhood violence leads to consistent and graded increases in the four NCDs that accounted for nearly 60 percent of the 53 million deaths globally in 2010—cardiovascular disease, cancer, chronic lung disease, and diabetes (Lozano and others 2012; Norman and others 2012). In both HICs and LMICs, childhood violence has been associated with major risk factors for these diseases, including alcohol abuse, tobacco use, physical inactivity, and obesity (Anda and others 2010). Beyond health effects, serious psychosocial effects of childhood violence that are observed decades later include severe problems with finances, family, jobs, anger, and stress (Hillis and others 2004).

### Basic Science Evidence

The biological underpinnings of the empirical associations between exposure to violence and subsequent major causes of mortality in adulthood have been established through basic science. Recent evidence demonstrates that traumatic stress, such as that associated with violence in childhood, impairs brain architecture (both structure and function), immune status, metabolic systems, and cellular inflammatory responses (Anda and others 2010). It is clear that early exposure to toxic stress in childhood confers lasting damage at the most basic levels of the nervous, endocrine, and immune systems, and that such exposures can alter the physical structure of DNA (epigenetic effects) (Danese and McEwen 2012). Important research summarizing the effects of early childhood experiences suggests that those multifaceted gene-environment interactions that cause negative health consequences after exposure to chronic stress also appear to confer positive health consequences after exposure to early environments that are engaging and nurturing (Heim and Binder 2012). Epidemiologic research complements these findings, demonstrating that early nurturing in the home leads to sustained positive economic and psychosocial consequences up to five decades later (Hillis and others 2010).

## ECONOMIC BURDEN OF INTERPERSONAL VIOLENCE

Given the high prevalence of interpersonal violence and its extensive consequences, the associated economic impact is substantial. However, no comprehensive framework for estimating the total economic burden of violence exists.

### Framework for Estimating the Costs of Violence

Challenges in creating such a framework include "weaknesses in the knowledge base both in economic costing and in violence prevention, difficulty in creating a universal algorithm for diverse settings, and disagreements in types of costs to include" (IOM and NRC 2012, 7). Although no methodology exists to enumerate the full impact of violence, costs that are commonly considered include *direct costs*, which arise proximal to the violent event, and *indirect costs*, which result from consequences, externalities, or lost opportunities (IOM and NRC 2012). In general, direct costs typically include those associated with medical care, psychological care, property damage, policing, incarceration, and residential treatment; indirect costs are those commonly associated with lost wages and decreased productivity. Current approaches that largely confine estimates of health-related costs to proximal consequences lead to marked underestimates because they fail to incorporate costs of HIV/AIDS, chronic diseases, and other conditions attributable to violence.

A comprehensive approach to estimating costs will strengthen global efforts to elevate the urgency of violence prevention (WHO 2004). Comparisons across countries of the costs of interpersonal violence are complicated by variations in definitions, types of costs, discount rates, comparable data, and methodology. Reports vary greatly in the types of costs they include, whether such costs are disaggregated, and whether they include costs associated with both victimization and perpetration. Although the absolute costs appear to be higher in HICs than LMICs, the relative costs of violence as a proportion of government spending are often high in both types of economies (table 5.3).

Reports of direct and indirect societal costs of interpersonal violence in general vary widely, ranging from US$75.2 million (2013 dollars) for homicide in New Zealand in 1992 to US$579.4 billion (2013 dollars) for homicide, child abuse, sexual and other assault, and robbery in the United States in 1993 (Fanslow and others 1997; Miller, Cohen, and Wiersema 1996). Estimates of the costs of both interpersonal and collective violence in the Americas show that direct and indirect economic costs ranged from 5.1 percent of 1997 gross domestic product (GDP) in Peru to 24.9 percent of 1997 GDP in El Salvador (Buvinic, Morrison, and Shifter 1999). Other estimates found that interpersonal violence accounted for 4.0 percent of GDP in Jamaica in 2006, 1.2 percent in Brazil in 2004, and 0.4 percent in Thailand in 2005 (Butchart and others 2008; Ward and others 2009).

Reports that estimate the national costs of child maltreatment are largely from HICs, whereas those that address IPV also include LMICs. In HICs, for example,

**Table 5.3** Summary of Costs of Interpersonal Violence, by Types of Violence

| Study | Country | Costs included (time frame) | Discount rate | Total costs (per year) | Costs converted to 2013 U.S. dollars* | Violence-associated costs as percentage of national health expenditures | Violence-associated costs as percentage of GDP |
|---|---|---|---|---|---|---|---|
| *Interpersonal violence in general* | | | | | | | |
| Miller, Cohen, and Wiersema 1996 | United States | Victim costs: medical and mental health care, victim services, productivity and quality of life losses (1993) (lifetime) | n.a. | US$358.0 billion for homicide, child abuse, sexual and other assault, and robbery (1993) | US$577.2 billion | n.a. | n.a. |
| Bellis and others 2012 | England and Wales | For homicide, wounding, assault, and sexual assault: criminal justice system, health and victim services, foregone output, and physical and emotional costs (lifetime) | n.a. | £29.9 billion (2008–09) | US$53.8 billion | n.a. | n.a. |
| Mayhew 2003 | Australia | For homicide, assault, and sexual assault: medical costs, lost wages, intangible costs such as pain, suffering, and reduced quality of life (annual) | n.a. | $A2.6 billion (2001) | US$1.8 billion | n.a. | n.a. |
| Fanslow and others 1997 | New Zealand | Lost earnings, legal fees, incarceration, and policing costs associated with homicide (annual) | n.a. | $NZ83.0 million, averaging $NZ1 million per homicide (1992) | US$74.9 million, averaging US$900 thousand per homicide | n.a. | n.a. |
| Buvinic, Morrison, and Shifter 1999 | Peru | For both interpersonal violence and collective violence: health impacts; private and public expenditures on police and security services; citizens' willingness to pay to live without violence; and value of goods lost, ransoms, and bribes (annual) | n.a. | n.a. | n.a. | n.a. | 5.1 percentage of 1997 GDP |
| Buvinic, Morrison, and Shifter 1999 | Brazil | For both interpersonal violence and collective violence: health impacts; private and public expenditures on police and security services; citizens' willingness to pay to live without violence; and value of goods lost, ransoms, and bribes (annual) | n.a. | n.a. | n.a. | n.a. | 10.5 percentage of 1997 GDP |
| Buvinic, Morrison, and Shifter 1999 | Venezuela, RB | For both interpersonal violence and collective violence: health impacts; private and public expenditures on police and security services; citizens' willingness to pay to live without violence; and value of goods lost, ransoms, and bribes (annual) | n.a. | n.a. | n.a. | n.a. | 11.8 percentage of 1997 GDP |

*table continues next page*

**Table 5.3** Summary of Costs of Interpersonal Violence, by Types of Violence (continued)

| Study | Country | Costs included (time frame) | Discount rate | Total costs (per year) | Costs converted to 2013 U.S. dollars* | Violence-associated costs as percentage of national health expenditures | Violence-associated costs as percentage of GDP |
|---|---|---|---|---|---|---|---|
| Buvinic, Morrison, and Shifter 1999 | Mexico | For both interpersonal violence and collective violence: health impacts; private and public expenditures on police and security services; citizens' willingness to pay to live without violence; and value of goods lost, ransoms, and bribes (annual) | n.a. | n.a. | n.a. | n.a. | 12.3 percentage of 1997 GDP |
| Buvinic, Morrison, and Shifter 1999 | Colombia | For both interpersonal violence and collective violence: health impacts; private and public expenditures on police and security services; citizens' willingness to pay to live without violence; and value of goods lost, ransoms, and bribes (annual) | n.a. | n.a. | n.a. | n.a. | 24.7 percentage of 1997 GDP |
| Buvinic, Morrison, and Shifter 1999 | El Salvador | For both interpersonal violence and collective violence: health impacts; private and public expenditures on police and security services; citizens' willingness to pay to live without violence; and value of goods lost, ransoms, and bribes (annual) | n.a. | n.a. | n.a. | n.a. | 24.9 percentage of 1997 GDP |
| Butchart and others 2008 | Brazil | Lifetime medical and productivity losses associated with self-directed and interpersonal violence (lifetime) | 3 percent | R$16.1 billion (2004) | US$6.4 billion | 0.4 percent | 1.2 percentage of 2004 GDP |
| Butchart and others 2008 | Jamaica | Lifetime medical and productivity losses associated with self-directed and interpersonal violence (lifetime) | 3 percent | J$29.6 billion (2006) | US$530.0 million | 12.0 percent | 4.0 percentage of 2006 GDP |
| Butchart and others 2008 | Thailand | Lifetime medical and productivity losses associated with self-directed and interpersonal violence (lifetime) | 3 percent | B15.7 billion (2005) | US$453.3 million | 4.0 percent | 0.4 percentage of 2005 GDP |
| *Child maltreatment* | | | | | | | |
| Fang and others 2012 | United States | Childhood health care, adult medical, lost productivity, child welfare, criminal justice, and special education costs (lifetime) | 3 percent | • US$124.0 billion lifetime costs from new cases of fatal and nonfatal child maltreatment (2010) | US$132.5 billion | n.a. | n.a. |

*table continues next page*

**Table 5.3** Summary of Costs of Interpersonal Violence, by Types of Violence (continued)

| Study | Country | Costs included (time frame) | Discount rate | Total costs (per year) | Costs converted to 2013 U.S. dollars* | Violence-associated costs as percentage of national health expenditures | Violence-associated costs as percentage of GDP |
|---|---|---|---|---|---|---|---|
| | | | | • US$210,012 average lifetime costs per victim of nonfatal child maltreatment<br>• US$1,272,900 average lifetime costs per death (2010 dollars) | | | |
| Habetha and others 2012 | Germany | Costs associated with health care, social, and educational services; foster care; productivity losses (lifetime) | n.a. | €11.1 billion (2008) | US$9.7 billion | n.a. | n.a. |
| Mendonca, Alves, and Cabral Filho 2002 | Recife, Brazil | Hospital costs (annual) | n.a. | n.a. | n.a. | Violence against children and adolescents accounted for 65.1 percent of hospital admissions and 77.9 percent of all hospital costs in the state of Pernambuco (1999) | n.a. |
| *Intimate partner violence* | | | | | | | |
| CDC 2003 | United States | Medical and mental health care costs; lost productivity (annual) | n.a. | US$5.8 billion (1995) | US$8.9 billion | n.a. | n.a. |
| Day 1995 | Canada | Costs of health care, policing, legal fees, incarceration, lost earnings, and psychological trauma (lifetime) | n.a. | Can$1.2 billion (1992) | US$1.7 billion | n.a. | n.a. |
| Morrison and Orlando 1999 | Chile | Lost productive capacity of abused women (annual) | n.a. | Ch$1.6 billion (1996) | US$5.8 million | n.a. | 2.0 percentage of 1996 GDP |
| Morrison and Orlando 1999 | Nicaragua | Lost productive capacity of abused women (annual) | n.a. | C$29.5 million (1996) | US$5.2 million | n.a. | 1.6 percentage of 1996 GDP |

*table continues next page*

**Table 5.3** Summary of Costs of Interpersonal Violence, by Types of Violence (continued)

| Study | Country | Costs included (time frame) | Discount rate | Total costs (per year) | Costs converted to 2013 U.S. dollars* | Violence-associated costs as percentage of national health expenditures | Violence-associated costs as percentage of GDP |
|---|---|---|---|---|---|---|---|
| International Center for Research on Women 2009 | Bangladesh | Costs of health care, justice, and lost productivity (annual) | n.a. | n.a. | n.a. | n.a. | 4.5 percentage of 2007 per capita gross national income |
| International Center for Research on Women 2009 | Morocco | Costs of health care, justice, and lost productivity (annual) | n.a. | n.a. | n.a. | n.a. | 22.0 percentage of 2007 per capita gross national income |
| International Center for Research on Women 2009 | Uganda | Costs of health care, justice, and lost productivity (annual) | n.a. | n.a. | n.a. | n.a. | 4.0 percentage of 2007 per capita gross national income |
| Roldós and Corso 2013 | Ecuador | Costs of medical and legal services, and productivity losses (annual) | n.a. | US$109.0 million (2012) | US$110.6 million | n.a. | n.a. |
| *Youth violence* | | | | | | | |
| Miller, Fisher, and Cohen 2001 | Pennsylvania, United States | Total victim costs, including quality of life and productivity losses of juvenile violence (lifetime) | 2.5 percent | US$5.4 billion (1993) | US$8.7 billion | n.a. | n.a. |

*Note:* * Conversions to 2013 U.S. dollars using Department of Labor Consumer Price Index Inflation Calculator; GDP = gross domestic product; n.a. = not applicable.

Fang and others (2012) estimated the U.S. total lifetime economic burden resulting from new cases of child maltreatment in 2008 to be US$135 billion (2013 dollars); an analysis using similar methods showed total costs of US$19.0 billion (2013 dollars) in Germany (Habetha and others 2012). HIC estimates of the annual direct and indirect costs of IPV against women exceeded US$8.9 billion in the United States and US$1.7 billion (all 2013 dollars) in Canada (CDC 2003; Day 1995). For LMICs, costs of the lost productive capacity of abused women as a percentage of GDP were equivalent to 2.0 percent in Chile, 1.6 percent in Nicaragua, and 22.0 percent in Morocco (table 5.3) (ICRW 2009; Morrison and Orlando 1999). Although adolescents and young adults commit a disproportionate share of all violence and, therefore, account for a high proportion of its cost, youth violence has been the subject of few economic cost studies (WHO 2004).

## Risk and Protective Factors for Violence

Violence results from the interplay of risk factors and protective factors. In table 5.4 these risk factors are organized by levels of the ecological model, which examines the relationship between individual and contextual factors and considers violence as the product of these

**Table 5.4** Risk for Perpetrating Violence

| Level of the ecological model | Risk factors |
|---|---|
| Individual | • Early exposure to violence and adverse events, including child maltreatment and intimate partner violence |
| | • Male gender |
| | • Youth |
| | • Neuropsychological deficits, including attention-deficit hyperactivity disorder and learning disabilities |
| | • Personality disorders |
| | • Alcohol and substance misuse |
| | • History of violence |
| Household | • Intimate partner violence |
| | • Household members with criminal records |
| | • Harsh, cold, or inconsistent parenting |
| | • Low socioeconomic status |
| Peer group | • Association with others who use and endorse the use of violence |
| Community | • High residential mobility |
| | • High unemployment |
| | • High population density |
| | • Poverty |
| | • Drug trade |
| | • Inadequate victim care services |
| Societal | • Rapid social change |
| | • Economic inequality |
| | • Gender inequality |
| | • Policies that sustain or increase inequalities |
| | • Patriarchal norms that prioritize men's power over women and adults' power over children |
| | • Societal norms that support violence |
| | • Poor rule of law |
| | • Weak criminal justice system |
| | • Availability of lethal means, for example, firearms |

*Source:* Krug and others 2002.

multiple levels of influence on behavior (Dahlberg and Krug 2001). Identifying these factors is important, because increasing protection and decreasing risk underlie effective prevention. Several cross-cutting risk factors for perpetrating violence are described in table 5.4. Many of these factors also increase an individual's likelihood of being a victim; for example, young men ages 15 to 44 are most likely to be both victims and perpetrators in any country. Additional factors, such as having a disability (Hughes and others 2012), increase the risk of becoming a victim but not a perpetrator.

The recognition that different types of interpersonal violence share common risk factors, often occur in combination, and may be causal factors for one other is important (Reza, Mercy, and Krug 2001). For example, child maltreatment is a risk factor for youth violence and IPV. Three cross-cutting risk factors bear particular mention because they represent factors that, if successfully addressed by prevention initiatives, could have substantial impact: parenting, substance abuse (particularly alcohol), and the availability of lethal means.

Harsh, cold, and inconsistent parenting has been linked to youth violence (van der Merwe, Dawes, and Ward 2012), IPV (Ireland and Smith 2009), and the increased risk of abusing one's own children (Thornberry, Knight, and Lovegrove 2012). In contrast, children who receive warm, consistent parenting tend to have better outcomes (Eisenberg and others 2005; Smith, Landry, and Swank 2010).

Substance abuse, and particularly alcohol abuse, is implicated in a number of ways in both victimization and perpetration of violence (Monteiro 2007; WHO 2006). Maternal use of alcohol during pregnancy can result in fetal alcohol spectrum disorders, with their attendant executive functioning disorders (Mattson and others 2013), which increase the risk of aggression in affected children. Alcohol use also reduces self-control and the ability to process information (Giancola 2000), making it more likely both that drinkers will use violence in response to perceived threats and that they will be vulnerable to victimization (Klosterman and Fals-Stewart 2006). Alcohol misuse has been implicated across all forms of violence, including perpetration of child maltreatment (Gilbert and others 2009) and elder abuse (Lachs and Pillemer 2004), and in both victimization and perpetration of youth violence (van der Merwe, Dawes, and Ward 2012) and IPV (Jewkes 2002).

Access to lethal means of perpetrating interpersonal violence, such as firearms and sharp objects, contributes substantially to the likelihood that such violence will result in death or serious injury (Beaman and others 2000). In the United States, the presence of a firearm in the home is associated with an increased risk of homicides, especially among women (Miller, Azrael, and Hemenway 2013). The same authors report that in cross-national comparisons of HICs, higher homicide rates have been associated with greater access to firearms.

## INTERVENTIONS AND THEIR APPLICABILITY TO LOW- AND MIDDLE-INCOME COUNTRIES

Public health interventions aim to prevent violence from occurring. Prevention efforts addressing common underlying risk factors have the potential to decrease several different forms of violence simultaneously. Such efforts include two broad groups of interventions:

- The first group targets documented risk and protective factors (for example, enhancing support for parents, reducing the availability and abuse of alcohol, and reducing access to lethal means) in well-defined target groups, such as adolescents. This group includes specific violence prevention programs implemented at the community, state and provincial, and national levels.
- The second group consists of policies and programs that address the social determinants of violence, including efforts to improve the conditions of daily life and to promote more equitable distribution of power, money, and resources.

Policy makers understand that a single intervention or policy will not solve the whole problem, nor will one sector solve it alone; as with automobile safety, the solutions will be incremental and will require multisectoral collaboration among policy makers in criminal justice, public health, education, and other areas.

The design, targeting, monitoring, and evaluation of both groups of interventions are enabled by the availability of timely and reliable surveillance information about outcomes of interest, including homicides, nonfatal injuries treated in emergency departments, and self-reported violence recorded through surveys. Indeed, one program that has significantly reduced violence-related injuries in Cardiff, Wales, is based on the systematic sharing of anonymous data from hospital emergency rooms and the police to better identify high-risk locations for violence (Florence and others 2013). Such locations become the focus of situation-specific interventions to reduce risks, for example, by increasing the presence of police patrols at high-risk times where alcohol is served, altering practices around the serving of alcohol (such as the mandatory use of plastic barware), and instituting crowd control at public transportation stops.

## Specific Violence Prevention Programs

Most of the scientific evidence for specific prevention programs to date is from HICs. Although conditions differ in LMICs, table 5.5 shows seven categories of violence prevention programs in HICs that are scientifically credible, along with the types of violence they prevent and considerations for their applicability in LMICs.

### Developing Safe, Stable, and Nurturing Relationships between Parents or Caregivers and Children

Interventions that support the development of safe, stable, and nurturing relationships between parents or caregivers and children in their early years can prevent child maltreatment and reduce childhood aggression (Bilukha and others 2005; Kaminski and others 2008). Emerging evidence suggests that such relationships can also reduce violence in adolescence and early adulthood; theoretical grounds exist for assuming they decrease IPV and self-directed violence in later life (Caldera and others 2007; Olds and others 1998; Walker and others 2011). In addition, these relationships offer the potential to prevent problem behaviors, such as substance misuse, eating disorders, and unsafe sex, which are important risk factors for NCDs; STIs, including HIV/AIDS; and unintentional injuries.

Although most evidence for the effectiveness of parenting programs comes from HICs (Knerr, Gardner, and Cluver 2013; Mikton and Butchart 2009), several initiatives to evaluate such programs in LMICs have recently been established, for example, the Children and Violence Evaluation Challenge Fund. In addition, parenting programs are quite widely implemented in LMICs to support early child development, raising the possibility that violence prevention components could be integrated into those programs.

### Developing Life Skills in Children and Adolescents

Social development programs to build social, emotional, and behavioral competencies can prevent violence (Hahn and others 2007; Hawkins and others 1999; Klevens and others 2009). Preschool enrichment programs that provide children with academic and social skills at an early age appear promising (Baker-Henningham and others 2012; Nelson, Westhues, and MacLeod 2003). However, outcomes vary greatly across programs, and relatively few programs have been evaluated for their effects on violence (Durlak, Weissberg, and Pachan 2010).

School-based programs can address gender norms and attitudes with the aim of preventing dating violence. The Safe Dates program in the United States (Foshee and others 2005) and the Youth Relationship Project in Canada (Wolfe and others 2009) are evidence-based approaches that could be adapted to LMICs. Life skills and social development training programs are popular in LMICs. Some include evaluations of effectiveness (for example, PREPARE in South Africa). However, because programs are typically delivered in schools, they depend on the readiness of the educational system to implement the program and reinforce its effects. Oversight and management structures must be in place before such programs are implemented.

### Reducing the Availability and Harmful Use of Alcohol

Alcohol availability can be regulated by restricting the hours of sale and reducing the number of alcohol retail outlets (Cohen 2007; Duailibi and others 2007; Nemtsov 1998). Reduced hours of sales have been associated with reduced violence, and higher outlet densities have been associated with higher levels of violence. Empirical evidence has shown that higher prices for alcohol can decrease consumption and reduce mortality attributed to alcohol (Zhao and others 2013). Moreover, economic modeling suggests that price increases can reduce violence (Markowitz and Grossman 1998, 2000). Brief interventions and longer-term treatment for problem drinkers have been shown to reduce child maltreatment and IPV (Dinh-Zarr and others 2004). Interventions in and around drinking establishments that target crowding, management practice, physical design, staff training, and access to late night transportation also show promise in reducing violence (Bellis and Hughes 2008; Graham and Homel 2008).

Although most evidence for the effectiveness of interventions in preventing violence comes from HICs, several success stories come from LMICs, including the reduced trading hours in Brazil (Duailibi and others 2007). Given that LMICs show some of the greatest increases in alcohol consumption, more outcome evaluations of strategies to address alcohol-related violence in these settings are urgently needed. Two areas that should be explored are the effectiveness of (1) minimum drinking-age laws and (2) efforts to regulate the marketing of alcohol. However, in many LMICs, a large proportion of alcohol consumed is produced at home. In such settings, establishing policies to regulate alcohol production and sale is an important prerequisite for effective prevention (WHO and Liverpool John Moores University 2006). As WHO Member States, all LMICs are committed to implementing the global plan of action on alcohol and health (WHO 2010). That plan includes the interventions described.

**Table 5.5** Overview of Violence Prevention Strategies Showing Evidence for Effectiveness and Applicability in Low- and Middle-Income Countries

| Intervention | Type of violence | | | | | LMIC applicability |
|---|---|---|---|---|---|---|
| | Child maltreatment | Intimate partner violence | Sexual violence | Youth violence | Elder abuse | |
| *Developing safe, stable, and nurturing relationships between children and their parents and caregivers* | | | | | | |
| Parent training, including home visitation by nurses | ● | | | ○ | | These programs are likely to be highly applicable in LMICs. Few such programs in LMICs have been evaluated for violence prevention outcomes; several such studies are underway. Programs are resource-intensive and need to be adapted to the requirements of and assets available in LMICs. |
| Parent-child programs | ○ | | | ○ | | |
| *Developing life skills in children and adolescents* | | | | | | |
| Preschool enrichment programs | | | | ○ | | Most programs are delivered in schools and depend on the school system to deliver the program and reinforce its effects. Oversight and management structures must be in place before such programs are implemented. |
| Social development programs | | | | ● | | |
| School-based programs to address gender norms and attitudes | | ● | ○ | | | |
| *Reducing the availability and harmful use of alcohol* | | | | | | |
| Regulation of alcohol sales | | | ○ | ○ | | Alcohol is an established risk factor for all types of violence. Some LMICs have seen rapid increases in alcohol consumption. Strategies to address alcohol may eventually be relevant to LMICs where alcohol is currently not available. |
| Increases in alcohol prices | | | ○ | | | |
| Interventions for problem drinkers | | ● | | | | |
| Well-managed and well-designed drinking environments | | | | | | |
| *Reducing access to lethal means* | | | | | | |
| Restrictive firearm licensing and purchase policies | | | | ○ | | There is limited evidence of the effectiveness of programs and policies in reducing access to lethal means of perpetrating violence in LMICs. Emerging evidence from LMICs that have changed policies will shed light on the effectiveness of strategies for firearm injury prevention. |
| Enforced bans on carrying firearms in public | | | | ○ | | |
| *Promoting gender equality to prevent violence against women* | | | | | | |
| Microfinance combined with gender equity training | | ○ | | | | Strong evidence for the effectiveness of such programs is limited to outcome evaluation studies in low-resource, rural communities in South Africa. Several outcome evaluation studies of similar programs are underway in other LMICs. |
| Life skills interventions | | ○ | | | | |

*table continues next page*

**Table 5.5** Overview of Violence Prevention Strategies Showing Evidence for Effectiveness and Applicability in Low- and Middle-Income Countries (continued)

| Intervention | Type of violence | | | | | | LMIC applicability |
|---|---|---|---|---|---|---|---|
| | Child maltreatment | Intimate partner violence | Sexual violence | Youth violence | Elder abuse | | |
| *Changing cultural and social norms that support violence* | | | | | | | |
| Social marketing to modify social norms | | ○ | ○ | | | | Programs that aim to change social norms supportive of violence through standalone mass-media campaigns are popular in LMICs. However, there is no evidence that such standalone programs are effective. They should be delivered in combination with other programs that address risk and protective factors more directly. |
| *Instituting victim identification, care, and support programs* | | | | | | | |
| Screening and referral | | ○ | | | | | Stark differences exist in access to services (for example, between high- and low-income groups, and between urban and rural settings). The shortage of highly trained, well-supervised staff has been a barrier to the implementation of services in LMICs. However, in the psychosocial arena, new approaches using community health workers are promising. |
| Advocacy support programs | | ● | | | | | |
| Psychosocial interventions | | | ○ | | | | |
| Protection orders | | ○ | | | | | |

*Source:* WHO 2009.
*Note:* LMICs = low- and middle-income countries; ● = well supported by evidence (multiple randomized controlled trials with different populations); ○ = emerging evidence.

### Reducing Access to Lethal Means

Evidence from North America is the primary basis of two systematic reviews and one meta-analysis that summarize the effects of various strategies to prevent firearm-related violence. One systematic review (Hahn and others 2005) concluded that the evidence is insufficient to determine whether firearm laws have any effect on violence. Such laws include bans on specified firearms or ammunition, restrictions on the acquisition of firearms, waiting periods for acquisition, firearms registration, licensing of owners, "shall issue" carry laws that allow people who pass background checks to carry concealed weapons, child access prevention laws, and zero tolerance laws for firearms in schools. Another systematic review (Koper and Mayo-Wilson 2009) found that directed police patrols focusing on illegal gun carrying can prevent gun crimes (including murders, shootings, robberies in which guns are used, and armed assaults). One meta-analysis (Makarios and Pratt 2012) suggests that bans on the sale of firearms had small effects, and law enforcement strategies had moderate effects in reducing gun violence.

More recent evidence suggests that the use of street outreach workers to mediate conflicts and provide social support, such as job referrals and access to social services in the U.S. context, may be effective in reducing youth homicides and firearm offenses (Webster and others 2012). In addition, studies from Brazil and South Africa have found that stricter licensing and reduced circulation of firearms accounted for significant decreases in firearm-related injuries (Marinho de Souza and others 2007; Matzopoulos, Thompson, and Myers 2014). These reports therefore suggest, from a limited evidence base, that some strategies addressing access to firearms show promise, but additional research is needed.

Public health can make a critical contribution to preventing firearm injuries and deaths by collecting data and evidence. A range of strategies exists for reducing firearm-related violence, but further research and evidence are needed to assess their effectiveness (IOM and NRC 2013). Strategies identified by the Institute of Medicine (IOM) and others as being in particular need of additional research include the following:

- Increasing efforts to control access to firearms by individuals at risk of harming themselves or others (for example, the safe storage of guns, waiting periods, and background checks)
- Changing how firearms are used (for example, where firearms may be carried and provision of safety education)
- Reducing the lethality of guns (for example, designing firearms to make them safer and addressing magazine size).
- Evaluating strategies to reduce the use of military firearms in the aftermath of war or conflict, including strategies to disarm former combatants, disband armed groups, and reintegrate former combatants into civilian society.

Sound data and evidence on firearm injuries are needed to determine what programs and policies actually work in preventing these injuries while preserving the rights of legitimate gun owners.

### Promoting Gender Equality to Prevent Violence against Women

Several outcome evaluation studies demonstrate the effectiveness of multisector interventions to prevent violence against women by promoting gender equality. The Intervention with Microfinance and Gender Equity in South Africa, which combines microloans and gender equity training, reduced rates of self-reported violence by more than 50 percent (Pronyk and others 2006). The Stepping Stones program implemented in Asia and Sub-Saharan Africa is a life skills training program that addresses gender-based violence, relationship skills, assertiveness training, and communication about HIV/AIDS and has shown promising results (Jewkes and others 2008; Paine and others 2002). The popularity of microfinance and conditional cash transfer programs in LMICs, into which violence prevention objectives could be integrated, further underscores their applicability.

### Changing Cultural and Societal Norms That Support Violence

Interventions that challenge cultural and social norms supporting violence are widely used, and their relatively low cost makes them a popular option. Such interventions are often restricted to standalone mass-media campaigns that are intended to raise awareness about the harmful effects of violence, thereby reducing the likelihood of future acts of violence. No evidence shows that such campaigns are effective; however, some evidence suggests that programs combining awareness-raising efforts with other mechanisms to change norms (for example, social development and life skills training and legislation) are effective. In South Africa, the Soul City initiative used television (through a soap opera series), radio, and nationally distributed information booklets to raise awareness of new IPV laws. The intervention increased the proportion of people who saw such violence as unacceptable (Usdin and others 2005).

**Implementing Victim Identification, Care, and Support Programs**

Interventions to identify victims of interpersonal violence and to provide effective care and support are critical for protecting health and breaking cycles of violence from one generation to the next. Evidence of effectiveness is emerging in several areas:

- Screening tools to identify victims of IPV and refer them to appropriate services (Ramsay and others 2002)
- Psychosocial interventions, such as trauma-focused cognitive behavioral therapy, to reduce mental health problems associated with violence (Bass and others 2013; Kornør and others 2008)
- Protection orders, which prohibit perpetrators of IPV from contacting victims (Holt and others 2003), to reduce repeat victimization.

Several trials have shown that advocacy support programs—which offer services such as counseling, safety planning, and referral—increase victims' safety behaviors and reduce the risk of further harm (McFarlane and others 2006).

**Policies and Programs to Address the Social Determinants of Violence**

Violence is strongly associated with social determinants, such as employment, income equity, rapid social change, and access to education. The expectation that policies and programs can prevent violence by addressing social determinants derives from ecological studies that use cross-sectional and time-series methods to document associations between social determinants and violence. Comprehensive violence prevention strategies should do more than just address the risk factors targeted by the specific programs; such strategies should be integrated with policies directed at the inequities that fuel violence. This integration is particularly important in LMICs, where daily living conditions can undermine the opportunities for positive early child development. For example, the context can include economic and social policies that exacerbate gaps between rich and poor and between men and women.

## ECONOMIC EVALUATION OF INTERVENTIONS

Economic evaluation provides a way to compare gains resulting from an intervention, which has its own costs and risks. Given the high prevalence of interpersonal violence and its direct and indirect costs, identifying effective, low-cost interventions to reduce violence is an urgent priority. However, the same challenges that complicate measuring the costs of violence also complicate measuring the benefits associated with its prevention (Barnett 1993; WHO 2004). Despite widely varying methodologies, most studies show that behavioral, legal, and regulatory interventions are cost-effective (WHO 2004). Evidence addressing specific types of violence, largely from HICs, has identified a variety of cost-effective interventions to prevent child maltreatment, IPV, and youth violence (table 5.6). Despite the disproportionate effects of violence in LMICs, economic evaluations of interventions are rare; therefore, systematic research to measure the economic benefits of violence prevention efforts in LMICs would fill a critical gap.

## IMPLEMENTATION OF PREVENTION STRATEGIES

The gap between the science and the practice of violence prevention is growing. Although numerous effective programs, policies, and innovations have been identified, they are unlikely to have a substantial public health impact unless they are widely disseminated, implemented with quality and scale, and sustained over the long term (Rhoades, Bumbarger, and Moore 2012). Moreover, the benefits of their implementation must also be monitored. The infrastructure needed to support the dissemination, scaling up, and sustenance of effective programs and policies is slowly emerging.

Given the rapid expansion of and increasing demand for evidence-based violence prevention innovations, especially in LMICs, building an infrastructure that can more effectively move innovations from research to action is increasingly important. That infrastructure requires attention to three interrelated sets of functions and activities that should be coordinated across global, country, and local levels: prevention synthesis and translation, prevention support, and prevention delivery (Wandersman and others 2008).

**Prevention Synthesis and Translation**

The greater the extent to which innovations for violence prevention are accessible (both from informational and financial perspectives), user-friendly, and clearly communicated, the more likely it is that effective approaches will be successfully disseminated and implemented (Clancy and Cronin 2005). The seven-part series on *Violence Prevention: The Evidence* is an example of an effort to synthesize and translate the scientific evidence into easily understandable and accessible

**Table 5.6** Summary of Economic Evaluations of Interventions to Prevent Interpersonal Violence, by Type of Violence

| Type of violence | Intervention type | Intervention details | Cost-effectiveness |
|---|---|---|---|
| Child maltreatment | Home visiting | Nurse-family partnerships provide home visiting for low-income mothers to improve prenatal health-related behaviors, provide more responsible and competent care of infants and toddlers, and improve parents' economic self-sufficiency (Lee and others 2012). Location: United States | Net benefit (in 2011 dollars) for each program participant was US$13,181 (US$13,617 in 2013 dollars); benefit-to-cost ratio was US$2.37 for every US$1.00 spent (US$2.46 in 2013 dollars). |
| | Parent-child interaction therapy | Empirical treatment for conduct disorders is based on behavioral interventions to improve parent-child interaction (Lee and others 2012). Location: United States | Net benefit (in 2011 dollars) for each program participant was US$5,617 (US$5,820 in 2013 dollars); benefit-to-cost ratio was US$4.62 for every $1.00 spent (US$4.79 in 2013 dollars). |
| | Educational and family support | The Child-Parent Center Program is a program for economically disadvantaged children and parents that provides a stable early learning environment and educational and support services for parents (Temple and Reynolds 2007). Location: Chicago, Illinois | Range of benefit-to-cost ratio (in 2002 dollars) was US$5.98 (US$7.76 in 2013 dollars) to US$10.15 (US$13.18 in 2013 dollars) for every US$1.00 spent. |
| Intimate partner violence (IPV) | Microfinance with gender and human immunodeficiency virus/acquired immune deficiency syndrome (HIV/AIDS) training | The Intervention with Microfinance for AIDS and Gender Equity (IMAGE) provides a combination of microfinance with gender and HIV/AIDS training for women to improve health, income, behavioral skills, communication, and norms (Jan and others 2011). Location: Rural South Africa | Cost per disability-adjusted life year averted for the initial scale-up was US$2,307 (in 2004 dollars; US$2,852 in 2013 dollars). |
| | Education for primary care providers | Training allows clinicians to increase their identification and referral of survivors of IPV (Norman and others 2010). Location: United Kingdom | Incremental cost-effectiveness ratio was £2,450 per quality-adjusted life year (in 2005 pounds) ($4,228 in 2013 dollars). |
| | Shelters for victims | Shelters provide a safe haven for women and child victims of IPV, including support and safety planning (Chanley, Chanley, and Campbell 2001). Location: Arizona | Net social benefit was US$3.4 million dollars (in 1999 dollars); minimum benefit-to-cost ratio was US$4.60 for every US$1.00 spent (US$6.45 in 2013 dollars). |
| Youth violence | Anonymized information sharing between police and hospital emergency department | The Cardiff model provides information to direct targeted prevention measures. Youth were among those most likely to benefit (Florence and others 2013). Location: Cardiff, United Kingdom | The cumulative social benefit-to-cost ratio was £82 (in 2003 pounds) for every £1.00 spent (US$163 in 2013 dollars). |
| | Multicomponent, long-term school and family-based program | Fast Track, a program for at-risk children in grades 1–10, includes tutoring, parent support, child social-skills training, and home visits (Foster, Jones, and the Conduct Problems Prevention Research Group 2006). Location: Durham, North Carolina; Nashville, Tennessee; Seattle, Washington; and rural central Pennsylvania | The intervention was not cost-effective at a threshold of US$50,000 willingness to pay (in 2004 dollars; US$61,817 in 2013 dollars) for an act of interpersonal violence. |

*table continues next page*

**Table 5.6** Summary of Economic Evaluations of Interventions to Prevent Interpersonal Violence, by Type of Violence (continued)

| Type of violence | Intervention type | Intervention details | Cost-effectiveness |
|---|---|---|---|
| | Mobilization of community stakeholders to implement evidence-based systems | Communities That Care (CTC) mobilizes stakeholders to collaborate on preventing adolescent substance use, delinquency, and interpersonal violence (Kuklinski and others 2012). Location: 24 communities in seven states | Very cost beneficial in the United States; net present benefit of CTC was US$5,250 per youth (in 2004 dollars; US$6,491 in 2013 dollars), with a benefit-to-cost ratio of US$5.30 for every US$1.00 spent (US$6.55 in 2013 dollars). |
| | Educational incentives | Incentives included four years of cash and other incentives to induce disadvantaged high school students to graduate (Greenwood and others 1996). Location: California | For every US$1.0 million (in 1993 dollars; $1.62 million in 2013 dollars), 258 serious crimes were prevented. |
| | Parent training and family therapy | The intervention included training for parents and therapy for families with young school-age children who have shown aggressive behavior (Greenwood and others 1996). Location: California | For every US$1.0 million (in 1993 dollars; US$1.62 million in 2013 dollars), 157 serious crimes were prevented. |
| | Supervision | The intervention included monitoring and supervising high school–age youth who have exhibited delinquent behavior (Greenwood and others 1996). Location: California | For every US$1.0 million (in 1993 dollars; US$1.62 million in 2013 dollars), 72 serious crimes were prevented. |
| | Home visiting and day care | The intervention included home visits by child care professionals from birth through the first two years of childhood, followed by four years of day care (Greenwood and others 1996). Location: California | For every US$1.0 million (in 1993 dollars; US$1.62 million in 2013 dollars), 11 serious crimes were prevented. |

briefing documents that demonstrate the effectiveness of interventions to prevent interpersonal and self-directed violence (Liverpool John Moores University 2013; WHO 2009).

### Prevention Support

Synthesizing and translating information about violence prevention innovations, although important, are likely to be insufficient to change prevention practices. Countries, districts, and communities seeking to apply violence prevention innovations need the capacity to be successful in scaling up effective programs with fidelity (Wandersman and others 2008). A growing body of research suggests that providing support in the form of specialized training, monitoring of fidelity, technical assistance, and coaching, along with improving the skills and motivation of implementing organizations, increases the use and successful implementation of innovations (Fixsen and other 2005; Mihalic and Irwin 2003; Wandersman and others 2008).

An example of a well-functioning prevention support system in the United States is the state of Pennsylvania's Evidence-Based Prevention and Intervention Support Center (EPISCenter) at the University of Pennsylvania (Rhoades, Bumbarger, and Moore 2012). The EPISCenter uses flexible, targeted, and research-based technical assistance to develop the capacity of communities to support the implementation of evidence-based violence prevention programs.

### Prevention Delivery

The successful implementation of evidence-based innovations requires that they be carried out and sustained in organizational settings (Wandersman and others 2008). Organizations' capacities to deliver the violence prevention innovations include maintaining a well-functioning organization; recruiting and maintaining well-trained staff members; developing community support; working with other organizations; and improving skills in selecting, implementing, and sustaining an innovation over time (Mihalic and Irwin 2003; Wandersman and others 2008). The Parent Centre in South Africa and Raising Voices in Uganda are two examples of organizations in LMICs that are seeking to sustain the implementation of interventions to prevent violence against women and children (Butchart and Hendricks 2000; The Parent Centre 2013; Raising Voices 2013).

## CONCLUSIONS

The primary rationale for addressing interpersonal violence as a public health problem has been its role in causing physical injury and homicide. Evidence has shown that interpersonal violence also plays an important role in the etiology of mental illness, chronic disease, and even infectious diseases such as HIV/AIDS. Unfortunately, such wide-ranging effects remain largely invisible to public health leaders, policy makers, and the public. Violence is often hidden, victims rarely come into contact with official or service agencies, and many of the health and social consequences are not evident until years after exposure. Greater awareness of these impacts is now leading to actions that can reduce the enormous health and social burden of violence.

Many LMICs face daunting challenges, including the HIV/AIDS epidemic, ongoing wars and conflicts, cardiovascular and other chronic diseases, suicide, and traffic injuries. Given the effects of violence on these outcomes, preventing interpersonal violence can become a powerful lever that, if successfully engaged, will allow LMICs to more effectively address a broad range of challenges.

The study of violence crosses many domains, and collaboration across different government sectors and across different disciplines and professions is critical, both to fully understand the problem and to effectively prevent it. Violence affects almost every government sector, including justice and law enforcement, social services, protection of women and children, education, transportation, finance, health care and public health, labor, tourism, foreign affairs, interior affairs, commerce, and tourism. The disciplines that have important contributions to make include law, psychology, sociology, social work, medicine and almost every medical specialty, anthropology, engineering, business, architecture and design, and urban planning. Given this influence, the involvement of foundations, multilateral agencies, and corporations in programs to prevent violence is also expanding.

Progress in preventing interpersonal violence is advancing rapidly, and clearly the global public health community's increased understanding and capacity to prevent interpersonal violence will make a difference. The lessons learned during their brief experience with violence prevention efforts are consistent with the lessons from the community's much longer experience with the prevention of infectious and chronic diseases. Violence can be prevented if citizens, their governments, and the global community start now, act wisely, and work together.

## NOTE

Disclaimer: The findings and conclusions in this chapter are those of the authors and do not necessarily represent the official position of the Centers for Disease Control and Prevention or the World Health Organization (WHO).

World Bank Income Classifications as of July 2014 are as follows, based on estimates of gross national income per capita for 2013:

- Low-income countries (LICs) = US$1,045 or less
- Middle-income countries (MICs) are subdivided:
  a) Lower-middle-income = US$1,046 to US$4,125
  b) Upper-middle-income (UMICs) = US$4,126 to US$12,745
- High-income countries (HICs) = US$12,746 or more.

## REFERENCES

Anda, R. F., A. Butchart, V. J. Felitti, and D. W. Brown. 2010. "Building a Framework for Global Surveillance of the Public Health Implications of Adverse Childhood Experiences." *American Journal of Preventive Medicine* 39 (1): 93–98.

Andersson, N., A. Cockcroft, and B. Shea. 2008. "Gender-Based Violence and HIV: Relevance for HIV Prevention in Hyperendemic Countries of Southern Africa." *AIDS* 22 (S4): S73–86.

Baker-Henningham, H., S. Scott, K. Jones, and S. Walker. 2012. "Reducing Child Conduct Problems and Promoting Social Skills in a Middle-Income Country: Cluster Randomised Controlled Trial." *British Journal of Psychiatry* 201 (2): 101–18.

Barnett, W. S. 1993. "Economic Evaluation of Home Visiting Programs." *The Future of Children* 3 (3): 93–112.

Bass, J. K., J. Annan, S. McIvor Murray, D. Kaysen, S. Griffiths, and others. 2013. "Controlled Trial of Psychotherapy for Congolese Survivors of Sexual Violence." *New England Journal of Medicine* 368 (23): 2182–91.

Beaman, V., J. L. Annest, J. A. Mercy, M. Kresnow, and D. A. Pollock. 2000. "Lethality of Firearm-Related Injuries in the United States Population." *Annals of Emergency Medicine* 35 (3): 258–66.

Bellis, M. A., and K. Hughes. 2008. "Comprehensive Strategies to Prevent Alcohol-Related Violence." In *Institute for the Prevention of Crime Review Volume 2: Towards More Comprehensive Approaches to Prevention and Safety*, edited by R. Hastings and M. Bania, 137–68. Ottawa: ON: Institute for Prevention of Crime.

Bellis, M. A., K. Hughes, C. Perkins, and A. Bennett. 2012. *Protecting People, Promoting Health: A Public Health Approach to Violence Prevention for England*. Liverpool, U.K.: Department of Health and National Health Service.

Bilukha, O., R. A. Hahn, A. Crosby, M. T. Fullilove, A. Liberman, and others. 2005. "The Effectiveness of Early Childhood Home Visitation in Preventing Violence: A Systematic Review." *American Journal of Preventive Medicine* 28 (2): S11–39.

Borwankar, R., R. Diallo, and A. E. Sommerfelt. 2008. *Gender-Based Violence in Sub-Saharan Africa: A Review of Demographic and Health Survey Findings and Their Use in National Planning*. Washington, DC: United States Agency for International Development.

Bott, S., A. Guedes, M. Goodwin, and J. A. Mendoza. 2012. *Violence against Women in Latin America and the Caribbean: A Comparative Analysis of Population-Based Data from 12 Countries*. Washington, DC: Pan American Health Organization.

Buchanan, C., ed. 2013. *Gun Violence, Disability and Recovery*. Sydney: Surviving Gun Violence Project.

Butchart, A., D. Brown, A. Khanh-Huynh, P. Corso, N. Florquin, and others. 2008. *Manual for Estimating the Economic Costs of Injuries Due to Interpersonal and Self-Directed Violence*. Geneva: World Health Organization.

Butchart, A., and K. Engstrom. 2002. "Sex- and Age-Specific Effects of Economic Development and Inequality on Homicide Rates in 0 to 24 Year Olds: A Cross-Sectional Analysis." *Bulletin of the World Health Organization* 80 (October): 797–805.

Butchart, A., and G. Hendricks. 2000. "The Parent Centre." In *Behind the Mask: Getting to Grips with Crime and Violence in South Africa*, edited by T. Emmett and A. Butchart, 147–76. Pretoria: Human Sciences Research Council.

Buvinic, M., A. R. Morrison, and M. Shifter. 1999. "Violence in the Americas: A Framework for Action." In *Too Close to Home: Domestic Violence in the Americas*, edited by A. R. Morrison and M. L. Biehl, 3–34. New York: Inter-American Development Bank.

Caldera, D., L. Burrell, K. Rodriguez, S. S. Crowne, C. Rohde, and others. 2007. "Impact of a Statewide Home Visiting Program on Parenting and on Child Health and Development." *Child Abuse and Neglect* 31 (8): 829–52.

Capaldi, D. M., N. B. Knoble, J. W. Shortt, and H. K. Kim. 2012. "A Systematic Review of Risk Factors for Intimate Partner Violence." *Partner Abuse* 3 (2): 231–80.

CDC (Centers for Disease Control and Prevention). 2003. *Costs of Intimate Partner Violence against Women in the United States*. Atlanta: National Center for Injury Prevention and Control.

CDC, INURED (Interuniversity Institute for Research and Development), and the Comité de Coordination. 2014. *Violence against Children in Haiti: Findings from a National Survey, 2012*. Port-au-Prince, Haiti: Centers for Disease Control and Prevention.

Chanley, S. A., J. J. Chanley, and H. E. Campbell. 2001. "Providing Refuge: The Value of Domestic Violence Shelter Services." *American Review of Public Administration* 31 (4): 393–413.

Clancy, C. M., and K. Cronin. 2005. "Evidence-Based Decision Making: Global Evidence, Local Decisions." *Health Affairs* 24 (1): 151–62.

Cohen, A. B. 2007. "Sobering Up: The Impact of the 1985–1988 Russian Anti-Alcohol Campaign on Child Health." Unpublished paper, Tufts University, Boston, MA.

Cooper, C., A. Selwood, and G. Livingston. 2008. "The Prevalence of Elder Abuse and Neglect: A Systematic Review." *Age and Aging* 37 (2): 151–60.

Dahlberg, L. L., and E. G. Krug. 2002. "Violence: A Global Public Health Problem." In *World Report on Violence and Health,* edited by E. G. Krug, L. L. Dahlberg, J. A. Mercy, A. B. Zwi, and R. Lozano, 1–21. Geneva: World Health Organization.

Danese, A., and B. McEwen. 2012. "Adverse Childhood Experiences, Allostasis, Allostatic Load, and Age-Related Disease." *Physiology and Behavior* 106 (1): 29–39.

Day, T. 1995. "The Health Related Costs of Violence against Women: The Tip of the Iceberg." Centre for Research on Violence against Women and Children Publication Series, University of Western Ontario, London, Ontario.

Devries, K., C. Watts, M. Yoshihama, L. Kiss, L. B. Schraiber, and others. 2011. "Violence against Women Is Strongly Associated with Suicide Attempts: Evidence from the WHO Multi-Country Study on Women's Health and Domestic Violence against Women." *Social Science and Medicine* 73 (1): 79–86.

Dinh-Zarr, T. B., C. Goss, E. Heitman, E. Roberts, and C. DiGuiseppi. 2004. "Interventions for Preventing Injuries in Problem Drinkers." *Cochrane Database of Systematic Reviews* 3 (3): CD001857.

Duailibi, S., W. Ponicki, J. Grube, I. Pinsky, R. Laranjeira, and M. Raw. 2007. "The Effect of Restricting Opening Hours on Alcohol-Related Violence." *American Journal of Public Health* 97 (12): 2276–80.

Durlak, J. A., R. P. Weissberg, and M. Pachan. 2010. "A Meta-Analysis of After-School Programs That Seek to Promote Personal and Social Skills in Children and Adolescents." *American Journal of Community Psychology* 45 (3–4): 294–309.

Eisenberg, N., Q. Zhou, T. L. Spinrad, C. Valiente, R. A. Fabes, and others. 2005. "Relations among Positive Parenting, Children's Effortful Control, and Externalizing Problems: A Three-Wave Longitudinal Study." *Child Development* 76 (5): 1055–71.

Fang, X., D. S. Brown, C. S. Florence, and J. A. Mercy. 2012. "The Economic Burden of Child Maltreatment in the United States and Implications for Prevention." *Child Abuse and Neglect* 36 (2): 156–65.

Fanslow, J., C. Coggan, B. Miller, and R. Norton. 1997. "The Economic Cost of Homicide in New Zealand." *Social Science and Medicine* 45 (7): 973–97.

Fisher, J., M. Cabral de Mello, V. Patel, A. Rahman, T. Tran, and others. 2012. "Prevalence and Determinants of Common Perinatal Mental Disorders in Women in Low- and Lower-Middle-Income Countries: A Systematic Review." *Bulletin of the World Health Organization* 90 (2): 139–49.

Fixsen, D. L., S. F. Naoom, K. A. Blase, R. M. Friedman, and F. Wallace. 2005. *Implementation Research: A Synthesis of the Literature.* Tampa, FL: University of South Florida, Louis de la Parte Florida Mental Health Institute, The National Implementation Research Network.

Florence, C., J. Shepherd, I. Brennan, and T. R. Simon. 2013. "An Economic Evaluation of Anonymised Information Sharing in a Partnership between Health Services, Police and Local Government for Preventing Violence-Related Injury." *Injury Prevention* 20 (2): 108–14. doi:10.1136/injuryprev-2012-040622.

Foshee, V. A., K. E. Bauman, S. T. Ennett, C. Suchindran, T. Benefield, and others. 2005. "Assessing the Effects of the Dating Violence Prevention Program 'Safe Dates' Using Random Coefficient Regression Modeling." *Prevention Science* 6 (3): 245–57.

Foster, E. M., D. Jones, and the Conduct Problems Prevention Research Group. 2006. "Can a Costly Intervention Be Cost Effective? An Analysis of Violence Prevention." *Archives of General Psychiatry* 63 (11): 1284–91.

Giancola, P. 2000. "Executive Functioning: A Conceptual Framework for Alcohol-Related Aggression." *Experimental and Clinical Psychopharmacology* 8 (4): 576–97.

Gilbert, R., C. S. Widom, K. Browne, D. Fergusson, E. Webb, and S. Janson. 2009. "Burden and Consequences of Child Maltreatment in High-Income Countries." *The Lancet* 373 (9657): 68–81.

Gore, F. M., P. J. N. Bloem, G. C. Patton, J. Ferguson, V. Joseph, and others. 2011. "Global Burden of Disease in Young People Aged 10–24 Years: A Systematic Analysis." *The Lancet* 377 (9783): 2093–102.

Graham, K., and R. Homel. 2008. *Raising the Bar: Preventing Aggression in and around Bars, Pubs and Clubs.* Devon, U.K.: Willan Publishing.

Greenwood, P. W., K. E. Model, C. P. Rydell, and J. Chiesa. 1996. *Diverting Children from a Life of Crime: Measuring Costs and Benefits.* Santa Monica, CA: Rand.

Habetha, S., S. Bleich, J. Weidenhammer, and J. M. Fegert. 2012. "A Prevalence-Based Approach to Societal Costs Occurring in Consequence of Child Abuse and Neglect." *Child and Adolescent Psychiatry and Mental Health* 6: 35. doi:10.1186/1753-2000-6-35.

Hahn, R. A., O. Bilukha, A. Crosby, M. T. Fullilove, A. Liberman, and others. 2005. "Firearms Laws and the Reduction of Violence: A Systematic Review." *American Journal of Preventive Medicine* 28 (2S1): 40–71.

Hahn, R. A., D. Fuqua-Whitley, H. Wethington, J. Lowy, A. Crosby, and others. 2007. "Effectiveness of Universal School-Based Programs to Prevent Violent and Aggressive Behavior: A Systematic Review." *American Journal of Preventive Medicine* 33 (2S): S114–29.

Hawkins, J. D., R. F. Catalano, R. Kosterman, R. Abbott, and K. G. Hill. 1999. "Preventing Adolescent Health-Risk Behaviors by Strengthening Protection during Childhood." *Archive of Pediatrics and Adolescent Medicine* 153 (3): 226–34.

Heim, C., and E. B. Binder. 2012. "Current Research Trends in Early Life Stress and Depression: Review of Human Studies on Sensitive Periods, Gene-Environment Interactions, and Epigenetics." *Experimental Neurology* 233 (1): 102–11.

Hillis, S. D., R. F. Anda, S. R. Dube, V. J. Felitti, P. A. Marchbanks, and J. S. Marks. 2004. "The Association between Adverse

Childhood Experiences and Adolescent Pregnancy, Long-Term Psychosocial Outcomes, and Fetal Death." *Pediatrics* 113 (2): 320–27.

Hillis, S. D., R. F. Anda, S. R. Dube, V. J. Felitti, P. A. Marchbanks, and others. 2010. "The Protective Effect of Family Strengths in Childhood against Adolescent Pregnancy and Its Long-Term Psychosocial Consequences." *Permanente Journal* 14 (3): 18–27.

Holt, V. L., M. A. Kernic, M. E. Wolf, and F. P. Rivara. 2003. "Do Protection Orders Affect the Likelihood of Future Partner Violence and Injury?" *American Journal of Preventive Medicine* 24 (1): 16–21.

Hughes, K., M. A. Bellis, L. Jones, S. Wood, G. Bates, and others. 2012. "Prevalence and Risk of Violence against Adults with Disabilities: A Systematic Review and Meta-Analysis of Observational Studies." *The Lancet* 80 (9845): 899–907. doi:10.1016/S0410-6736(11)61851-5.

ICRW (International Center for Research on Women). 2009. "Intimate Partner Violence: High Costs to Households and Communities." Policy Brief, ICRW, Washington, DC.

IOM (Institute of Medicine). 2013. *Evaluation of PEPFAR.* Washington, DC: National Academics Press.

IOM and NRC (National Research Council). 2012. *Social and Economic Costs of Violence.* Washington, DC: National Academies Press.

———. 2013. *Priorities for Research to Reduce the Threat of Firearm-Related Violence.* Washington, DC: National Academies Press.

Ireland, T., and C. Smith. 2009. "Living in Partner-Violent Families: Developmental Links to Antisocial Behavior and Relationship Violence." *Journal of Youth and Adolescence* 38 (3): 323–39.

Jan, J., G. Ferrari, C. H. Watts, J. R. Hargreaves, J. C. Kim, and others. 2011. "Economic Evaluation of a Combined Microfinance and Gender Training Intervention for the Prevention of Intimate Partner Violence in Rural South Africa." *Health Policy and Planning* 26 (5): 366–72.

Jewkes, R. K. 2002. "Intimate Partner Violence: Causes and Prevention." *The Lancet* 359 (9315): 1423–29.

Jewkes, R. K., M. Nduna, J. Levin, N. Jama, K. Dunkle, and others. 2008. "Impact of Stepping Stones on Incidence of HIV and HSV-2 and Sexual Behaviour in Rural South Africa: Cluster Randomised Controlled Trial." *British Medical Journal* 337: a506. doi:10.1136/bmj.a506.

Kaminski, J. W., L. A. Valle, J. H. Filene, and C. L. Boyle. 2008. "A Meta-Analytic Review of Components Associated with Parent Training Program Effectiveness." *Journal of Abnormal Child Psychology* 36 (4): 567–89.

Kessler, R. C., K. A. McLaughlin, J. G. Green, M. J. Gruber, N. A. Sampson, and others. 2010. "Childhood Adversities and Adult Psychopathology in the WHO World Mental Health Surveys." *British Journal of Psychiatry* 197 (5): 378–85.

Kissin, D. M., L. Zapata, R. Yorick, E. N. Vinogradova, G. V. Volkova, and others. 2007. "HIV Seroprevalence in Street Youth, St. Petersburg, Russia." *AIDS* 21 (17): 2333–40.

Klevens, J., J. W. Martinez, B. Le, C. Rojas, A. Duque, and others. 2009. "Evaluation of Two Interventions to Reduce Aggressive and Antisocial Behavior in First and Second Graders in a Resource-Poor Setting." *International Journal of Educational Research* 48 (5): 307–19.

Klosterman, K. C., and W. Fals-Stewart. 2006. "Intimate Partner Violence and Alcohol Use: Exploring the Role of Drinking in Partner Violence and Its Implications for Intervention." *Aggression and Violent Behavior* 11 (6): 587–97.

Knerr, W., F. Gardner, and L. Cluver. 2013. "Improving Positive Parenting Skills and Reducing Harsh and Abusive Parenting in Low- and Middle-Income Countries: A Systematic Review." *Prevention Science* 14 (4): 352–63.

Koper, C. S., and E. Mayo-Wilson. 2009. "Police Strategies to Reduce Illegal Possession and Carrying of Firearms: Effects on Gun Crime." *Campbell Systematic Reviews* 8 (11). doi:10.4073/csr.2012.11.

Kornør, H., D. Winje, Ø. Ekeberg, L. Weisæth, I. Kirkehei, and others. 2008. "Early Trauma-Focused Cognitive-Behavioural Therapy to Prevent Chronic Post-Traumatic Stress Disorder and Related Symptoms: A Systematic Review and Meta-Analysis." *BMC Psychiatry* 8: 81.

Krug, E. G., L. I. Dahlberg, J. A. Mercy, A. B. Zwi, and R. Lozano, eds. 2002. *World Report on Violence and Health.* Geneva: World Health Organization.

Kuklinski, M. R., J. S. Briney, J. D. Hawkins, and R. F. Catalano. 2012. "Cost-Benefit Analysis of Communities That Care Outcomes at Eighth Grade." *Prevention Science* 13 (2): 150–61.

Lachs, M. S., and K. Pillemer. 2004. "Elder Abuse." *The Lancet* 364 (9441): 1263–72.

Lee, S., S. Aos, E. Drake, A. Pennucci, M. Miller, and L. Anderson. 2012. "Return on Investment: Evidence-Based Options to Improve Statewide Outcomes, April 2012." Document No. 12-04-1201, Washington State Institute for Public Policy, Olympia, WA.

Liverpool Johns Moores University. 2013. "Violence Prevention Evidence Base." Database, Centre for Public Health, Liverpool John Moores University, Liverpool, U.K. http://www.preventviolence.info/EvidenceBase.

Lozano, R., M. Naghavi, K. Foreman, S. Lim, K. Shibuya, and others. 2012. "Global and Regional Mortality from 235 Causes of Death for 20 Age Groups in 1990 and 2010: A Systematic Analysis for the Global Burden of Disease Study 2010." *The Lancet* 380 (9859): 2095–128.

Machtinger, E. L., J. E. Haberer, T. C. Wilson, and D. S. Weiss. 2012. "Recent Trauma Is Associated with Antiretroviral Failure and HIV Transmission Risk Behavior among HIV-Positive Women and Female-Identified Transgenders." *AIDS and Behavior* 16 (8): 2160–70. Epub 2012/03/20.

Machtinger, E. L., T. C. Wilson, J. E. Haberer, and D. S. Weiss. 2012. "Psychological Trauma and PTSD in HIV-Positive Women: A Meta-Analysis." *AIDS and Behavior* 16 (8): 2091–100.

Makarios, M. D., and T. C. Pratt. 2012. "The Effectiveness of Policies and Programs That Attempt to Reduce Firearm

Violence: A Meta-Analysis." *Crime and Delinquency* 58 (2): 222–44.

Marinho de Souza, M. de F., J. Macinko, A. P. Alencar, D. C. Malta, and O. L. de Morais Neo. 2007. "Reductions in Firearm-Related Mortality and Hospitalizations in Brazil after Gun Control." *Health Affairs* 26 (2): 575–84.

Markowitz, S., and M. Grossman. 1998. "Alcohol Regulation and Domestic Violence towards Children." *Contemporary Economic Policy* 16 (3): 309–20.

———. 2000. "The Effects of Beer Taxes on Physical Child Abuse." *Journal of Health Economics* 19 (2): 271–82.

Mattson, S. N., S. C. Roesch, L. Glass, B. N. Deweese, C. D. Coles, and others. 2013. "Further Development of a Neurobehavioral Profile of Fetal Alcohol Spectrum Disorders." *Alcoholism: Clinical and Experimental Research* 37 (3): 517–28.

Matzopoulos, R. G., M. L. Thompson, and J. E. Myers. 2014. "Firearm and Non-Firearm Homicide in Five South African Cities: A Retrospective Population-Based Study." *American Journal of Public Health* 104 (3): 455–60.

Mayhew, P. 2003. "Counting the Costs of Crime in Australia." *Trends and Issues in Crime and Criminal Justice,* no. 247. Australian Institute of Criminology, Canberra.

McFarlane, J. M., J. Y. Groff, J. A. O'Brien, and K. Watson. 2006. "Secondary Prevention of Intimate Partner Violence: A Randomized Controlled Trial." *Nursing Research* 55 (1): 52–61.

Mendonca, R. N., J. G. Alves, and J. E. Cabral Filho. 2002. "Hospital Costs Due to Violence against Children and Adolescents in Pernambuco State, Brazil, during 1999." *Cad Saude Publica* 18 (6): 1577–81.

Mihalic, S., and K. Irwin. 2003. "Blueprints for Violence Prevention: From Research to Real World Settings: Factors Influencing the Successful Replication of Model Programs." *Youth Violence and Juvenile Justice* 1: 307–29.

Mikton, C., and A. Butchart. 2009. "Child Maltreatment Prevention: A Systematic Review of Reviews." *Bulletin of the World Health Organization* 87 (5): 353–61.

Miller, M., D. Azrael, and D. Hemenway. 2013. "Firearms and Violent Death in the United States." In *Reducing Gun Violence in America*, edited by D. W. Webster and J. S. Vernick, 1–20. Baltimore, MD: Johns Hopkins University Press.

Miller, T. R., M. A. Cohen, and B. Wiersema. 1996. *Victim Costs and Consequences: A New Look*. National Institute of Justice Research Report, National Institute of Justice, United States Department of Justice, Washington, DC.

Miller, T. R., D. A. Fisher, and M. A. Cohen. 2001. "Costs of Juvenile Violence: Policy Implications." *Pediatrics* 107 (1): e3.

Monteiro, M. 2007. *Alcohol and Public Health in the Americas: A Case for Action*. Washington, DC: Pan American Health Organization.

Morrison, A. R., and M. B. Orlando. 1999. "Social and Economic Costs of Domestic Violence: Chile and Nicaragua." In *Too Close to Home: Domestic Violence in the Americas*, edited by A. R. Morrison and B. E. Orlando, 51–80. New York: Inter-American Development Bank.

Nelson, G., A. Westhues, and J. MacLeod. 2003. "A Meta-Analysis of Longitudinal Research on Preschool Prevention Programs for Children." *Prevention and Treatment* 6 (1): 31A. doi:10.1037/1522-3736.6.1.631a.

Nemtsov, A. V. 1998. "Alcohol-Related Harm and Alcohol Consumption in Moscow before, during and after a Major Anti-Alcohol Campaign." *Addiction* 93 (10): 1501–10.

Norman, R., A. Spencer, S. Eldridge, and G. Feder. 2010. "Cost Effectiveness of a Programme to Detect and Provide Better Care for Female Victims of Intimate Partner Violence." *Journal of Health Services and Research Policy* 15 (3): 143–49.

Norman, R. E., M. Byambaa, R. De, A. Butchart, J. Scott, and others. 2012. "The Long-Term Health Consequences of Child Physical Abuse, Emotional Abuse, and Neglect: A Systematic Review and Meta-Analysis." *PLoS Med* 9 (11): e1001349. doi:10.1371/journal.pmed.1001349.

Norton, R., and O. Kobusingye. 2013. "Injuries." *New England Journal of Medicine* 368 (18): 1723–30.

Olds, D., C. R. Henderson, R. Cole, J. Eckenrode, H. Kitzman, and others. 1998. "Long-Term Effects of Nurse Home Visitation on Children's Criminal and Antisocial Behavior: 15-year Follow-Up of a Randomized Controlled Trial." *Journal of the American Medical Association* 280 (14): 1238–44.

Paine, K., G. Hart, M. Jawo, S. Ceesay, M. Jallow, and others. 2002. "Before We Were Sleeping, Now We Are Awake: Preliminary Evaluation of the Stepping Stones Sexual Health Programme in The Gambia." *African Journal of AIDS Research* 1 (1): 41–52.

The Parent Centre. 2013. "The Parent Centre: Helping Children through Parents." http://www.theparentcentre.org.za/.

Pinheiro, P. S. 2006. *World Report on Violence against Children*. Geneva: United Nations.

Pronyk, P. M., J. R. Hargreaves, J. C. Kim, L. A. Morison, G. Phetla, and others. 2006. "Effect of a Structural Intervention for the Prevention of Intimate-Partner Violence and HIV in Rural South Africa: A Cluster Randomised Trial." *The Lancet* 368 (9551): 1973–83.

Raising Voices. 2013. "Raising Voices: Preventing Violence against Women and Children." http://raisingvoices.org/about.

Ramsay, J., J. Richardson, Y. H. Carter, L. L. Davidson, and G. Feder. 2002. "Should Health Professionals Screen Women for Domestic Violence? Systematic Review." *British Medical Journal* 325 (7359): 314.

Reed, R., M. Fazel, L. Jones, C. Panter-Brick, and A. Stein. 2012. "Mental Health of Displaced and Refugee Children Resettled in Low-Income and Middle-Income Countries: Risk and Protective Factors." *The Lancet* 379 (9812): 250–65.

Reza, A., J. A. Mercy, and E. G. Krug. 2001. "The Epidemiology of Violent Deaths in the World." *Injury Prevention* 7 (2): 104–11.

Reza, A., M. J. Breiding, G. Gulaid, J. A. Mercy, C. Blanton, and others. 2009. "Sexual Violence and Its Health Consequences for Female Children in Swaziland: A Cluster Survey Study." *The Lancet* 373 (9679): 1966–72.

Rhoades, B. L., B. K. Bumbarger, and J. E. Moore. 2012. "The Role of a State-Level Prevention Support System in Promoting High-Quality Implementation and Sustainability of Evidence-Based Programs." *American Journal of Community Psychology* 50 (3): 386–401.

Robbins, C. L., L. Zapata, D. M. Kissin, N. Shevchenko, R. Yorick, and others. 2010. "Multicity HIV Seroprevalence in Street Youth, Ukraine." *International Journal of STDs and AIDS* 21 (7): 489–96.

Roldós, M. I., and P. Corso. 2013. "The Economic Burden of Intimate Partner Violence in Ecuador: Setting the Agenda for Future Research and Violence Prevention Policies." *Western Journal Emergency Medicine* 14 (4): 347–53.

Rosenberg, M. L., A. Butchart, J. Mercy, V. Narasimhan, H. Waters, and others. 2006. "Interpersonal Violence." In *Disease Control Priorities in Developing Countries*, 2nd ed., edited by D. T. Jamison, J. G. Breman, A. R. Measham, R. G. Alleyne, M. Claeson, and others, 755–70. Washington, DC: Oxford University Press and World Bank.

Silverman, J. G., M. R. Decker, D. M. Cheng, K. Wirth, N. Saggurti, and others. 2011. "Gender-Based Disparities in Infant and Child Mortality Based on Maternal Exposure to Spousal Violence: The Heavy Burden Borne by Indian Girls." *Archives of Pediatric and Adolescent Medicine* 165 (1): 22–27.

Silverman, J. G., R. Michele, M. R. Decker, L. Heather, M. S. McCauley, and others. 2009. "Regional Assessment of Sex Trafficking and STI/HIV in Southeast Asia: Connections between Sexual Exploitation, Violence, and Sexual Risk." United Nations Development Programme Regional Center, Colombo. http://www.undp.org/content /dam/undp/library/hivaids/English/SexTrafficking.pdf.

Smith, K. W., S. H. Landry, and P. R. Swank. 2010. "The Influence of Early Patterns of Positive Parenting on Children's Preschool Outcomes." *Early Education and Development* 11 (2): 147–69.

Stöckl, H., K. Devries, A. Rotsein, N. Abrahams, J. Campbell, and others. 2013. "The Global Prevalence of Intimate Partner Homicide: A Systematic Review." *The Lancet* 382 (9895): 859–65.

Stoltenborgh, M. A., M. H. van Ijzendoorn, E. M. Euser, M. J. Bakermans-Kranenburg. 2011. "Global Perspective on Child Sexual Abuse: Meta-Analysis of Prevalence around the World." *Child Maltreatment* 16 (2): 79–101.

Stoltenborgh, M. A., M. J. Bakermans-Kranenburg, M. H. van Ijzendoorn, and L. R. Alink. 2013a. "Cultural-Geographical Differences in the Occurrence of Child Physical Abuse? A Meta-Analysis of Global Prevalence." *International Journal of Psychology* 48 (2): 81–94.

Stoltenborgh, M. A., M. J. Bakermans-Kranenburg, and M. H. van Ijzendoorn. 2013b. "The Neglect of Child Neglect: A Meta-Analytic Review of the Prevalence of Neglect." *Social Psychiatry and Psychiatric Epidemiology* 48 (3): 345–55.

Temple, J. A., and A. J. Reynolds. 2007. "Benefits and Costs of Investments in Pre-School Education: Evidence from the Child-Parent Centers and Related Programs." *Economics of Education Review* 26 (1): 126–44.

Tharp, A. T., S. Degue, L. A. Valle, K. A. Brookmeyer, G. M. Massetti, and others. 2012. "A Systematic Qualitative Review of Risk and Protective Factors for Sexual Violence Perpetration." *Trauma, Violence, and Abuse* 14 (2): 133–67.

Thornberry, T. P., K. E. Knight, and P. J. Lovegrove. 2012. "Does Maltreatment Beget Maltreatment? A Systematic Review of the Intergenerational Literature." *Trauma, Violence and Abuse* 13 (3): 135–52.

UN (United Nations). 2006. *Secretary General's In-Depth Study on All Forms of Violence against Women*. New York: United Nations.

———. 2015. *Transforming Our World: The 2030 Agenda for Sustainable Development; Resolution Adopted by the General Assembly*. 70/1. New York: United Nations. http://www.un.org/ga/search/view_doc.asp?symbol=A /RES/70/1&Lang=E.

UNICEF (United Nations Children's Fund). 2010. *Child Disciplinary Practices at Home: Evidence from a Range of Low- and Middle-Income Countries*. New York: UNICEF.

UNICEF, CDC (Centers for Disease Control and Prevention), and KNBS (Kenya National Bureau of Statistics). 2012. *Violence against Children in Kenya: Findings from a 2010 National Survey*. Nairobi: UNICEF Kenya Country Office.

UNICEF, CDC, and the Muhimbili University of Health and Allied Science. 2012. *Violence against Children in Tanzania: Findings from a National Survey 2009*. Dar es Salaam, Tanzania: UNICEF Tanzania.

Usdin, S., E. Scheepers, S. Goldstein, and G. Japhet. 2005. "Achieving Social Change on Gender-Based Violence: A Report on the Impact Evaluation of Soul City's Fourth Series." *Social Science and Medicine* 61 (11): 2434–45.

van der Merwe, A., A. Dawes, and C. L. Ward. 2012. "The Development of Youth Violence: An Ecological Understanding." In *Youth Violence in South Africa: Sources and Solutions*, edited by C. L. Ward, A. van der Merwe, and A. Dawes. Cape Town, South Africa: UCT Press.

Walker, S. P., S. M. Chang, M. Vera-Hernandez, and S. Grantham-McGregor. 2011. "Early Childhood Stimulation Benefits Adult Competence and Reduces Violent Behavior." *Pediatrics* 127 (5): 849–57.

Wandersman, A., J. Duffy, P. Flaspohler, R. Noonan, K. Lubell, and others. 2008. "Bridging the Gap between Prevention Research and Practice: The Interactive Systems Framework for Dissemination and Implementation." *American Journal of Community Psychology* 41 (3–4): 171–81.

Ward, E., T. McCartney, D. W. Brown, A. Grant, A. Butchart, and others. 2009. "Results of an Exercise to Estimate the Costs of Interpersonal Violence in Jamaica." *West Indian Medical Journal* 58 (5): 446–51.

Webster, D. W., J. M. Whitehill, J. S. Vernick, and F. C. Curriero. 2012. "Effects of Baltimore's *Safe Streets* Program on Gun Violence: A Replication of Chicago's *CeaseFire* Program." *Bulletin of the New York Academy of Medicine* 90 (1): 27–40.

WHO (World Health Organization). 2004. *The Economic Dimensions of Interpersonal Violence*, edited by H. Waters, A. Hyder, Y. Rajkotia, S. Basu, J. A. Rehwinkel, and others. Geneva: WHO. http://whqlibdoc.who.int/publications/2004/9241591609.pdf.

——. 2006. "Youth Violence and Alcohol Fact Sheet" (accessed June 30, 2013). http://www.who.int/violence_injury_prevention/violence/world_report/factsheets/ft_youth.pdf.

——. 2008. *Preventing Violence and Reducing Its Impact: How Development Agencies Can Help*. Geneva: WHO.

——. 2009. *Violence Prevention: The Evidence. Overview*. Geneva: WHO.

——. 2010. *Global Strategy to Reduce the Harmful Use of Alcohol*. Geneva: WHO.

——. 2013. *Global and Regional Estimates of Violence against Women: Prevalence and Health Effects of Intimate Partner and Non-Partner Sexual Violence*. Geneva: WHO.

——. 2014. "Global Health Estimates Summary Tables: Deaths by Cause, Age and Sex, by WHO Region." WHO, Geneva. http://www.who.int/healthinfo/global_burden_disease/en/.

WHO (World Health Organization) and Liverpool John Moores University. 2006. "Interpersonal Violence and Alcohol." WHO Policy Briefing. Geneva: WHO.

http://www.who.int/violence_injury_prevention/violence/world_report/factsheets/pb_violencealcohol.pdf.

Wolfe, D. A., C. Crooks, P. Jaffe, D. Chiodo, R. Hughes, and others. 2009. "A School-Based Program to Prevent Adolescent Dating Violence: A Cluster Randomized Trial." *Archives of Pediatrics and Adolescent Medicine* 163 (8): 692–99.

Zapata, L. B., D. M. Kissin, C. L. Robbins, E. Finnerty, H. Skipalska, and others. 2011. "Multi-City Assessment of Lifetime Pregnancy Involvement among Street Youth, Ukraine." *Journal of Urban Health* 88 (4): 779–92.

Zapata, L. B., D. M. Kissin, O. Bogoliubova, R. V. Yorick, J. M. Kraft, and others. 2013. "Orphaned and Abused Youth Are Vulnerable to Pregnancy and Suicide Risk." *Child Abuse and Neglect* 37 (5): 310–19.

Zhao, J., T. Stockwell, G. Martin, S. Macdonald, K. Vallance, and others. 2013. "The Relationship between Minimum Alcohol Prices, Outlet Densities and Alcohol-Attributable Deaths in British Columbia, 2002–2009." *Addiction* 108 (6): 1059–69. doi:10.1111/add.12139.

ZIMSTAT (Zimbabwe National Statistics Agency), UNICEF (United Nations Children's Fund), and CCORE (Collaborating Centre for Operational Research and Evaluation). 2012. *National Baseline Survey on Life Experiences of Adolescents in Zimbabwe 2011*. Preliminary Report. ZIMSTAT, Harare, Zimbabwe.

# Chapter 6

# Occupation and Risk for Injuries

Safa Abdalla, Spenser S. Apramian, Linda F. Cantley, and
Mark R. Cullen

## INTRODUCTION

The world of work has changed dramatically. Globalization
affects the structure of workplaces, the way work is
performed, and occupational safety and health (OSH).
Despite great strides in improving OSH during the past
century, an estimated 317 million nonfatal occupational
injuries and 321,000 occupational fatalities occur globally
each year, that is, 151 workers sustain a work-related
accident every 15 seconds (ILO 2013a). Poor workplace
safety and health place a substantial economic burden on
individuals, employers, and society. Estimates from the
International Social Security Association (ISSA) suggest
that costs associated with nonfatal workplace accidents
alone equal approximately 4 percent of world gross domestic product (GDP) each year (ISSA 2014; SafeWork 2012).

Although virtually every job entails some risk for
injury, the magnitude of risk varies widely across jobs,
sectors, geographic regions, and individuals. Occupational
injury rates have been rising in low- and middle-income
countries (LMICs), but declining in high-income
countries (HICs), although the effect of globalization has
been mixed. The steady decline in Australia, North
America, and Western Europe is due, at least in part, to
the export of labor-intensive and often more dangerous
industrial production to regions where salaries are lower,
workplace regulations are less stringent, and working
conditions are generally poorer. However, in HICs the
number of small firms and informal sector jobs has
grown markedly. These firms and jobs are underserved

by OSH regulations and enforcement; are difficult to
reach with traditional OSH services; and have greater, but
largely hidden, risk for accident and injury. Consequently,
although the true burden of occupational injury in HICs
remains uncertain, an estimated 6.9 million worker injuries occurred in the European Union (EU) during 2006
and 8.5 million occurred in the United States during
2007 (Chau and others 2014; Leigh and Marcin 2012).
Occupational injuries and fatalities take an even greater
toll in LMICs, where a large portion of the population
works in the informal sector or in high-hazard sectors,
including agriculture, construction, fishing, and mining,
with associated costs as high as 10 percent of GDP.

The great recession of 2007–09 had a negative effect
on OSH in many countries. Corporations downsized,
restructured, and outsourced or transferred work to
third-party employers, temporary employment agencies,
or independent contractors. As of 2011, 22.3 million
fewer adults and 6.4 million fewer youths participated in
the labor force than anticipated according to global
trends before the downturn. From 2007 to 2010, the
ratio of jobs to population declined sharply—from 61.2
percent in 2007 to 60.2 percent in 2010 (ILO 2012c)—
and the number of workers in precarious or vulnerable
employment reached an estimated 1.52 billion, an
increase of nearly 23 million since 2009 and 136 million
since 2000. Latin America and the Caribbean, the Middle
East, South Asia, South-East Asia and the Pacific, and
Sub-Saharan Africa experienced the largest increase in

Corresponding author: Safa Abdalla, Stanford University, Palo Alto, California, United States; sabdalla@stanford.edu.

vulnerable employment. Women were disproportionately affected in the Middle East, North Africa, and Sub-Saharan Africa.

This chapter discusses the many changes in work and work-related injuries in seven sections. Following this introduction, the second section reviews the current state of occupational injury and safety in HICs, with an emphasis on recent developments and observations, and the third focuses on the situation in LMICs, again with an emphasis on recent developments. The fourth section reviews the effect of global supply chains on global business practices. The fifth section discusses the economic effects of these changes and interventions used in ameliorating the problems raised, drawing heavily from observations in the preceding sections to the extent possible. The sixth section provides a brief synopsis of the contributions that workplace physical, chemical, and biologic exposures may make to the occurrence of acute and chronic medical conditions. A final section provides conclusions.

## OCCUPATIONAL INJURY IN HICs

Several developments have the potential to raise occupational injury rates. In HICs, temporary work and other forms of flexible employment have risen, including contingent work, home-based work, part-time contracts, unregulated work, and other nontraditional work. Most of these arrangements are precarious; they are unstable, offer little social protection, and pay low wages. Consistent evidence has shown that workers in precarious or vulnerable work arrangements experience more health and safety hazards and poorer health and safety outcomes than do other workers. Labor statistics often capture only precarious workers in temporary employment, underestimating the true burden of precarious employment on OSH (Benavides and others 2006; Virtanen, Janlert, and Hammarström 2011). Temporary workers have twice the risk for occupational injury as permanent workers, but the reasons for this higher risk are poorly defined. They are likely to include less job experience, less recognition of workplace hazards, and inadequate or ineffective safety training (Virtanen, Janlert, and Hammarström 2011). Despite substantially higher rates of occupational injury, temporary workers have lower absence rates, perhaps fearing the loss of their job (Benavides and others 2006; Virtanen, Janlert, and Hammarström 2011).

Economic and employment growth in many regions relies to a great extent on small and medium enterprises (SMEs). More than 90 percent of businesses in the EU and the United States employ fewer than 20 employees, and SMEs account for an estimated 82 percent of all occupational injuries (Ecorys 2012). SMEs are extremely diverse, covering many sectors and work activities and often offering flexible work environments. Given their small size, many SMEs have limited resources and lack formal OSH programs and training. Results from a national survey of U.S. firms with fewer than 250 employees found that few had an employee safety committee, 50 percent had no formal safety policies, and only 60 percent provided safety training to new employees (NFIB 2002). Moreover, a survey of major health insurers in Germany indicated that SMEs in the manufacturing sector had reduced their OSH management since the economic recession, a concerning trend (Kraemer 2010).

Employees of small business enterprises are exposed to higher health and safety risks than are employees of larger enterprises (Fabiano, Currò, and Pastorino 2004; Sinclair, Cunningham, and Schulte 2013). They also have much greater difficulty assessing and controlling these risks (Eakin, Champoux, and MacEachen 2010; Sørensen, Hasle, and Bach 2007).

Furthermore, most OSH laws and regulatory agencies are designed for large enterprises in the formal economy and either exempt or do not cover the informal economy and SMEs. Hence, there is little reporting on these sectors or enforcement of laws and regulations even in HICs. Employees who work in small enterprises far outnumber those who work in larger enterprises in many countries, so addressing these gaps is critical (Hasle and Limborg 2006).

The substantial increase in outsourcing in recent decades has shifted some work to workers' homes and other informal settings. Whereas many home-based workers are self-employed, others may work under some form of outsourcing arrangement and fall under the broad umbrella of precarious employment.

Studies examining the health and safety effects of outsourcing or subcontracting and home-based work have reported poorer OSH outcomes, using a range of measures (Quinlan and Bohle 2008). Questions regarding the mechanisms by which outsourcing and home-based work negatively affect health remain, but several factors may contribute (table 6.1).

There is no universally accepted definition of migrant workers. However, evidence from several press investigations and published reports suggests that regardless of their legal status, migrant workers experience various forms of exploitation at work, although conditions are typically worse for undocumented workers (McKay, Craw, and Chopra 2006). Migrant workers are less likely to receive workplace health and safety training in many sectors. When such training is provided, language barriers may prevent workers from understanding basic safety procedures or knowing how or where to report safety or health concerns.

**Table 6.1** Negative OSH Consequences Potentially Arising from Home-Based and Outsourced Work

| Contributing factor | Hazard |
| --- | --- |
| Economic and reward pressure | • Work intensification and compromised OSH |
| Disorganization of management systems | • Limited worker training or supervision |
| | • Poorly designed work settings |
| | • Inadequate safety protocols |
| | • Obscured mechanisms for workers to raise concerns |
| Dispersed workforce with complex management structures | • Less regulatory oversight and enforcement |
| | • Workforce logistically difficult for inspectorates to reach |
| | • Less worker understanding of employer OSH obligations and worker rights |

*Source:* Lippel 2005.
*Note:* OSH = occupational safety and health.

Although migrant workers face similar workplace hazards as local workers in similar sectors and jobs, their safety and health may be at greater jeopardy for reasons specific to their situation. Migrant workers are more likely to be employed in hazardous work, work longer hours with fewer breaks, perform shift work, and be temporary workers or subcontractors and are less likely to report accidents (Premji, Lippel, and Messing 2008; Premji and others 2010). Migrant workers are often overqualified for the work they perform in host countries, and workplace injury may limit their occupational mobility, perpetuating the education–job mismatch. There is a great need to address barriers to suitable employment and to improve health and safety strategies targeting recent immigrants.

## Workplace Hazards

Research conducted in HICs is the predominant source of information about the contribution of workplace hazards (physical, psychosocial, and work organization) and individual factors (gender, age, and health status) to occupational injury risk as well as ways to mitigate risk.

### Physical Exposures

Physical exposures related to job tasks, workplace environment, use of tools and materials, machine operation, and machine-paced work affect workers in different occupations and employment sectors (Chau and others 2009; Vandergrift and others 2012). The following physical workplace exposures are strongly associated with injury risk:

- Manual handling
- Forceful exertions
- Highly repetitive motions with short work cycles

- Awkward postures of the neck, trunk, and extremities
- Whole-body or segmental vibration
- Mechanical contact stress from work positions or handling of tools and equipment
- High levels of ambient noise
- Extreme temperatures
- Work performed from heights
- Work performed around operating machinery.

Although many jobs in HICs continue to require manual labor, exposure to workplace physical hazards is not limited to manual workers. Results from the 2010 European Working Conditions Survey indicate that 33 percent of European workers handle heavy loads for at least 25 percent of their working time and 23 percent are exposed to workplace vibration (Eurofound 2010). Additionally, 30 percent of European workers are exposed to tiring positions 25–75 percent of their working time, and 16 percent of workers are exposed to tiring positions 100 percent of their working time (Eurofound 2010).

In the United States, approximately 27 percent of working adults are exposed continually to repetitive motion, 25 percent spend more than half of their time at work either bending or twisting, an estimated 10 percent are exposed to cramped workspaces that require them to assume awkward postures every day, and 2.7 percent are exposed to whole-body vibration (Tak and Calvert 2011). Workplace physical hazards clearly persist in HICs, underscoring the importance of mitigating these hazards even as countries move toward becoming largely service-based economies.

### Psychosocial Exposures

Significant changes in technology and management ideologies, combined with increases in global competition, are responsible for the trend toward more difficult, faster, more productive labor with less control over tasks (Green 2005). Workplace psychosocial hazards arising from evolving work demands, in conjunction with changing economic and social contexts of work, are emerging threats to physical and mental health (EU OSHA 2007; NIOSH 2002). Evidence has been amassed suggesting an association between stressors and the risk for work-related injury (Glasscock and others 2006; Kim and others 2009; Nakata and others 2006) and musculoskeletal disorder (MSD) (Bongers and others 2006; da Costa and Vieira 2010; Ghaffari and others 2008).

Psychosocial stressors include the following:

- Work intensification
- Highly monotonous work
- Time pressure or deadlines
- Significant mental workload
- Ambiguous or conflicting roles
- Lack of decision-making authority
- Machine-paced work or piecework
- Isolation
- Weak supervisor support
- Demand or reward imbalance
- Job insecurity.

Physical and psychosocial workplace exposures increase the risk for injury and MSD. In combination, they create even greater risk (Lapointe and others 2009; Magnavita and others 2011), with important implications for OSH interventions.

## Work Organization

The modern 24-hour society has greatly affected the timing of work hours. The development of new technologies and global economic competition require that goods and services be made available at all hours of the day and night (Costa 2010). The traditional schedule of regular, mainly daytime working hours has given way to a variety of work patterns for many workers in HICs. Results from the 2000 European Working Conditions Survey indicate that only 25 percent of employed workers and less than 10 percent of self-employed workers have traditional work schedules. The vast majority work irregular hours, including some combination of compressed work hours, variable work hours, shift work or night work, weekend work, part-time work, and on-call work (Costa and others 2004). A large body of evidence suggests that shift work and night work interfere with circadian rhythms, decrease efficiency, and strain social and family relationships (Costa and Di Milia 2010).

Workers with rotating shifts often experience sleep deficits and fatigue, which decrease their mental agility, reduce performance efficiency, and increase error rates. Evidence suggests that night workers have higher risk for injury than do day workers, with successive night shifts further elevating the risk (Folkard and Tucker 2003). Increased risk for injury has also been associated with working overtime, long hours, and 12-hour shifts (Dembe, Delbos, and Erickson 2008; Folkard and Lombardi 2006). Shorter sleep duration and longer work hours are independently associated with the risk for work-related injury, mainly because fatigue impairs cognitive functioning and slows response time (Lombardi and others 2010). The understanding of the effect of fatigue on performance is complicated by the existence of individual differences in vulnerability to fatigue. These differences may be critical for workers in round-the-clock operational settings (Van Dongen, Caldwell, and Caldwell 2011).

As women increasingly participate in the labor force and men assume a progressively larger role in domestic duties in most HICs, in combination with substantial changes in family composition and labor force demographics, balancing work and family demands has become more challenging (Valcour 2007). Work–life conflict has been associated with adverse outcomes, including work-related MSDs (Hämmig and others 2011), sleep disorders and fatigue (Wirtz, Nachreiner, and Rolfes 2011), and reduced labor force participation and its economic consequences (Jansen and others 2010). Associations between work–life conflict and adverse outcomes extend beyond the high-risk sectors. For example, in the retail sector, Sunday work significantly increases the risk for accidents (Wirtz, Nachreiner, and Rolfes 2011). Workplace interventions that reduce conflicts between work and private life and address other risk factors are needed to prevent workplace injury and MSDs.

## Individual Factors

Individuals have varying susceptibilities to workplace injury, and this variability is related to occupational and individual characteristics (Clarke 2011; Schulte and others 2012). Many reports have found a consistently elevated risk for injury among younger workers (Breslin and others 2007; Breslin, Smith, and Moore 2011) and workers with lower educational attainment (Breslin 2008; Strong and Zimmerman 2005).

The increased risk for injury among novice workers compared to their longer-tenured counterparts remains despite adjustment for confounders, including age, sex, and job (Kubo and others 2013; Morassaei and others 2013). The reasons include a combination of unfamiliarity with job tasks or work environment, failure to recognize workplace hazards, ineffective or inadequate safety training, and differential exposure to more hazardous tasks at the beginning of a job (Breslin and Smith 2006; Morassaei and others 2013).

Workers with lower levels of education appear to be particularly vulnerable, possibly because of their greater exposure to physical demands or other hazards (Breslin 2008). Additional evidence suggests that experienced (and older) workers plan ahead in order to limit fatigue and avoid stressful emergency situations much more than do their less experienced coworkers (Pueyo, Toupin, and Volkoff 2011). Experienced workers also engage in more verbal communication with their colleagues.

These findings illustrate the potential benefit to be gained from targeted job training.

## Gender

The gender gap in labor force participation is closing globally. Women's participation has held steady at roughly 52 percent for the past few decades, and men's participation has declined from 81 percent in 1990 to 77 percent in 2010. A wide gap remains in some regions. Women's participation has fallen well below 50 percent in Northern Africa, Western Asia, and Southern Asia (UN DESA 2010). Although women predominantly and increasingly work in the services sector, the proportion of women employed in traditionally male-dominated sectors such as manufacturing has risen.

Injury and fatality statistics by industry suggest that women are at lower risk for workplace injury (Lin, Chen, and Luo 2008, 2011). However, many of these reports fail to account for the differential distribution of men and women among jobs or even tasks within jobs. Evidence is emerging that women are at elevated risk for acute injury and MSD, controlling for job and individual confounders (Taiwo and others 2009; Tessier-Sherman and others 2014). Qualitative research also suggests that male workers—in traditionally male- and female-dominated jobs—have more control over their job and often receive more safety training than do their female coworkers (Kelsh and Sahl 1996; Turgoose and others 2006). Further, research examining gender differences in the performance of repetitive tasks suggests that identical, force-demanding tasks may be considerably more strenuous for females than for males (Nordander and others 2008), which could increase the risk for injury and MSD among women.

These findings, combined with the increasing labor force participation of women globally and the large proportion of women in precarious employment, suggest that future attention should focus specifically on understanding the physical, psychosocial, and training needs of women.

## Age

Among younger workers, differential distribution by type of job, workplace environment, and organizational structure plays an important role in their elevated risk for injury, because younger workers are more likely to work in more hazardous jobs (Breslin and Smith 2005) and are overrepresented in small enterprises, which have limited OSH resources (Eakin, Champoux, and MacEachen 2010; Headd 2000). Moreover, almost half of working adolescents receive no safety training, suggesting that workplaces where young workers are employed pay less attention to OSH (Knight, Castillo, and Layne 1995).

As life expectancy increases, the population ages, and many workers extend their working life beyond traditional retirement age, interest in the consequences of injury among older workers has grown (Smith and others 2014). Although older workers may have a lower risk for injury (Chau and others 2014; Smith and others 2014), they may suffer worse consequences if they are injured, requiring longer periods for recovery and higher associated costs (Pransky, Loisel, and Anema 2011; Silverstein 2008).

However, little is known about the changing OSH needs of workers beyond ages 55–60 years, because most occupational analyses denote 55+ as the oldest age category (Farrow and Reynolds 2012). More research is crucial to inform OSH for aging workers.

## Health

A few reports have linked chronic health problems to occupational injury, but substantial gaps remain in the evidence. Several reports suggest that hearing impairment increases the risk for occupational accidents and injury (Cantley and others 2015; Girard and others 2009). Diabetes, chronic heart disease, and depression may also confer increased risk for acute occupational injury, although the evidence is more limited (Kubo and others 2014; Palmer, Harris, and Coggon 2008).

## Employment Sector

Globalization has subjected the manufacturing sector in HICs to intense international competition. As a result, high-hazard technologies have moved to LMICs, and the services sector has become increasingly important. Although occupational injury is a risk in the services sector, the riskiest sectors are agriculture, forestry, fishing, construction, manufacturing, and transportation. These sectors account for approximately half of the serious accidents at work and the largest share of fatal accidents. According to estimates from the Survey of Occupational Injuries and Illnesses conducted by the U.S. Bureau of Labor Statistics, among the 2.8 million nonfatal occupational injuries reported by private industry in 2012, 75 percent occurred in service-providing industries, which employed approximately 82 percent of the private industry workforce. The remaining 25 percent occurred in goods-producing industries, which employed 18 percent of the private industry workforce (BLS 2013).

### Agriculture, Forestry, and Fishing

Work in the agricultural, forestry and fishing sector is among the most hazardous, and comparatively weaker health and safety regulations, in combination with growing numbers of immigrant workers and a paucity of surveillance data, have resulted in widespread under-recognition of worker injury risk. And although occupational health and safety research is limited overall for this sector, research for the forestry and fishing subsectors is particularly sparse. Recognizing the dual needs for more accurate surveillance data and development and implementation of effective OSH interventions, a formal research and public health practice agenda for this sector is underway (NIOSH 2008).

Agricultural production not only employs the largest number of workers worldwide (about 1.3 billion), but also consistently ranks as one of the most hazardous sectors It has high rates of both fatal and nonfatal injuries and fatality rates several times higher than the average for all industries combined in the EU and North America (BLS 2014; Frank and others 2004; Vijayvergiya, Bohra, and Jhanwar 2012).

Agricultural injuries are less well documented in developing countries, where the vast majority of this workforce is located (Lehtola and others 2008). Even in HICs, which have only 9 percent of the global agricultural workforce, many agricultural accidents and injuries are not captured because of the high rates of self-employment and large number of small farms, temporary workers, and migrant workers.

The unique nature of many farms helps explain the increased risk for injury among agricultural workers. Many farms are small and family owned, with economic pressures fostering use of less-expensive methods and equipment that may increase injury risk. Many farms are also family homes, where children and young adults live and work at least part-time and safety training is likely learned through personal experience and from family members rather than through more structured processes. Farm work is seasonal and labor intensive; workers are exposed to adverse weather conditions and subjected to concentrated periods of work that lead to time pressures, stress, and fatigue, which are linked to increased risk for accidents and injuries. Leading risk factors for agriculture-related injuries and fatalities include operation of farm equipment and machinery, work with animals, work performed at heights, and falling objects (Pfortmueller and others 2013). Tractor use is associated with a large number of fatalities.

### Construction

Construction is one of the most physically demanding and dangerous sectors in both LMICs and HICs. Workers are regularly exposed to ergonomic and safety hazards from manual handling, power tools and equipment, noise, confined spaces and electricity, work performed from heights, excavation, irregular work hours, and exposure to weather extremes. A construction worksite is also complex and dynamic. Often it comprises multiple employers with potentially divergent safety cultures and a high proportion of self-employed workers, adding to the challenge of effectively disseminating safety information and interventions for effective uptake. This sector also employs a disproportionate number of immigrants, independent contractors, on-call or day laborers, contract workers, temporary workers, and young workers—all subgroups with higher injury risk, which presents major challenges for OSH in this sector (CPWR 2013).

In HICs, construction workers have higher-than-average risk for injury and MSD, and the leading causes of injury involve contact with objects and overexertion. More than half of injuries sustained by self-employed workers require five or more days away from work compared to only a quarter of the injuries sustained by workers employed by firms (HSE 2014a).

In HICs, construction workers have a three- to four-fold risk for a fatal accident at work compared to workers in other sectors, while in LMICs the risk is as much as sixfold (ILO 2014b). Even among HICs, however, fatality rates differ, although the reasons for this disparity are poorly understood (Mendeloff and Staetsky 2014).

### Manufacturing

Although the manufacturing sector comprises a diverse array of industries worldwide, the majority of manufacturing jobs are labor intensive. Workers who are engaged in transforming materials, substances, or components into products are at risk for injury from physical exertion; contact with machinery and equipment; long work hours; changing work shifts; slips, trips, and falls (STFs); and new methods or organization that may increase job strain.

The manufacturing sector employs approximately 10 percent of the workforce in both the United Kingdom and the United States but accounts for a disproportionate number of injuries. In the United Kingdom, the manufacturing sector accounts for 18 percent of nonfatal workplace injuries requiring more than seven days away from work and 17 percent of major specified injuries. STFs on the same level (29 percent), contact with machinery (14 percent), and a blow by an object (13 percent) are the most frequently cited causes of major or specified injury (HSE 2014b).

### Wholesale and Retail Trade

Although workers in the wholesale and retail trade sector are generally perceived as having lower risks for injury than are workers in other sectors, many trade jobs are physically demanding, which places workers at risk for back and upper-extremity disorders. Given the large number of workers and continued growth in this sector, a wide range of workplace hazards may pose a risk for injury among a considerable number of workers. In addition, psychosocial and organizational factors may contribute to the burden of injury. Historically, the causes of and potential interventions for safety hazards within this sector have received little attention, but this is one of eight sectors for which a research agenda has been developed to address existing gaps (Anderson and others 2010).

### Health Care and Social Services

The health care and social services sector is a large employer in HICs, with projections suggesting continued growth as populations age. Workers in this sector are mainly female and experience high rates of injury, especially musculoskeletal injury. Injuries resulting from overexertion and STFs are particularly problematic (Bell and others 2008; Collins, Bell, and Gronqvist 2010). Frequent lifting, transferring, and repositioning of patients are leading causes of musculoskeletal injury among health care workers in both acute and longer-term care settings, whereas STFs are particularly prevalent among facility support workers and community health workers (Drebit and others 2010). Because sharps injuries are extremely common among these workers, targeted preventive efforts have been undertaken in recent years.

### Transportation and Warehousing

The transportation and warehousing sector, which enables the movement of passengers and goods via air, rail, water, and road, is vitally important to the economies in HICs and encompasses a very diverse group of workers, jobs, and job-related hazards. The risk for accidents causing human injury and fatality is widely recognized. However, the range of hazards—including

risks associated with the handling of dangerous substances, the performance of physical jobs in isolation, long and variable working hours, frequent need for vigilance, and psychosocial and organizational factors—that combine to increase injury risk among workers in this sector are less recognized. Exposure to whole-body vibration and prolonged sitting or standing, interspersed with the physically strenuous work of loading and unloading goods, increase the risk for MSDs, especially back disorders. The shift in manufacturing from inventory-based systems to leaner, just-in-time production processes has created very narrow margins for timely delivery. Transport workers are also exposed to high levels of noise in and around vehicles.

## OCCUPATIONAL INJURY IN LMICs

According to the latest estimates from the 2013 Global Burden of Disease (GBD) study, more than 80 percent of occupational injury related deaths in the world occur in LMICs (Murray and others 2014), where the death rate is higher than in HICs. Occupational risk factors for injuries are also the leading cause of occupational fatalities among men and women ages 15–49 years (figure 6.1) and the leading cause of disability-adjusted life years (DALYs) resulting from occupational risks in LMICs. Almost half of these deaths and DALYs are attributable to transport injuries.

Covering only unintentional injuries, these estimates exclude workplace violence, which is increasingly being documented in LMICs. Table 6.2 summarizes the literature on the incidence of physical violence in the workplace.

LMICs clearly need to address the alarmingly protracted trend in occupational injuries. However, intricately related factors—economic adversity, competing priorities, resource mismanagement, workforce migration, conflict and internal displacement, and urban-to-rural influx, among other factors—foster a dearth of financial and human resources devoted to such efforts, while crafting an industrial landscape that features a vulnerable workforce. Those factors, in turn, underpin most of the challenges facing implementation of OSH in LMICs. Although some of these challenges are not unique to LMICs, their pervasiveness impedes a simplistic transfer of potentially successful occupational health interventions from HICs. An overview of these challenges follows.

Evidence on the proximal work- and worker-related risk factors in LMICs suggests that they are not substantially different from those documented in HICs. Table 6.3 gives some examples of risk factors.

**Figure 6.1** Mortality Attributable to Occupational Risks in Low- and Middle-Income Countries, 2010

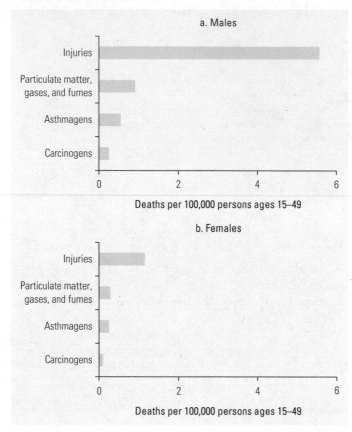

**a. Males**

| | |
|---|---|
| Injuries | |
| Particulate matter, gases, and fumes | |
| Asthmagens | |
| Carcinogens | |

Deaths per 100,000 persons ages 15–49

**b. Females**

| | |
|---|---|
| Injuries | |
| Particulate matter, gases, and fumes | |
| Asthmagens | |
| Carcinogens | |

Deaths per 100,000 persons ages 15–49

*Source:* Based on Global Burden of Disease Study 2013 estimates (Murray and others 2014).

Many LMICs have health and safety legislation in place, but capacity for enforcement is weak (ILO 2012b). A common feature in several LMICs is a slower increase and sometimes a decrease in the ratio of trained labor inspectors to workers. This situation suggests inadequate institutional capacity to enforce provisions for safe work environments, although comparisons over time are limited by the poor quality of the data. Moreover, underfunding of government departments mandated with statutory inspection, as reported in Zambia (ILO 2012a), weakens the infrastructure required for carrying out inspections.

The World Health Organization (WHO) and its partners have called for integrating occupational health with primary health care (WHO 2001, 2012). However, health care workers are too few in number and poorly distributed, particularly in LMICs, where the crisis is fed by inadequate infrastructure, insufficient investment in health care and training, and outmigration of health care workers (Chen and others 2004).

Trade unions can be strong partners and advocates for worker safety. Recent agreements have been signed in the Asia-Pacific region to increase the participation of trade unions in promoting safe workplaces by organizing campaigns and participating in national OSH strategies and plans, among other activities (ILO 2014a). However, trade union density is low in some countries in Latin America and the Caribbean, and Sub-Saharan Africa (Hayter and Stoevska 2011). This situation limits

**Table 6.2** Exposure to Physical Violence in the Workplace in Some Low- and Middle-Income Countries

| Region and location | Study | Study population | Number exposed | Year | Percentage per year |
|---|---|---|---|---|---|
| *Asia* | | | | | |
| Taiwan, China | Chen and others 2008 | Nurses, nurse aides, and clerks in a psychiatric hospital | 222 | 2003 | 35 |
| | Pai and Lee 2011 | Registered clinical nurses | 521 | — | 19.6 |
| Thailand | Kamchuchat and others 2008 | Nurses | 545 | 2005 | 3.1 |
| | Sripichyakan, Thungpunkum, and Supavititpatana 2003 | Health care workers | 1,090 | 2001 | 11.0 |
| *Middle East and North Africa* | | | | | |
| Egypt, Arab Rep. | Abbas and others 2010 | Nurses in Ismailia governorate | 970 | 2010 | 3.0 |
| *Latin America and the Caribbean* | | | | | |
| Brazil | Alonso Castillo and others 2006 | Working women ages 18–60 | 109 | — | 39.0 |
| | Palácios and others 2003 | Health care workers | 1,569 | 2001 | 6.0 |

*table continues next page*

**Table 6.2** Exposure to Physical Violence in the Workplace in Some Low- and Middle-Income Countries (continued)

| Region and location | Study | Study population | Number exposed | Year | Percentage per year |
|---|---|---|---|---|---|
| Mexico | Alonso Castillo and others 2006 | Working women ages 18–60 | 669 | — | 16.0 |
| Peru | Schlick and others 2014 | Children and adolescents attending night school in Cusco | 375 | 2010 | 3.0 |
| *Sub-Saharan Africa* | | | | | |
| Kenya | El Ghaziri and others 2014 | Nurses and midwives | 227 | 2007 | 8.8 |
| Mozambique | Couto, Lawoko, and Svanstrom 2009 | Conductors and drivers | 504 | — | 32.0 |
| | Caldas and others 2003 | Health care workers | 396 | 2001 | 8.0 |
| Nigeria | El Ghaziri and others 2014 | Nurses and midwives | 159 | 2008–10 | 32.1 |
| | Azodo, Ezeja, and Ehikhamenor 2011 | Oral health care professionals in Southern Nigeria | 175 | 2009 | 6.0 |
| South Africa | Steinman 2003 | Health care workers | 1,018 | 2001 | 13.0 |
| Tanzania | El Ghaziri and others 2014 | Nurses and midwives | 146 | 2009 | 22.0 |
| Other Sub-Saharan African countries[a] | El Ghaziri and others 2014 | Nurses and midwives | 85 | 2007 | 21.0 |

*Note:* — = not available.
a. Central African Republic, Eritrea, Ethiopia, Malawi, Namibia, Togo, Uganda, Zambia, Zimbabwe, and others.

**Table 6.3** Risk Factors for Workplace Injury and Violence in Various Worker Populations in LMICs

| Population | Risk factors of occupational injury | Study |
|---|---|---|
| Miners in Zimbabwe | Underground work, long working hours, targets per shift (work pressure), inadequate personal protective equipment | Chimamise and others 2013 |
| Machine operators in Ethiopia | Work pressure, malfunctioning machines, unfamiliar techniques, unfamiliar tasks, failure to wear gloves | Ahmed 2008 |
| Textile factory workers in Ethiopia | Lack of training, sleep disturbance, job stress, long hours, manual work, work requiring visual concentration | Aderaw, Engdaw, and Tadesse 2011; Yessuf Serkalem, Moges Haimanot, and Ahmed Ansha 2014 |
| All workers in a representative household sample in Vietnam | Regular or daily alcohol consumption | Phung and others 2008 |
| Health care workers in Cairo University hospitals | Time on the job | Zawilla and Ahmed 2013 |
| Nurses in Mulago National Hospital in Uganda | Lack of training on needlestick injuries, long working hours, recapping of needles, failure to wear gloves | Nsubuga and Jaakkola 2005 |
| Commercial motorcyclists in Nigeria | Lack of formal education, alcohol consumption | Adogu, Ilika, and Asuzu 2009 |
| Workers in Thailand | Low income, long working hours, heat stress | Berecki-Gisolf and others 2013; Tawatsupa and others 2013 |
| Workers in a commune in Vietnam | Overlapping employment (full-time in industry, part-time in agriculture) | Marucci-Wellman and others 2011 |

*table continues next page*

**Table 6.3** Risk Factors for Workplace Injury and Violence in Various Worker Populations in LMICs (continued)

| Population | Risk factors of occupational injury | Study |
|---|---|---|
| Nurses in the Philippines (needlestick injuries) | Night shifts | de Castro and others 2010 |
| Nurses and midwives in Sub-Saharan Africa (workplace violence) | Risky client characteristics, long working shifts | El Ghaziri and others 2014 |
| Frontline workers in 60 factories in China | Educational level, mental stress, previous injury, working hours | Yu and others 2012 |
| Cleaners in the city council's health services department in Zimbabwe | Lack of preemployment training | Gonese and others 2006 |

*Note:* LMICs = low- and middle-income countries.

the scope for workers to engage in organized action to promote their safety (although high union density does not necessarily mean strong bargaining power).

Employers in SMEs can be an important informal source of information on OSH for their employees. In Ghana, a positive perception of organizational support was associated with a positive perception and practice of safety and a lower rate of injury among workers (Gyekye and Salminen 2007). Yet some employers, especially in small enterprises, have little knowledge of OSH and rarely adopt OSH practices, although the evidence is limited (Hu and others 1998).

Estimating and tracking the burden of occupational injuries in LMICs is crucial but challenging. Many countries lack an acceptably complete system for registering fatalities. The informal sector is usually excluded from the mandatory reporting of occupational injuries, and injuries often are not reported even where formal channels of reporting exist, for example, sharps injuries among health care workers (Hanafi and others 2011; Mbaisi and others 2013; Shiao and others 2009). Health facility data and some national surveys in LMICs collect data on injuries, but these data often are of poor quality or incomplete, failing either to identify their relation to work or to analyze and report on this dimension. Attempts to estimate the global burden are useful for highlighting the problem internationally, but they may not be fit for supporting local decision making or for tracking trends at the subnational level.

The informal sector grew tangibly over the past four decades in many LMICs. In most countries in Sub-Saharan Africa with time-series data, the share of informal sector employment (including both informal and formal jobs in the informal sector and informal jobs in the formal sector) in total nonagricultural employment is rising. A similar trend is seen in Latin America and in Southern and South-East Asia. Notable exceptions are Mexico, South Africa, and Thailand and countries in Western Asia (Charmes 2012). Informality levels also vary, ranging from one-half of nonagricultural employment in North Africa to almost three-quarters in Sub-Saharan Africa (ILO 2002). Some regional differences are evident in the contribution of the informal sector to GDP. The highest level is in Sub-Saharan Africa, where the informal sector contributes almost two-thirds of GDP and one-half of nonagricultural gross value added. Agriculture alone comprises up to 60–65 percent of total informal employment except in Latin America and the Middle East and North Africa, where construction and manufacturing constitute the bulk of nonagricultural informal employment (Charmes 2012).

The relation between informal employment and occupational injury risk is difficult to characterize mainly because of scarce data on occupational injuries and working conditions in the informal setting. Many workers in informal employment are poor, work in adverse physical conditions, and lack social insurance protection and benefits that could mitigate the consequences of occupational injury (Muntaner and others 2010). Table 6.4 highlights some of the risks in informal employment situations.

The few studies on this topic have found that informal sector workers did not have higher injury rates than formal sector workers. For example, a study in Costa Rica reported a relative risk of only 1.06 (Mora and others 2011), while in Nicaragua, injury rates in the informal sector were half those in the formal sector. These reports likely reflect high levels of underreporting among informal workers rather than lower injury rates (Noe and others 2004). In Vietnam, work-related injuries were 72 percent more frequent among informal workers (falling to 45 percent when adjusting for sociodemographic factors) than among formal workers, but the role of chance could not be ruled out statistically (Phung and others 2008). Severe injuries were even found to be more frequent among formal workers.

**Table 6.4** Occupational Hazards Identified in Various Informal Industries in LMICs

| Informal industry | Hazard | Study |
|---|---|---|
| Agriculture | Hand tools (spades and sickles), machinery (harvester and threshers), venomous animals, pesticides, falls, exposure to sun and heat | Loewenson 1998; Mohan and Patel 1992 |
| Street vending | Traffic injuries, fire, assault, weather extremes | Alfers 2009; Alfers and Abban 2011 |
| Textile | Fire, chemicals | Regoeng 2003 |
| Auto repair | Fire, chemical solvents and acids, mechanical injury | Buhlebenlosi and others 2013; Regoeng 2003 |
| Waste management and recycling | Medical waste including syringes, broken glass | Cunningham, Simpson, and Keifer 2012 |
| Welding | Radiation | Buhlebenlosi and others 2013 |
| Carpentry | Sharp tools | Regoeng 2003 |
| Manufacturing | Sharp tools, exposure to sun and heat, chemicals | Loewenson 1998 |
| Domestic work | Violence (verbal, physical, sexual); repetitive strain, household chemicals | Alfers 2011 |

*Note:* LMICs = low- and middle-income countries.

However, the severity of injury was defined by type of health care received. Thus, the finding probably reflects differential access to health care, because case fatality was higher among informal workers. These studies did not account for differences in the duration of actual exposure to injury risk.

OSH in the informal sector is particularly challenging. The magnitude of the injury problem is difficult to measure because of lack of routine mandatory reports. This prohibits injury from taking its deserved position on the list of priorities for policy makers and, in turn, contributes to the shortage of resources devoted to addressing it. Minimal contact with the health and safety authorities suggests that monitoring and enforcing safe working conditions are almost impossible tasks (Muntaner and others 2010). The informal economy, dominated by agriculture, construction, and manufacturing, often relies on low-cost manual technologies. Potentially effective control measures such as engineering controls and elimination or substitution of hazards may be too costly and thus problematic to implement in LMICs.

Personal safety measures, such as the use of personal protective equipment, can therefore be a principal means of OSH in such settings. Workers in the informal sectors reportedly have high levels of knowledge about hazards and personal protection methods, but compliance with health and safety precautions can be exceptionally challenging in the absence of enforcement. For example, 73 percent of the Jua Kali informal sector in Kenya knew that eye injury could be prevented by the use of personal protective equipment. However, only about 12 percent said that they actually used such equipment, mainly because of a perception of low risk and a sense that the equipment interferes with work precision (Chepkener 2013). Similarly, 90 percent of welders in Southwestern Nigeria were aware of protective eye gear, but less than half owned them and only 10 percent actually used them, citing similar reasons for nonuse (Ajayi and others 2011). Among vegetable farmers in Ghana who use chemicals in farming, almost three-quarters did not use protective cover when handling insecticides and about 80 percent disposed of empty containers unsafely (Ntow and others 2006). Sugarcane crushers in India thought that hand injuries sustained during work were just "bad luck" or "God's will," more than 60 percent blamed injuries on carelessness, a minority thought that safe machines were needed, and less than 33 percent indicated that they would use protective equipment even if it were provided for free (David and Goel 2001).

Economic hardship and conflict have long fueled cross-border labor migration and rural-urban migration in Africa, Asia, and Latin America. Temporary workers, farm laborers, female traders, and professionals have been moving between countries of West Africa along gradients of economic opportunity, mainly to Côte d'Ivoire and Ghana and more recently to Nigeria, slowing their pace at times of economic and political crises in those countries (Adepoju 2005). Political turmoil and poverty in Zimbabwe led many Zimbabweans to enter neighboring South Africa, where they found work as farm laborers (Vigneswaran 2007). In Latin America, Argentina attracts the most significant amount of immigration from within the region. The most significant migration corridors are Paraguay–Argentina, Bolivia–Argentina, and Colombia–República Bolivariana de Venezuela. Other corridors of lesser importance are Peru–Argentina and Peru–Chile

(Texido and Warn 2013). In China, rural-urban migration has been on the rise and forms the bulk of internal migration (Wang 2008).

Similar to migrant workers in HICs, migrant workers in LMICs are at risk for social exclusion, exploitation by employers, informal employment, and poor working conditions (ILO 2013c; Marilda and Maciel 2014; Texido and Warn 2013; Vigneswaran 2007). In China, where access to public services relies on the *hukou* system of household registration, internal migrants who leave their place of registration cannot use health insurance and other benefits and services (Mou and others 2013). Rural migrants may lack proper training for the job (Pringle and Frost 2003) and work long hours in poor conditions with low wages and limited benefits (ILO 2011b). Studies suggest that migrant workers in China have a higher rate of injury than do registered urban residents and are more likely to engage in hazardous occupations (Xia and others 2012).

The percentage of children at work—a special subset of informal workers—in LMICs ranges widely from 2.5 percent of children ages 7–14 years in Costa Rica and India to as high as 74 percent in Benin (World Bank 2014). The percentage of working children who do not attend school also varies widely, from around 2 percent to 89 percent, but does not exceed 50 percent in most LMICs. The vast majority of working children are employed in agriculture. Others are employed in a range of industries—fisheries, domestic work, mining and manufacturing, and construction—where adults are also employed, and some are soldiers in war-affected zones. The problem of child workers is waning worldwide but is still alarming in Sub-Saharan Africa, where one in five children is working (ILO 2013b). Child workers are at higher risk for injuries and may suffer greater consequences because their bodies are still growing. Working children often emulate unsafe behaviors of adults, lack adequate safety training, are at higher risk for exploitation, and endure long working hours and minimal pay, often superimposed on a background of deprivation (ILO 2011a). Eliminating child labor remains the ultimate international goal, but a child's work in LMICs can be instrumental for the family's livelihood and sometimes the child's own education. Until child labor has been eliminated, efforts to mitigate hazardous working conditions for children are needed (Siddiqi and Patrinos 1995).

In summary, LMICs bear the brunt of global occupational fatality and disability, yet many lack the resources and infrastructure to tackle them effectively. Challenges related to workforce shortages, compliance of employees and employers with OSH, lack of sound data, and predominance of a vulnerable and hard-to-reach informal workforce preclude the direct transfer of successful interventions from HICs to LMICs. Therefore, progress in OSH is inseparable from overall progress in many domains: economy, governance systems, data systems, education, employment prospects, and social justice. Addressing the problem will require community-based public health initiatives that transcend the traditional well-demarcated workplace, scale up participatory intervention, invest in the local workforce, and improve the quality and use of data.

## THE GLOBAL SUPPLY CHAIN

Over the past three decades, globalization has changed the way goods are manufactured and exchanged internationally. International supply chains offer a flow of materials from natural resource to final product in a manner that is cost-efficient and easily scalable to produce high-quality goods for affordable prices. The supply chain is governed by a focal company, often a multinational, which receives goods and materials from suppliers that use subcontractors to develop raw materials into finished products (Ustailieva, Eeckelaery, and Nunes 2012).

Firms in the EU and the United States have developed global supply chains spanning a variety of industries, ranging from apparel and toys to electronics (Locke 2013). Lambert and Cooper (2000, 70) define the members of a supply chain as "all companies/organizations with whom the focal company interacts directly or indirectly through its suppliers or customers, from point of origin to point of consumption." Many foreign manufacturers of U.S. goods (contract manufacturers) are not just subcontractors; they are supply-chain facilitators, providing U.S. firms with everything from production facilities and engineering expertise to logistics (Eltschinger 2007). One advantage of using foreign factories is the unmatched scalability of their labor. A sense of how globalized the supply chain has become can be gained by considering a Nike cross-trainer shoe: the outer rubber sole is refined in the Republic of Korea; processed into large rubber sheets in Taiwan, China; and shipped to an assembly plant in Indonesia, where it is attached to the shoe (Locke 2013). Intermediate exports grew from US$2.867 trillion in 2000 to US$7.723 trillion in 2012, and the share of intermediate goods as a percentage of total nonfuel exports is 55 percent, the highest in global history (WTO 2013). The number of intermediate goods integrated into global supply chains has reached a record high.

Industrial nations (prominently the United States and EU countries) continue to outsource a significant portion of the goods and services of their primary (agriculture, fishing, and mining) and secondary (manufacturing) sectors to LMICs, creating economic benefits and reducing the number of fatal occupational accidents occurring in HICs (Takala and Hämäläinen 2009). Their integration into global supply chains has provided LMICs with promising economic opportunities and a prominent place in the world economy, while providing HICs with low-cost labor (Rivoli 2009).

Focal companies have a clear profit incentive to acquire low-cost ready-for-market goods. In turn, suppliers contracted by the focal company strive to keep costs low and to deliver products quickly and reliably because of volatility in production orders and intense competition with rival firms. Because the contracted factories in LMICs tend to be under intense economic pressure to deliver intermediate products at a low cost, work-related injuries and occupational hazards persist. In order to respond to large fluctuations in the quantity of production in a short span of time, temporary employment has become very common in factories in LMICs (Smith, Sonnenfeld, and Pellow 2006).

The majority of workers integrated into global supply chains are migrants who move from poor rural areas to the rapidly developing and industrializing urban areas within their country seeking employment with higher pay, because rural job opportunities are often sparse and pay below subsistence-level wages (Welford and Frost 2006). From 1995 to 2000, 79 million migrant workers in China alone moved to prominent manufacturing cities in search of higher-paying employment (Wang and others 2011). Most of these migrant workers are young (ages 17–39 years), have little to no formal education, and lack experience in an industrial environment. Consequently, they tend to have a poor understanding of workplace risks and labor rights. They are placed in the highly hazardous workplaces of construction, mining, and manufacturing often without training, resulting in high rates of injury, sickness, and death at the workplace. The excessive competition for temporary work means that they are reluctant to report minor injuries on the job for fear of losing employment. These subcontracted laborers have one and a half times the occupational accident risk of their full-time counterparts (Quinlan 1999).

This growth of contract work is not a temporary trend. Rather, the number of workers with precarious employment is rising in LMICs, leading to a global gap in OSH standards and regulation (Nossar, Johnstone, and Quinlan 2003; Quinlan, Mayhew, and Bohle 2001). In China, 80 percent of the recorded on-site deaths were of migrant workers (Wang and others 2011). Currently, 50–70 percent of workers in LMICs define their employment as "vulnerable"—work that is low in pay, lacks security and safety, and provides few to no labor rights (Locke 2013).

Additionally, there is little to no professional OSH oversight to ensure the safety of workers, especially among large manufacturing plants in China, where 15,000–20,000 workers are at risk for injury at any given moment (Brown 2007). Moreover, these employees are hired and fired on short notice. This rise in nonpermanent labor has been associated with poorer OSH outcomes in developing areas such as Bangladesh, China, Lebanon, South Africa, and Thailand, as well as Central America (Baldwin 2011). Finally, forced overtime in excess of 6-day, 72-hour work weeks is all too common (Locke and Romis 2007), resulting in increased risk for accidents and repetitive motion injuries (Brown 2007).

Another issue of concern is the limited availability and accessibility of OSH training and education in source countries undergoing rapid industrialization (Ahasan 2003). The occupational health services coverage in China, for example, is estimated to be in the 10 percent range, whereas in HICs, the average is in the 20–50 percent range (Barboza, Lattman, and Rampell 2012). Moreover, the intergovernmental organization overseeing the occupational health services of manufacturers in LMICs—the International Labour Organization (ILO)—has reported less than 1 percent of occupational accidents in nations such as China and India because occupational records in these countries are either nonexistent or inconsistently maintained (Hämäläinen, Takala, and Saarela 2006).

## Regulation of Occupational Health

Fragmented production in the global supply chain has resulted in the establishment of a flurry of regulatory bodies meant to control the OSH and labor rights of each supplier. However, the complexity of the chain often prohibits effective regulation. In the twentieth century, OSH and labor rights were regulated at the national level for many LMICs. The ILO and WHO provided similar regulation at the international level, publishing reports on worker conditions and employment demographics for each sector globally. However, a previous effort to include social clauses within global trade agreements was struck down by WHO when both LMICs and HICs voiced their strong dissent (Locke 2013). Thus, the advent of the global supply chain left a void in the regulation of OSH and labor rights, because authority was dispersed in a complex web of buyers and sellers. Compounding this situation are the economic incentives for governments to ignore factory OSH violations in order to keep the cost of production low (Locke 2013).

To bridge the gap in OSH oversight, nongovernmental organizations (NGOs)—privately owned laborwatch groups—have emerged as so-called regulators of the working conditions of factories by articulating international expectations for OSH conditions, wages, and gender equality. These organizations conduct random audits of factories and publish reports on their performance.

NGOs have been unable to regulate suppliers or the focal company itself. Monitoring alone has had marginally small results, according to a case study by Locke and Romis (2007) that analyzed audits from more than 800 factories in Nike's 51-country supply chain.

A newer development in global supply chain regulation is the notion of corporate social responsibility; the focal company has a direct responsibility to protect the interests of society by upholding OSH and labor equality standards throughout its supply chain. Many multinational corporations, such as Adidas, Apple, Gap, Nike, and Walmart, have defined criteria that their suppliers must meet and then conducted factory audits as part of a yearly report analyzing current labor conditions in their supply chain (Apple 2014; Burke, Scheuer, and Meredith 2007; Gap 2012; Verbeek and Ivanov 2013; Yu 2007). Little research has been conducted on the effectiveness of these initiatives (Ustailieva, Eeckelaery, and Nunes 2012). The paradoxical demand for both high OSH standards and low-cost labor creates conflicting incentives for recording occupational injuries (Brown 2007).

## Common OSH Risks

The distinctive economic incentives and pressures operating in the global supply chain give rise to numerous OSH risks. Although the specific risks are not unique to the global supply chain, the combination of hazards presents particular challenges. To examine the OSH risks engendered by the global supply chain, this section reviews the common sources of risk in the microelectronics and textile goods workplaces, prominent industries using the supply chain of LMICs.

## Electronics Industry

The electronics industry is one of the fastest-growing sectors in the world, with a vast network of suppliers (Locke 2013). Beginning in the 1980s, prominent multinational firms in Canada and the United States, such as Apple, IBM, Lucent, Maxtor, and 3Com, gradually adapted their supply chain management to a new form of outsourcing that granted licenses to suppliers from factories across the globe, prominently China, Malaysia, Mexico, and Singapore (Locke 2013). The contract manufacturers that received the most business were Flextronics, Hon Hai/Foxconn Technology Group, and Jabil, all of which have factories in LMICs around the world (Locke 2013). Many of these companies generate electronic products spanning the "6 Cs": computers, communications equipment, consumer products, car parts, content (e-book readers), and health care products (Ngai and Chan 2012). Today, 75 percent of computer products are manufactured by contract manufacturers as opposed to original equipment manufacturers (Brown 2009). By 2000, the most successful of these companies had production facilities in as many as seven countries, mostly LMICs (Locke 2013).

The magnitude of employment that these contract manufacturers manage can be illustrated by Foxconn: in 2013, it employed 1.4 million workers in China alone (Chan, Pun, and Selden 2013). The common structure of a factory in the global supply chain is a large assembly line consisting of hundreds of workers performing a single 20- to 30-second operation repetitively until their shift ends (Sandoval and Bjurling 2014). This level of repetition is mentally taxing (Butollo, Kusch, and Laufer 2009) and is accompanied by reports of suicides and attempted suicides (Ngai and Chan 2012). The common OSH risks in the electronics manufacturing industry include fatigue resulting from long work shifts and physically demanding work with very few or no breaks and no proper safety equipment (Sandoval and Bjurling 2014).

Serious occupational injuries are common in electronics factories. According to a study that gathered 500 audit reports from 276 factory suppliers of Hewlett-Packard from June 2004 to January 2009, 59 percent of the factories were in violation of legal working hours, 40 percent were in violation of emergency preparation, 32 percent were in violation of hazardous material storage, and 22 percent were in violation of occupational safety (Locke 2013). Of these suppliers' workers, 95 percent were performing repetitive tasks while standing in an assembly line, and most were female migrants (Locke 2013). A similar study published by a coalition of NGOs, referred to as ProcureITfair, found that workers for the Excelsior Electronics plant in Dongguan, China—a computer and digital electronics manufacturing facility for Apple, Intel, and Sony components at the time of investigation—were working for 10–12 hours on a poorly ventilated shop floor and inhaling industrial alcohol, cleaning agents and thinners at the printed circuit board processing area (Butollo, Kusch, and Laufer 2009; ProcureITfair 2008). According to statistics gathered from Shenzhen factories that were released by mainland authorities, an average of 13 workers lose a finger or an arm daily, and 1 worker perishes onsite every 4.5 days (Murdoch and Gould 2004).

Another serious issue is the unsafe handling of flammable materials, leading to deadly factory fires. On Foxconn's campus in Chengdu, three workers perished in a polishing department fire (Sandoval and Bjurling 2014). In Zhejiang Province, a factory fire killed five workers (Murdoch and Gould 2004).

## Textile, Clothing, and Footwear Industry

On April 24, 2013, the Rana Plaza factory building collapsed in Dhaka, Bangladesh, killing 1,129 workers and injuring more than 2,000, making it the deadliest industrial disaster to date (Adler-Milstein, Champagne, and Haas 2014). Just five months before the Rana Plaza disaster, 112 workers were killed in a factory fire in Dhaka at Tazreen Fashions, an apparel supplier for Disney, ENYCE, Sean Combs, Sears/Kmart, and Walmart (Adler-Milstein, Champagne, and Haas 2014). Between 1990 and 2010, 33 major fires occurred in garment factories, as well as 200 smaller fires in Bangladesh alone, injuring more than 5,000 workers (Brown 2010). These textile factories—stationed in poorly structured high-rise buildings—lack safety exits and proper electrical wiring (Adler-Milstein, Champagne, and Haas 2014). Table 6.5 shows a select number of fire accidents that occurred in Bangladeshi garment factories from 2000 to 2006.

The ready-made garment sector in Bangladesh accounts for 78 percent of the country's export earnings (Ahamed 2013). Since liberalizing its economy in the 1980s, Bangladesh has integrated its ready-made garment industry, which includes mass-produced textile products, into the global supply chain, exporting more than US$5 billion worth of products each year (Akhter and others 2010; Rahman 2004). In 2009–10, Bangladesh's knitted and plain-weave garment industries grew 46 and 40 percent, respectively, as a direct result of rising production costs in China for brands such as H&M and Walmart (Jun and others 2012).

A recent study gathered data from audit reports of 210 factories supplying a major global apparel firm that span Bangladesh, China, the Dominican Republic, Honduras, and India (Locke 2013). The study revealed that the apparel firm's compliance program, regarded by private regulatory programs as the most effective in the industry, had an overall compliance rate of 51 percent. The criteria for compliance covered compensation, working conditions, and overtime hours. The worst compliance was found in the factories in South and East Asia, where 56 and 72 percent of the factories, respectively, were not approved.

China has the strongest presence in the supply chain of the footwear industry; 86 percent of all footwear sold in the United States comes from factories in Southern China (Locke 2013). Guangdong is the hub of the athletic footwear industry because of its well-designed ports, access to large numbers of cheap laborers, and lack of government regulation (Frenkel 2001). According to recent publications, work in the Chinese shoe manufacturing

**Table 6.5** Selected Fire Accidents in Garment Factories in Bangladesh, 2000–06

| Date | Place | Number killed | Number injured | Cause of fire | Cause of death |
|---|---|---|---|---|---|
| February 23, 2006 | KTS Textiles, Chittagong | 91 | 400 | Electric short circuit | Only exit locked; fire, suffocation, stampede |
| March 6, 2006 | Industry, Gazipur | 3 | — | Fire panic | Only exit blocked by boxes, smoke, stampede |
| March 2006 | Salem Fashion Wear Ltd. | 3 | 50 | Unknown | Stampede |
| May 3, 2004 | Misco Super Market, Dhaka | 9 | 50 | False fire alarm | Stampede |
| August 1, 2001 | Kafrul | 26 | 76 | Unknown | Smoke, stampede |
| August 8, 2001 | Mico Sweater Ltd., Mirpur | 28 | 100 | Unknown | Single exit locked |
| 2000 | Near the capital | 48 | 70 | Burst boiler | Trapped in locked, burning building |
| 2000 | Chowdhury Knitwear, Norshingdi | 53 | 100 | Short circuit | Fire, smoke, stampede |
| August 28, 2000 | A garment, Banani | 12 | 45 | Unknown | Suffocation, stampede |

*Source:* Akhter and others 2010.
*Note:* — = not available.

industry is fraught with excessive overtime, managerial neglect of OSH conditions, and sexual harassment (Locke 2013).

Much like trends in the electronics industry, contracted temporary work in the textile, clothing, and footwear industries has been growing, leading to dangerous OSH conditions for workers (Nossar, Johnstone, and Quinlan 2003). In a study examining the comparative dangers of contingent work in the clothing and manufacturing industries (Mayhew and Quinlan 1999), contracted employees in the clothing industry had three times the number of occupational injuries as did contracted workers in the manufacturing sector. One possible explanation for this disparity in injury experience is that garment workers are often paid by an incentive system that pushes them to work faster than their manufacturing counterparts, who are paid by the hour, and increases the risk for injury.

## OCCUPATIONAL INJURY INTERVENTIONS

Because working conditions significantly influence worker performance and productivity, optimizing the conditions for improved health and safety has far-reaching implications for individuals, employers, and economies globally. Identifying and implementing effective health and safety interventions at the policy level and in individual workplaces to foster sustainable and safe work environments are important. However, there is no one-size-fits-all strategy for reducing the risk for occupational injury. LMICs are especially diverse in their type and amount of resources, strength of their regulatory institutions, industrial profile, and levels of informality, among other relevant features. Therefore, the range of viable options for a country in Sub-Saharan Africa, for example, may not be the same as that for a country in Latin America. Nonetheless, considering comprehensive solutions that integrate multiple strategies for improving not only primary prevention, but also injury care, rehabilitation, workforce training, and data systems is important.

### Primary Prevention

Given the challenges in LMICs, prevention of occupational injury should consider two distinct but related questions: What is known to work? How can it be applied successfully and sustainably? These questions can be rephrased as technical measure effectiveness versus implementation or program effectiveness.

Because of resource constraints in LMICs, applying the more effective, but also more expensive, technical measures from the top of the hierarchy of hazard controls—elimination, engineering, administration, or personal protection (in order of decreasing effectiveness)—may not be feasible except perhaps in large, well-resourced enterprises. Very few studies have evaluated the effectiveness of technical measures in LMICs. In India, the use of protective eye equipment reduced the incidence of eye injury among agricultural workers (Chatterjee and others 2012), while the installation of mirrors above tandoor ovens showed potential for reducing burns among oven operators in Pakistan (Nasrullah and Awan 2012). These remain very isolated islands of evidence.

### Injury Care and Return to Work

Prehospital, hospital, and ambulatory care for occupational injury in some LMICs is part of the general capacity for trauma care. Although basic health units in the workplace or the community can manage minor trauma, a sophisticated prehospital and hospital trauma care system is crucial for saving lives and mitigating the effect of severe occupational injuries. Much room exists for improvement in such systems in LMICs (Baker and others 2013; Dunser, Baelani, and Ganbold 2006; Goosen and others 2003), but not without resources that could be beyond reach in such settings. In a nonrandom control study, Murad, Larsen, and Husum (2012) reported a lower injury mortality rate among patients managed by field-trained first responders than among those not managed by first responders. Applying a similar approach in workplaces or communities may be an affordable alternative for improving outcomes, particularly in the informal sector.

Access to rehabilitation services following injury cannot be dissociated from the general problem of limited access to quality health services in LMICs. Similar to emergency medical services, there is much room for building and improving rehabilitation services in LMICs (Haig and others 2009; Tinney and others 2007). Data on the duration of disability after injury in LMICs are very scarce, and such data are critically needed for an evaluation of initiatives that aim to minimize disability and enhance early return to work.

### Capacity Building and Retention

Scaling up training programs to develop a competent occupational health workforce, including primary health care workers, needs to be coupled with simultaneous and serious retention efforts. The disproportionate concentration of the health workforce in urban areas is a global phenomenon (Chen and others 2004), but it is accentuated in LMICs by the rural-to-urban influx as a result of poor investment in rural development. The most common reasons for "brain drain" are better remuneration, safer environment, and better living conditions in the receiving country and lack of facilities in the sending country. Adjusting training to local needs—for example, by providing enough training to enable locals to serve their own populations—coupled with efforts to improve working and living conditions, may curb outmigration in LMICs (WHO 2006a).

To overcome OSH resource scarcity, models have highlighted the use of intermediary organizations designed to bridge the gaps between public health and safety organizations and SMEs and to deliver occupational health and safety services (Soares and others 2012). Because SMEs are diverse and often insular, straightforward information is needed regarding OSH initiatives that can offer specific, tangible benefits and be readily adapted to their organizational structure. Through regular interactions with individual SMEs, intermediary organizations may offer the best opportunity to influence OSH decision making, providing short-, medium-, and long-range benefits (Gervais and others 2009).

## Data for Planning, Monitoring, and Evaluation

Effective and targeted prevention efforts are impossible without viable local data. A recent review of an audit of suppliers to Apple revealed that fewer than one in seven recorded any injury or health events in the past year (Apramian and Cullen 2015). The ILO guidelines for improving national reporting of occupational injuries acknowledge the challenges of expanding reporting to cover small enterprises, migrant workers, the self-employed, and the informal sector (Ehnes 2012). Among the recommended solutions are legalizing migrant work and creating administrative connections through which small enterprises are obliged to report to a national database, for example, in the same way they report information for tax purposes or social insurance.

However, more pragmatic solutions may be needed for these hard-to-reach groups. One possible solution is ensuring that occupational injury modules are part of periodic household or establishment surveys (Taswell and Wingfield-Digby 2008). Enhancing routine health information data with identifiers of the relation to work and the occupation and industry of the injured person is a promising approach. Marucci-Wellman and others (2013) tested an active surveillance system that builds on the health information system in one commune in Vietnam and compared its outcomes with those from a range of unenhanced and enhanced passive surveillance models also based on the existing system. Although active

surveillance performed better than passive surveillance, such an approach could be expensive and difficult to monitor and sustain. As a middle ground, passive surveillance that is enhanced with data on place and activity during injury, supplemented with active surveillance in high-risk settings, has been suggested.

Determining whether prevention programs that rely on participatory approaches, particularly those overseen by primary health care workers, could be a suitable platform for active surveillance will be useful. Ensuring the quality and completeness of data is crucial for the success of such approaches.

## Regulation and Enforcement

Governments in HICs protect workers against health and safety risks through OSH legislation, regulation, and enforcement via workplace inspections that may result in citations and penalties. These approaches are often considered the cornerstone of workplace safety and health risk management (Mischke and others 2013; Tompa, Trevithick, and McLeod 2007). However, these policies are lacking or inconsistently applied in many parts of the developing world.

Studies examining the effect of OSH inspections, citations, and penalties have shown varying results (Foley and others 2012; Friedman and Forst 2007; Levine, Toffel, and Johnson 2012). Some evidence shows that inspections resulting in penalties are associated with lower rates of lost workday injuries in the years immediately following inspections (Gray and Mendeloff 2005). Other evidence suggests that penalty inspections extend their influence beyond the injuries closely related to the specific regulations for which citations and penalties were levied (Gray and Mendeloff 2002; Mendeloff and Gray 2005); that is, penalties may prompt employers to enhance general safety efforts and to respond to cited deficiencies (Haviland and others 2010). Verbeek and Ivanov (2013) appraised systematic evidence for effectiveness of basic OSH interventions in settings similar to those prevailing in LMICs and found that enforcement of regulations reduced injury rates.

In the most comprehensive report to date, a Cochrane review assessed evidence on the enforcement of OSH regulations and the prevention of occupational diseases and injuries. Mischke and others (2013) found that inspections likely reduce the risk for injury in the long term, although the magnitude of effect remains unclear. Further, focused inspections appear to have greater effect than more general inspections, although the current evidence is low quality. Unfortunately, because inspections are costly and resources are limited, the enforcement or threat of enforcement fails to reach all workplaces equally.

Additionally, the changing political, economic, and legal landscape of work is creating new stressors and potential hazards with consequences that not yet understood. Although regulations and enforcement activities are designed to protect worker safety and health, employer obligations have not yet been fully realized (Niskanen and others 2010). Given the limited number and unequal distribution of labor inspectors worldwide, more effective mechanisms are needed to translate OSH regulations into widespread practice.

Achieving sustainably safe work environments within the organizational structure of supply chains will require both private voluntary and public mandatory regulation. The involvement of local government can be crucial to upholding proper labor standards and, historically, it has underused its own capacity to impose worker standards on foreign investors in global supply chains (Amengual 2011). However, the fluid, fast-evolving structure of international supply chains means that static governmental law alone cannot sufficiently protect worker rights and health.

Rather, a joint effort with NGOs and government intervention is necessary. An example of such joint regulation involves the protection of the rights of workers in *maquiladoras*—Mexican manufacturing plants that operate in a free-trade zone (Locke 2013). The NGO CEREAL (Centro de Reflexión y Acción Laboral, or Centre for Reflection and Action on Labour Issues), the Guadalajara Chamber of Commerce, and electronics suppliers in this zone developed a dispute system known as the Accord to handle issues regarding worker compensation and benefits. Workers file complaints within the courts of the Accord, and cases are resolved directly with the factory's human resources department, bypassing the slow, often ineffective, Mexican judicial system (Locke 2013). Before the Accord, workers were subject to government neglect largely because of a weak union presence in maquiladoras and a general lack of understanding of Mexican law. Since the advent of the Accord system, workers can file labor violation cases in court and have them resolved within a few months.

## Worker Training

Training workers as well as managers in hazard recognition and control, safe work practices to reduce risk, proper use of personal protective equipment, safety and health information, and emergency procedures is a widely recognized, essential component of OSH programs (Burke, Scheuer, and Meredith 2007; Redinger and Levine 1998).

Systematic reviews of research pertaining to the effectiveness of OSH training found strong evidence for positive effects on worker safety and health behaviors, but insufficient evidence that training alone improves health or safety outcomes (Amick and others 2010; Robson and others 2012). A review of evidence on the effectiveness of OSH interventions in agriculture, SMEs, and informal sector settings did not find educational interventions to be effective in reducing injury risk (Verbeek and Ivanov 2013). However, worker perceptions of safety training may positively affect safety by increasing worker recognition of potential risks, thereby enhancing workers' ability to identify near misses and increasing the likelihood that they will report injuries at all levels of severity (Lauver and Lester 2007). Contemporary learning theory suggests that incorporating structured dialogue and action-focused reflection into OSH training may enhance the effect of training on workers' engagement in safe work behaviors and confidence in their ability to handle unanticipated events safely (Burke and others 2006; Burke, Scheuer, and Meredith 2007).

Given the increasingly diverse workforce and demographic disparities in injury risk, OSH training programs need to target workers with language barriers and low literacy and incorporate cultural and societal aspects to be effective. Failing to address these aspects can deepen the OSH disparities (Steege and others 2014).

## Safety Climate and Safety Culture

A general belief holds that management commitment plays a fundamental role in developing a strong safety climate and culture and that strong management commitment to and support of safety enhance employee adherence to safe work practices and ultimately reduce workplace injuries.

However, evidence showing a direct link between safety culture and climate and injury outcomes is limited. Having a strong safety culture may have a positive effect on workers' use of safe behaviors, injury and illness rates, or reporting of injuries and illnesses, but the evidence is mixed or inconclusive (GAO 2012). A meta-analysis found support for an association between safety climate and safety performance, but also found a much weaker link between safety climate and injury (Clarke 2006).

Subsequent work examined the effect of government subsidies designed to improve occupational safety by changing safety culture. Research found that only half of the subsidized interventions evaluated were deemed successful in improving reporting of hazards, reducing unsafe behaviors, or reducing accidents, indicating the challenge of promoting organizational culture change (Hale and others 2010).

Factors associated with successfully improving safety culture included a planned, systematic approach that generates sufficient energy and support for deployment of multiple safety interventions, engagement and empowerment of workers in the learning and change process, and training and motivation of managers at all levels (Hale and others 2010). Evidence from the restaurant industry suggests that employees' perceptions of management's commitment to safety and safety training are separate dimensions of the work environment, the former a proximal predictor of future injury and the latter a more distal predictor (Huang and others 2012).

### Safety Incentive Programs

Safety incentive programs are popular and widespread, yet little research has been done regarding their effect on the occurrence and reporting of injuries (GAO 2012). Such rate-based and behavior-based incentive programs are intended to entice workers to work safely, but safety incentive programs may discourage injury reporting.

Studies evaluating incentive programs have reported varying conclusions about their effect on workplace safety. Some have reported that rate-based safety incentive programs have no effect on injury reporting (Brown and others 2005). Others have concluded that safety incentive programs reduce injuries (Alavosius and others 2009; Gangwar and Goodrum 2005), and still others have shown that workers whose employers enact policies involving discipline as a consequence of injury are less likely to report injuries for fear of punishment than are those whose workplaces have no such programs (Lipscomb and others 2013). The bulk of evidence is equivocal. These discrepancies may be due, in part, to the widely varying components of safety incentive programs. Some offer incentives for reporting near-miss incidents, reporting other safety concerns, or wearing protective equipment, and others reward work groups for having fewer injuries.

Behavioral interventions such as monetary incentives, praise and feedback, and team competition may reduce injuries in settings similar to those prevailing in LMICs, but the evidence is limited (Verbeek and Ivanov 2013). Effective implementation of behavioral interventions may require a greater degree of organizational regulation than currently exists in LMICs.

### Ergonomic Interventions

Because ergonomic hazards vary markedly between industries and jobs within specific industries, the optimal means to mitigate those hazards likewise vary. Despite this variation, ever-growing evidence suggests that participatory ergonomics may be an effective strategy for identifying and addressing workplace biomechanical, psychophysical, and psychosocial risk factors (Niu 2010); reducing injury and MSD risk (Cantley and others 2014); maximizing the involvement of workplace stakeholders; improving production, worker perceptions, worker morale, and job satisfaction (Dennerlein and others 2012; Vink, Koningsveld, and Molenbroek 2006); and embedding ergonomics within organizational processes (Driessen and others 2011; Pehkonen and others 2009; Törnström and others 2008).

However, critical prerequisites for a successful ergonomics program are a well-established system for identifying and assessing risk factors and implementing solutions; communicating effectively with workers and management; and actively engaging workers, management, and technical personnel in the ergonomics process (Broberg, Andersen, and Seim 2011; Niskanen and others 2010; Pehkonen and others 2009; Zink, Steimle, and Schröder 2008).

Evidence showing a positive effect of ergonomic hazard control on reducing injury risk across groups of workers and jobs has been rather limited and conflicting (Fujishiro and others 2005; McSweeney and others 2002; Palmer and others 2012). However, several studies have reported an association between reduced risk for MSDs and acute injuries associated with manual handling and ergonomic job modification (Carrivick and others 2005; Marras and others 2000; van der Molen and others 2005). A recent report illustrated the benefits of identifying ergonomic hazards and controlling risk for any type of acute injury or MSD among a population of manufacturing workers, and risk was reduced further with each hazard control implemented (Cantley and others 2014). Furthermore, the application of an ergonomics process for identifying and mitigating organizational and psychosocial demands that contribute to both injury and MSD risk at work has been the subject of some recent research (Bentley 2009).

The body of scientific evidence supports the financial case for ergonomic programs. Ergonomic programs have been shown to be cost-effective, particularly in manufacturing, and ergonomics best practices focus on integrated approaches to hazard control rather than on specific ergonomic tools and procedures (Amick and others 2009).

### Other Participatory Approaches

Some countries in Asia are increasingly using action-oriented participatory approaches to deliver OSH interventions, particularly in difficult-to-reach or difficult-to-regulate settings such as small enterprises and the informal economy (Kawakami 2007). Also widely deployed in HICs, this approach involves the target population in identifying hazards and developing and implementing safety interventions (figure 6.2), thus ensuring a more appropriate fit between an intervention and a particular workplace setting. Interventions using a participatory approach could even help eliminate hazards and substitute them with appropriate, low-cost, and safe alternatives. This approach promotes ownership, improving the potential for compliance and sustainability.

In Cambodia, the Work Improvement in Safe Home program focused on home workers and small businesses. OSH trainers mobilized by government, worker, and employer organizations assisted participants in identifying practical safety solutions using a simple action checklist (Kawakami and others 2011).

In a slightly different version in Thailand, primary care unit (national hospital system) staff members were retrained as OSH service providers, assessing OSH risk and giving low-cost improvement advice through participatory group discussions (Kawakami 2007). In Vietnam, the Worker Improvement in Neighborhood Development program has been extensively applied in agriculture. Supported by provincial government officials, farmers were trained to use illustrated checklists to propagate examples of good practice among established networks of their peers. The approach could potentially be used to address child labor in hazardous agricultural work (ILO 2012d). The program has expanded since the launch of Vietnam's first national OSH program in 2006.

A few studies have employed an uncontrolled pre- and post intervention design to test the effectiveness of these approaches. In Thailand, reductions in toluene and carbon monoxide levels were recorded following the application of participatory training in the informal sectors of artificial flower making and batik processing (Manothum and others 2009). Similar benefits were observed after applying the same approach in the informal weaving, ceramic, and blanket-making industries (Manothum and Rukijkanpanich 2010). Knowledge, attitude toward occupational safety, and use or provision of personal protective equipment were improved after participatory training of 525 welding workers in 25 SMEs in China. However, improvements in implementation of engineering controls were inadequate (Fu and others 2013).

## Prevention of Falls from Heights and Slips, Trips, and Falls

Falls from heights are a serious hazard for many workers, especially in the construction sector. Same-level STFs pose a substantial hazard for workers in nearly every sector, but especially in health care, food services, and wholesale and retail trade.

Much has been learned about the causes and prevention of injuries resulting from these hazards, and resources have been developed to assist employers and workers in recognizing and controlling them. However, barriers continue to limit the dissemination of knowledge and use of interventions in the field. For example, gaps in knowledge persist regarding how to use fall protection measures (Committee to Review the NIOSH Construction Research Program 2008).

Management systems designed to ensure the use of fall protection measures have been shown to reduce falls among construction contractors (Becker and others 2001). Implementing comprehensive STF prevention programs that include analysis of common causes of STFs, general awareness campaigns, workplace hazard assessments, changes in housekeeping products and procedures, consistent removal of ice and snow, changes in flooring, and provision of slip-resistant footwear for high-risk employees can substantially reduce the risk for STF injuries among hospital workers (Bell and others 2008). These results

**Figure 6.2** Steps for Promoting Participatory OSH Training in Workplaces in the Informal Economy

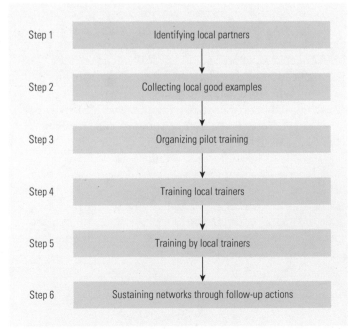

Step 1 — Identifying local partners

Step 2 — Collecting local good examples

Step 3 — Organizing pilot training

Step 4 — Training local trainers

Step 5 — Training by local trainers

Step 6 — Sustaining networks through follow-up actions

Source: Kawakami 2007.
Note: OSH = occupational safety and health.

should be readily transferable to other sectors at similar risk for STFs.

## Sector-Specific Interventions

### Health Care

Mechanical patient-lifting devices have been shown to reduce the back compressive forces on nursing personnel by approximately 60 percent, reduce the lifting required during patient transfers, and improve patient perceptions of comfort (Garg and Owen 1992; Zhuang and others 2000). Working with national and international researchers, the National Institute for Occupational Safety and Health in the United States conducted research into comprehensive safe patient-handling policies involving the use of mechanical lifts and repositioning aids, a zero-lift policy, and employee training on the use of lifting devices. This approach was highly effective in reducing back injury risk among health care workers of all ages and lengths of work experience, regardless of the type of facility (Collins and others 2004). Additionally, clinical use and scientific studies have documented the effectiveness of blunt-tip suture needles in reducing needlestick injuries, and multiple resources have been developed to disseminate this information to health care workers (CDC 2010; NIOSH 2007).

Very few controlled studies demonstrate the effectiveness of different measures in preventing sharps injuries in LMICs. Cross-sectional comparative effectiveness analysis conducted in the Alexandria University hospitals in the Arab Republic of Egypt found that factors such as access to safe injection devices, adherence to infection control guidelines, access to written protocols on prompt reporting, and training on safe injection practice were associated with a lower probability of needlestick injury (Hanafi and others 2011).

Studies on the effectiveness of educational programs elicited inconsistent results. In contrast to an educational program, an official imperative program with monetary penalty for unsafe practice reduced syringe recapping among nurses in the Islamic Republic of Iran (Dianati and others 2012). A controlled study in China and an uncontrolled study in Taiwan, China, among student and intern nurses showed improved practices and reporting of sharps injuries following education interventions (Wang and others 2003; Yang and others 2007). In Cairo University hospitals, education combined with improved access to safe injection devices in intensive care units was associated with a reduction in the incidence of sharps injuries (Zawilla and Ahmed 2013). Countries such as the Syrian Arab Republic also report improvements in injection practice and reductions in sharps injuries after implementation of multifaceted

strategies combining the provision of safe injection devices, development and circulation of national guidelines, education campaigns, and training of health care workers (WHO 2011).

### Construction Worksite Safety

A great deal has been learned about engineering solutions to address major safety issues, including fall protection equipment, nail gun safety, and protection from contact with overhead power lines. However, overcoming the barriers to knowledge dissemination is needed to facilitate wider recognition of hazards and implementation of available solutions (Committee to Review the NIOSH Construction Research Program 2008). Efforts to increase awareness of construction worksite hazards should target vulnerable work groups, including immigrant workers, young workers, and contract workers, who are at substantially higher risk for injuries and fatalities in this sector.

Little research has systematically examined the effect of safety culture and OSH management systems on reducing injury and improving working conditions in the construction industry. However, evidence suggests that when owners, contractors, contractor associations, insurance carriers, and appropriate unions collaborate to establish and promote a safety culture, the risk for injury and fatalities can be reduced.

To enhance the uptake of safety training among the many immigrant workers in this sector, using training workers from representative cultural groups to deliver safety training may be more effective than using professional trainers. To promote effective integration of health and safety management into construction project planning, communication, and control, a project funded by the U.K. Health and Safety Executive developed several integrated tools for use. These include a responsibility chart, an option evaluation chart, health and safety hazard workshops, drawings presenting safety information, red-amber-green lists, health and safety milestones, and a process for controlling design changes (Cameron and Hare 2008; Hale and others 2010).

### Agriculture

Various safety interventions have been implemented within the agriculture sector in HICs, but their effect remains poorly understood. Farm safety hazards in LMICs, where the vast majority of agricultural workers are employed, have received much less attention.

Results from a meta-analysis found no evidence that educational interventions were effective at reducing injury risk, which is consistent with evidence suggesting that training alone is insufficient to prevent injuries. In contrast to earlier reports, limited evidence was found that rollover protective structures on tractors reduced injuries (Lehtola and others 2008). However, the dearth of high-quality studies illustrates the continued need to develop and evaluate farm injury interventions, particularly in LMICs.

National coordination of efforts across agriculture sector stakeholders is under development in several countries, including New Zealand, Sweden, and the United States (Lundqvist and Svennefelt 2012, 2014). In addition, initiatives to address injuries and fatalities associated with tractors and other farm machinery have been developed, including an electronic system to warn farm equipment drivers when someone enters the hazardous zone near their vehicle (EU-OSHA n.d., "Case Studies").

Pesticide poisoning is a major hazard in the agriculture sector in LMICs. Occupational exposure causes unintentional harm, while easy access is a key factor in intentional self-harm. In accordance with expert opinion, the WHO recommends a range of promising interventions regarding the safe storage of pesticides in households, communal storage, training of farm workers and schoolchildren, training of pesticide vendors, and use of community leaders to disseminate information on safe handling of pesticides (WHO 2006b). The effectiveness of these measures is yet to be demonstrated.

Social marketing—the use of commercial marketing strategies to raise awareness and promote safe behavior—has been advocated for tackling unsafe behaviors among young people (Lavack and others 2008; Monaghan and others 2008; Smith 2006). Although they are difficult to evaluate, social marketing campaigns have been associated with a reduction in occupational injuries in Germany (Mustard 2007). The effectiveness of such campaigns in LMIC settings remains to be seen, but the campaigns are probably suitable as components of participatory programs.

### Machine Safety

Worker contact with machinery or equipment presents a major risk for severe injury, particularly in the manufacturing and mining sectors. Some recent risk mitigation efforts include the application of capacitance-sensing technology (Powers Jr., Anmons, and Brand 2009) and the use of intelligent video technology to detect worker presence in hazardous locations near machinery. Although these efforts show promising results for preventing future injuries (Ruff 2010), they are less readily transferable to LMICs.

### Fatigue

Although fatigue is widely accepted as a public and workplace safety concern, critical gaps exist in the understanding of strategies to mitigate its causes and adverse health and safety effects (Noy and others 2011; Williamson and others 2011). Because both work and nonwork activities can greatly affect fatigue, fatigue risk management requires the involvement of employers and workers alike.

Regulatory limits on hours worked are evolving into multidimensional fatigue risk management systems that incorporate additional risk mitigation strategies, such as education and training; regular monitoring of fatigue levels; and systematic assessment of the role of fatigue in accidents and injuries in many sectors, including transportation and health care (Gander and others 2011). Development of effective and comprehensive fatigue risk management systems will require enhanced understanding of the complex relationship between fatigue and safety, because risk may be greatest at intermediate levels of fatigue, when operators may be less attentive (Folkard and Åkerstedt 2004).

### Workplace Violence

International commitment to preventing workplace violence is mirrored in the ILO's code of practice for preventing violence in the services sector (ILO 2003). Most of the proposed interventions apply to service organizations such as health care institutions. Evidence from areas such as government policy and strategy development could apply to other sectors where risks are not clearly defined, such as street vending and domestic work. However, awareness-raising and prevention initiatives still need to be part of participatory occupational health approaches that target all sectors.

### Psychosocial Risk Management

The association between baseline psychosocial workplace stressors and ill health and injury was documented recently among construction and municipal utility workers before the performance of a random control trial of a workplace safety intervention (Bodner and others 2014). The results from this trial will be useful for informing future interventions.

An analysis of data from the European Survey of Enterprises on New and Emerging Risks identified six aspects associated with psychosocial risk management. Establishment size, industry, and country predicted the degree of psychosocial risk management. Larger enterprises were associated with better psychosocial risk management. Manufacturing and construction sectors were associated with the least comprehensive psychosocial risk management, while the education, health, and social work sectors were associated with the most comprehensive. Countries in Northern Europe offered more psychosocial risk management than did countries in Southern and Eastern Europe (van Stolk and others 2012). Although room exists for improvement globally, this trend toward taking systemic approaches to managing workplace psychosocial risks in Europe is encouraging.

### Diffusion of OSH Interventions to SMEs

Much effort has been focused on developing OSH management systems for large enterprises, but similar development, implementation, and evaluation have been lacking for smaller enterprises (Hale and others 2010; Robson and others 2007). Given the barriers to disseminating OSH information to SMEs across many employment sectors, smaller businesses may require assistance from external organizations and other sources to fulfill their responsibility to protect the health and safety of their workers.

To address this concern, several EU member states have launched programs to support OSH in SMEs. Adequate risk assessment is a key component of OSH, but it can be costly and difficult for small businesses that lack resources for the task. To address this problem, EU-OSHA introduced the Online Interactive Risk Assessment (OiRA) project to encourage and help micro and small businesses assess their workplace risks via a cost-free Web application designed for ease of use. Sector-specific OiRA tools are being developed (EU-OSHA n.d., "Safeguarding Europe's Micro and Small Enterprises").

### Cost-Effectiveness of OSH Interventions

Although some evidence highlighting the economic benefits of OSH interventions has emerged in recent years, substantial gaps remain. Existing analyses focus primarily on benefits achieved via ergonomic interventions in four sectors: administrative and support services, health care, manufacturing and warehousing, and transportation. Strong evidence supports the financial merits of ergonomic interventions for the manufacturing and warehousing sector, moderate evidence was found for the administrative and support services and health care sectors, and limited evidence was found for the transportation sector (Guimaraes, Ribeiro, and Renner 2012; Tompa and others 2010). Studies have found that ergonomic and other musculoskeletal injury prevention interventions in manufacturing and warehousing environments are cost-effective and improve health and safety outcomes, and paybacks are realized over a time period ranging from just over three months to slightly more than two years (Tompa and others 2009).

Implementation of a participatory ergonomics process consisting of both proactive and reactive components yielded a benefit-to-cost ratio of 10.6 for an auto parts manufacturer; although the number of worker compensation claims was not reduced, the duration of claims was shortened, suggesting a reduction in injury severity (Tompa, Dolinschi, and Laing 2009). Similarly, economic evaluation of a participatory ergonomics process implemented in a clothing manufacturing plant, which introduced primarily low-cost, low-tech interventions, showed a benefit-to-cost ratio of 5.5; significant reductions in first aid incidents, modified-duty episodes, and short- and longer-term sickness absences; and improvements in efficiency and product quality (Tompa, Dolinschi, and Natale 2013).

Economic evaluations of OSH interventions in SMEs are difficult to find, although SMEs represent a significant force in the global economy and the cost of injuries to these establishments could be catastrophic (Targoutzidi and others 2013). Economic evaluations may be lacking, in part, because smaller enterprises rarely have a separate budget for OSH and routinely collect only very limited OSH data, which makes complete economic analyses quite a challenge (Lahiri, Gold, and Levenstein 2005). In light of research suggesting that each near-miss or non-injury accident costs at least 654 euros (US$740), the infrequent collection of information by SMEs on these incidents suggests inadequate diffusion of information, making the business case for OSH interventions and another gap to be filled (Binch and Bell 2007; Targoutzidi and others 2013). To identify and address factors relevant to SMEs and encourage investment in OSH interventions, Targoutzidi and others (2013) recently developed several case study examples as a tool for SMEs to calculate the costs and consequences of OSH interventions.

If one recognizes that the economic benefits derived from OSH interventions may extend beyond traditional outcomes to include improved profitability and worker engagement, then considering a range of outcomes when evaluating OSH interventions is critical to ensure that the true benefits of interventions are understood (Verbeek, Pulliainen, and Kankaanpää 2009). SMEs often perceive that performing work more safely would be costly. For this reason, highlighting the business case for OSH could facilitate the broader diffusion of OSH interventions globally.

## OCCUPATION AND RISK FOR ACUTE AND CHRONIC MEDICAL DISEASES

There is a vast literature on the contributions that physical, chemical, and biologic exposures at work may make to the occurrence of acute and chronic medical conditions (Rosenstock and others 2005). Indeed, almost every pathological condition has one or more possible occupational causes. Some conditions may have myriad causes, although deciphering the role of workplace exposures in each case is problematic. For others, the consequences of workplace exposures are unique, such as the poisonings caused by lead, mercury, arsenic, and other heavy metals; the pneumoconioses caused by coal, silica, or asbestos; or the rare syndromes caused by dioxins and vinyl chloride. These latter causes can, at least in theory, be diagnosed individually.

Other consequences present as very common, such as chronic obstructive lung disease caused and exacerbated by exposure to irritant dusts, coronary artery disease caused by exposure to particulate matter or workplace stressors, or the more common forms of cancer caused by exposure to several dozen common carcinogens. In individuals with these common ailments, the contribution of work can be assessed only by looking at patterns of disease in the population in aggregate.

However, broad debate continues about the burden of chronic disease that may be attributed to work even in well-studied HICs, ranging from as little as 1–2 percent to perhaps as high as 10 percent (Sorensen and others 2011). Far fewer data are available on LMICs. Moreover, although acute overexposures to toxins are commonplace (WHO 2004), their role in morbidity and mortality is unlikely to approach that of injury, which is the reason this vast subject is relegated to a brief overview.

## Exposure Classes

More than 100,000 chemical substances and numerous biologic hazards are found in workplaces around the globe. The control of occupational disease has focused on three major categories of hazard—physical, biological, and chemical:

- **Physical hazards** include noise, heat and cold, ionizing and nonionizing radiations, and stressors such as vibrations. Although the range of effects of these factors remains incompletely studied, hearing loss (noise), cardiovascular disease (noise, heat), and cancer (ionizing radiation) are the major concerns even in HICs.
- **Biologic hazards** include both infectious and allergenic microbes, highly allergenic plant and animal products such as latex rubber, and agents with direct biologic activity such as tobacco leaves and some pharmaceuticals. In general, biologic hazards pose significant risks for the small fraction of any workforce sensitive to them. They probably contribute little to overall disease burden in either HICs or LMICs.

- **Chemical hazards** include pesticides, organic solvents, heavy metals, fibrogenic dusts, and plastics and other reactive chemicals.
- **Pesticides** include several classes of intentionally biocidal materials. Their poor control is an established cause of substantial physiologic effect on persons regularly exposed and may cause permanent neurological and other effects.
- **Organic solvents** remove oils and grease and dissolve chemicals. Ubiquitous in every metal-working or plastics operation, they are potent liver toxins. Isolated members of the group can cause leukemia (benzene), severe neuropathy (n-hexane), and heart disease (carbon disulfide).
- **Heavy metals** include both naturally occurring (arsenic) and human-extracted (lead, mercury) materials. Many of these materials are extremely toxic, and human epidemics associated with exposure are well described (Dorne and others 2011; Jaishankar and others 2014). The degree to which modest exposures contribute to overall morbidity and mortality, including cardiovascular disease, cancer, and renal diseases, among others, is uncertain.
- **Fibrogenic dusts** include silica—present in every ore and stone—coal, and asbestos. Although coal has proved less hazardous than the others, millions of workers have been exposed to these lethal dusts, which cause lung scarring and cancer. Part of their importance is the enormous economic scope of mineral mining, refining, and fabrication and the general absence of any acute reaction to exposure, leaving many with the erroneous impression that the reactions are little more than a nuisance. In the aggregate, these dusts have contributed measurably to the world's burden of chronic lung disease and cancer, despite progress in control of exposure in most HICs.
- **Plastics and other reactive chemicals**, including dyes, explosives, and pharmaceuticals, are becoming increasingly problematic in LMICs because many workers move from rural agricultural areas to cities and manufacturing environments. The biologic consequences of exposure to this large and heterogeneous class of materials have been studied, but their potential for adverse effects is difficult to ascertain. Although a few members of this class of agents, such as formaldehyde, are relatively ubiquitous, most are associated with specific processes and tasks. For this reason, population-level risks tend to be modest.

## Prevention

Although the fraction of chronic diseases to which workplace factors contribute remains unknown, there is compelling reason to believe that some progress on prevention has been made in HICs. All evidence suggests that high-level exposures of the sort historically associated with acute disease have become far less common in the past four to five decades. This improvement is likely the result of a combination of regulations enforced in all HICs; successful litigation against manufacturers of products known to cause harm, such as asbestos; and a far higher level of awareness of workplace hazards by employers and employees alike, especially in unionized sectors of the workforce. Jurisdictions with reporting laws, including the United Kingdom and many U.S. states, have documented the marked decline in these sentinel cases (Stocks and others 2015). Although exposure to noise, heat, and fine particulate matter continues to be very widespread, potentially adding to the still-high burden of cardiovascular disease, average exposures to metals, pesticides, and carcinogens have improved (Kauppinen and others 2013; Symanski, Kupper, and Rappaport 1998).

The same cannot yet be said for the situation in most LMICs. The picture is clouded by severe impediments to control, with strong parallels to the issues affecting injury control:

- Because HICs have banned certain harmful materials, such as asbestos or polychlorinated biphenyl, stockpiles have made their way into countries without such regulations, a cycle affectionately referred to as chemical "dumping."
- Few professionals are trained in occupational exposure or disease control, and those with training often take advantage of the better employment prospects at multinational companies and in HICs.
- Few employers and workers receive training.
- Personal protective equipment is either too expensive or unavailable.
- Regulations, including social programs such as workers' compensation, are weak, because governments try to woo foreign investors with a so-called "race to the bottom."
- Even where regulations exist, they are often unenforceable because of political reasons or the absence of trained inspectors and laboratories, among others.
- The absence of unions or laws protecting the rights of workers creates difficulty in enforcing safer work practices.

Combined with the dearth of research, the sparseness of strategies for controlling exposure or preventing acute and chronic diseases is not surprising. For this reason, the discussion combines control of these conditions with injury control, for which the need is more immediate, the risks are well documented and recognized, and the available information is at least slightly more tractable.

## CONCLUSIONS

The most effective means to prevent occupational injuries globally is far from certain, and universally effective intervention strategies are improbable. Nevertheless, sufficient evidence exists to recommend widespread implementation of several approaches.

Developing and retaining a competent health care workforce is critical for LMICs. Community-based initiatives to promote OSH in conjunction with public health have the potential for broader reach in regions with few resources for health care workers. Empowering workers to advance change through wider implementation of participatory approaches could speed the identification and mitigation of hazards across many regions and sectors. Targeted and effectively delivered training for vulnerable workers, such as young workers, inexperienced workers, immigrant workers, and workers in SMEs, is needed to reduce the burden of occupational injury among these subgroups of workers worldwide. Efforts to formalize segments of the informal workforce are also needed to protect these vulnerable workers.

## NOTE

World Bank Income Classifications as of July 2014 are as follows, based on estimates of gross national income (GNI) per capita for 2013:

- Low-income countries (LICs) = US$1,045 or less
- Middle-income countries (MICs) are subdivided:
  a) Lower-middle-income = US$1,046 to US$4,125
  b) Upper-middle-income (UMICs) = US$4,126 to US$12,745
- High-income countries (HICs) = US$12,746 or more.

## REFERENCES

Abbas, M. A., L. A. Fiala, A. G. Abdel Rahman, and A. E. Fahim. 2010. "Epidemiology of Workplace Violence against Nursing Staff in Ismailia Governorate, Egypt." *Journal of the Egyptian Public Health Association* 85 (1–2): 29–43.

Adepoju, A. 2005. "Migration in West Africa." Paper prepared for the Policy Analysis and Research Programme of the Global Commission on International Migration, Human Resources Development Centre, Lagos, September.

Aderaw, Z., D. Engdaw, and T. Tadesse. 2011. "Determinants of Occupational Injury: A Case Control Study among Textile Factory Workers in Amhara Regional State, Ethiopia." *Journal of Tropical Medicine* 2: 657275.

Adler-Milstein, S., J. Champagne, and T. Haas. 2014. "The Right to Organize, Living Wage, and Real Change for Garment Workers." In *Lessons for Social Change in the Global Economy*, edited by S. Garwood, S. Croeser, and C. Yakinthou, 13–36. Plymouth, U.K.: Lexington Books.

Adogu, P. O., A. L. Ilika, and A. L. Asuzu. 2009. "Predictors of Road Traffic Accident, Road Traffic Injury, and Death among Commercial Motorcyclists in an Urban Area of Nigeria." *Nigerian Journal of Medicine* 18 (4): 393–97.

Ahamed, F. 2013. "Improving Social Compliance in Bangladesh's Ready-Made Garment Industry." *Labour and Management in Development* 13: 1–26.

Ahasan, R. 2003. "Education and Training in Developing Countries." *Work Study* 52 (6): 290–96.

Ahmed, E. 2008. "The Risk Factors for Machine Injury of the Upper Limb Case-Crossover Study in Tikur Anbessa University Hospital, Addis Ababa, Ethiopia." *Ethiopian Medical Journal* 46 (2): 163–72.

Ajayi, I. A., A. O. Adeoye, C. O. Bekibele, O. H. Onakpoya, and O. J. Omotoye. 2011. "Awareness and Utilization of Protective Eye Device among Welders in a Southwestern Nigeria Community." *Annals of African Medicine* 10 (4): 294–99.

Akhter, S., A. Salahuddin, M. Iqbal, A. Malek, and N. Jahan. 2010. "Health and Occupational Safety for Female Workforce of Garment Industries in Bangladesh." *Journal of Mechanical Engineering* 41 (1): 65–70.

Alavosius, M., J. Getting, J. Dagen, W. Newsome, and B. Hopkins. 2009. "Use of a Cooperative to Interlock Contingencies and Balance the Commonwealth." *Journal of Organizational Behavior Management* 29 (2): 193–211.

Alfers, L. 2009. *Occupational Health and Safety for Informal Workers in Ghana: A Case Study of Market and Street Traders in Accra*. Durban, South Africa: School of Development Studies, University of KwaZulu-Natal.

———. 2011. *Occupational Health and Safety and Domestic Work: A Synthesis of Research Findings from Brazil and Tanzania*. London: Women in Informal Employment: Globalizing and Organizing (WIEGO).

Alfers, L., and R. Abban. 2011. *Occupational Health and Safety for Indigenous Caterers in Accra, Ghana*. London: WIEGO.

Alonso Castillo, M. M., F. Y. Musayon Oblitas, H. M. David, and M. V. Gomez Meza. 2006. "Drug Consumption and Occupational Violence in Working Women, a Multicenter Study: Mexico, Peru, Brazil." *Revista Latino-Americana de Enfermagem* 14 (2): 155–62.

Amengual, M. 2011. "Enforcement without Autonomy: The Politics of Labor and Environmental Regulation in Argentina." PhD dissertation, Massachusetts Institute of Technology, Cambridge, MA.

Amick, B. C. III, S. Brewer, J. M. Tullar, D. Van Eerd, D. C. Cole, and others. 2009. "Musculoskeletal Disorders." *Professional Safety* 54 (3): 24–28.

Amick, B. C. III, C. Kennedy, J. Dennerlein, S. Brewer, S. Catli, and others. 2010. "Systematic Review of the Role of Occupational Health and Safety Interventions in the Prevention of Upper Extremity Musculoskeletal Symptoms, Signs, Disorders, Injuries, Claims, and Lost Time." *Journal of Occupational Rehabilitation* 20 (2): 127–62.

Anderson, V. P., P. A. Schulte, J. Sestito, H. Linn, and L. S. Nguyen. 2010. "Occupational Fatalities, Injuries, Illnesses, and Related Economic Loss in the Wholesale and Retail Trade Sector." *American Journal of Industrial Medicine* 53 (7): 673–85.

Apple. 2014. "Supplier Responsibility 2014 Progress Report." Apple, Cupertino, CA.

Apramian, S., and M. Cullen. 2015. M.R. (unpublished review)

Azodo, C. C., E. B. Ezeja, and E. E. Ehikhamenor. 2011. "Occupational Violence against Dental Professionals in Southern Nigeria." *African Health Sciences* 11 (3): 486–92.

Baker, T., E. Lugazia, J. Eriksen, V. Mwafongo, L. Irestedt, and others. 2013. "Emergency and Critical Care Services in Tanzania: A Survey of Ten Hospitals." *BMC Health Services Research* 13: 140.

Baldwin, R. 2011. "Trade and Industrialisation after Globalisation's 2nd Unbundling: How Building and Joining a Supply Chain Are Different and Why It Matters." Working Paper 17716, National Bureau of Economic Research, Cambridge, MA.

Barboza, D., P. Lattman, and C. Rampell. 2012. "How the U.S. Lost Out on iPhone Work." *New York Times*, January 21.

Becker, P., M. Fullen, M. Akladios, and G. Hobbs. 2001. "Prevention of Construction Falls by Organizational Intervention." *Injury Prevention* 7 (Suppl 1): i64–67.

Bell, J. L., J. W. Collins, L. Wolf, R. Grönqvist, S. Chiou, and others. 2008. "Evaluation of a Comprehensive Slip, Trip, and Fall Prevention Programme for Hospital Employees." *Ergonomics* 51 (12): 1906–25.

Benavides, F. G., J. Benach, C. Muntaner, G. L. Delclos, N. Catot, and others. 2006. "Associations between Temporary Employment and Occupational Injury: What Are the Mechanisms?" *Occupational and Environmental Medicine* 63 (6): 416–21.

Bentley, T. 2009. "The Role of Latent and Active Failures in Workplace Slips, Trips, and Falls: An Information Processing Approach." *Applied Ergonomics* 40 (2): 175–80.

Berecki-Gisolf, J., B. Tawatsupa, R. McClure, S. A. Seubsman, and others. 2013. "Determinants of Workplace Injury among Thai Cohort Study Participants." *BMJ Open* 3 (7): e003079.

Binch, S., and J. L. Bell. 2007. *The Cost of Non-Injury Accidents: Scoping Study*. Research Report RR585. Suffolk, U.K.: Health and Safety Executive.

BLS (Bureau of Labor Statistics). 2013. "Workplace Injuries and Illnesses, 2012." Bureau of Labor Statistics, U.S. Department of Labor, Washington, DC.

———. 2014. "Census of Fatal Occupational Injuries Summary, 2013." Bureau of Labor Statistics, U.S. Department of Labor, Washington, DC.

Bodner, T., M. Kraner, B. Bradford, L. Hammer, and D. Truxillo. 2014. "Safety, Health, and Well-Being of Municipal Utility and Construction Workers." *Journal of Occupational and Environmental Medicine* 56 (7): 771–78.

Bongers, P. M., S. Ijmker, S. van den Heuvel, and B. M. Blatter. 2006. "Epidemiology of Work-Related Neck and Upper-Limb Problems: Psychosocial and Personal Risk Factors (Part I) and Effective Interventions from a Bio Behavioural

Perspective (Part II)." *Journal of Occupational Rehabilitation* 16 (3): 272–95.

Breslin, F. C. 2008. "Educational Status and Work Injury among Young People: Refining the Targeting of Prevention Resources." *Canadian Journal of Public Health* 99 (2): 121–24.

Breslin, F. C., D. Day, E. Tompa, E. Irvin, S. Bhattacharyya, and others. 2007. "Non-Agricultural Work Injuries among Youth: A Systematic Review." *American Journal of Preventive Medicine* 32 (2): 151–62.

Breslin, F. C., and P. Smith. 2005. "Age-Related Differences in Work Injuries: A Multivariate, Population-Based Study." *American Journal of Industrial Medicine* 48 (1): 50–56.

———. 2006. "Trial by Fire: A Multivariate Examination of the Relation between Job Tenure and Work Injuries." *Occupational and Environmental Medicine* 63 (1): 27–32.

Breslin, F. C., P. M. Smith, and I. Moore. 2011. "Examining the Decline in Lost-Time Claim Rates across Age Groups in Ontario between 1991 and 2007." *Occupational and Environmental Medicine* 68 (11): 813–17.

Broberg, O., V. Andersen, and R. Seim. 2011. "Participatory Ergonomics in Design Processes: The Role of Boundary Objects." *Applied Ergonomics* 42 (3): 464–72.

Brown, G. 2007. "Corporate Social Responsibility: Brings Limited Progress on Workplace Safety in Global Supply Chain." *Occupational Hazards* 69: 16–21.

———. 2009. "Global Electronics Industry: Poster Child of 21st Century Sweatshops and Despoiler." *EHSToday*, September 1.

———. 2010. "Fashion Kills: Industrial Manslaughter in the Global Supply Chain." *EHSToday*, September 1.

Brown, J. G., A. Trinkoff, K. Rempher, K. McPhaul, B. Brady, and others. 2005. "Nurses' Inclination to Report Work-Related Injuries: Organizational, Work-Group, and Individual Factors Associated with Reporting." *AAOHN Journal* 53 (5): 213–17.

Buhlebenlosi, F., N. Sibanda, P. Chaurura, and O. Chiwara. 2013. "Occupational Safety in the Urban Informal Sector of Gaborone, Botswana: A Situational Analysis." *International Journal of Scientific and Technology Research* 2 (12): 293.

Burke, M. J., S. A. Sarpy, K. Smith-Crowe, S. Chan-Serafin, R. O. Salvador, and others. 2006. "Relative Effectiveness of Worker Safety and Health Training Methods." *American Journal of Public Health* 96 (2): 315–24.

Burke, M. J., M. L. Scheuer, and R. J. Meredith. 2007. "A Dialogical Approach to Skill Development: The Case of Safety Skills." *Human Resource Management Review* 17 (2): 235–50.

Butollo, F., J. Kusch, and T. Laufer. 2009. "Buy It Fair: Guideline for Sustainable Procurement of Computers." World Economy, Ecology, and Development (WEED), Berlin; Local Governments for Sustainability Europasekretariat (ICLEI), Freiburg.

Caldas, A., Z. Aly, P. S. Capece, and Y. Adam. 2003. "Violence against Personnel in Some Healthcare Units in Maputo City." International Council of Nurses, International Labour Organization, and World Health Organization, Geneva.

Cameron, I., and B. Hare. 2008. "Planning Tools for Integrating Health and Safety in Construction." *Construction Management and Economics* 26 (9): 899–909.

Cantley, L. F., D. Galusha, M. R. Cullen, C. Dixon-Ernst, P. R. Rabinowitz, and others. 2015. "Association between Ambient Noise Exposure, Hearing Acuity, and Risk of Acute Occupational Injury." *Scandinavian Journal of Work, Environment, and Health* 41 (1): 75–83.

Cantley, L. F., O. A. Taiwo, D. Galusha, R. Barbour, M. D. Slade, and others. 2014. "Effect of Systematic Ergonomic Hazard Identification and Control Implementation on Musculoskeletal Disorder and Injury Risk." *Scandinavian Journal of Work, Environment, and Health* 40 (1): 57–65.

Carrivick, P. J., A. H. Lee, K. K. Yau, and M. R. Stevenson. 2005. "Evaluating the Effectiveness of a Participatory Ergonomics Approach in Reducing the Risk and Severity of Injuries from Manual Handling." *Ergonomics* 48 (8): 907–14.

CDC (Centers for Disease Control and Prevention). 2010. *Workbook for Designing, Implementing, and Evaluating a Sharps Injury Prevention Program*. Atlanta, GA: CDC.

Chan, J., N. Pun, and M. Selden. 2013. "The Politics of Global Production: Apple, Foxconn, and China's New Working Class." *New Technology, Work, and Employment* 28 (2): 100–15.

Charmes, J. 2012. "The Informal Economy Worldwide: Trends and Characteristics." *Margin: The Journal of Applied Economic Research* 6 (2): 103–32.

Chatterjee, S., D. Agrawal, A. Sahu, and D. Dewangan. 2012. "Primary Prevention of Ocular Injury in Agricultural Workers with Safety Eye Wear." Paper prepared for the Seventieth All India Ophthalmological Society Conference (AIOC), Cochin, India, February 2–5.

Chau, N., A. Bhattacherjee, B. M. Kunar, and L. Group. 2009. "Relationship between Job, Lifestyle, Age, and Occupational Injuries." *Occupational Medicine* 59 (2): 114–19.

Chau, N., D. Dehaene, L. Benamghar, E. Bourgkard, J.-M. Mur, and others. 2014. "Roles of Age, Length of Service, and Job in Work-Related Injury: A Prospective Study of 63,620 Person-Years in Female Workers." *American Journal of Industrial Medicine* 57 (2): 172–83.

Chen, L., T. Evans, S. Anand, J. I. Boufford, H. Brown, and others. 2004. "Human Resources for Health: Overcoming the Crisis." *The Lancet* 364 (9449): 1984–90.

Chen, W. C., H. G. Hwu, S. M. Kung, H. J. Chiu, and J. D. Wang. 2008. "Prevalence and Determinants of Workplace Violence of Health Care Workers in a Psychiatric Hospital in Taiwan." *Journal of Occupational Health* 50 (3): 288–93.

Chepkener, A. C. 2013. "Knowledge, Attitude, and Practice of Eye Safety among Jua Kali Industry Workers in Nairobi, Kenya." University of Nairobi.

Chimamise, C., N. T. Gombe, M. Tshimanga, A. Chadambuka, G. Shambira, and others. 2013. "Factors Associated with Severe Occupational Injuries at Mining Company in Zimbabwe, 2010: A Cross-Sectional Study." *Pan African Medical Journal* 14: 5.

Clarke, S. 2006. "The Relationship between Safety Climate and Safety Performance: A Meta-Analytic Review." *Journal of Occupational Health Psychology* 11 (4): 315–27.

———. 2011. "Accident Proneness: Back in Vogue." In *Occupational Health and Safety*, edited by R. Burke, C. Cooper, and S. Clarke, 95–118. London: Gower.

Collins, J. W., J. L. Bell, and R. Gronqvist. 2010. "Developing Evidence-Based Interventions to Address the Leading Causes of Workers' Compensation among Healthcare Workers." *Rehabilitation Nursing Journal* 35 (6): 225–35, 261.

Collins, J. W., L. Wolf, J. L. Bell, and B. Evanoff. 2004. "An Evaluation of a 'Best Practices' Musculoskeletal Injury Prevention Program in Nursing Homes." *Injury Prevention* 10 (4): 206–11.

Committee to Review the NIOSH Construction Research Program. 2008. *Construction Research at NIOSH: Reviews of Research Programs of the National Institute for Occupational Safety and Health.* Washington, DC: National Academies Press.

Costa, G. 2010. "Shift Work and Health: Current Problems and Preventive Actions." *Safety and Health at Work* 1 (2): 112–23.

Costa, G., T. Åkerstedt, F. Nachreiner, F. Baltieri, J. Carvalhais, and others. 2004. "Flexible Working Hours, Health, and Well-Being in Europe: Some Considerations from a SALTSA Project." *Chronobiology International* 21 (6): 831–44.

Costa, G., and L. Di Milia. 2010. "Introductory Overview—19th International Symposium on Shiftwork and Working Time: Health and Well-Being in the 24-H Society." *Chronobiology International* 27 (5): 889–97.

Couto, M. T., S. Lawoko, and L. Svanstrom. 2009. "Exposure to Workplace Violence and Quality of Life among Drivers and Conductors in Maputo City, Mozambique." *International Journal of Occupational and Environmental Health* 15 (3): 299–304.

CPWR (Center for Construction Research and Training). 2013. *The Construction Chart Book: The U.S. Construction Industry and Its Workers.* Silver Spring, MD: CPWR.

Cunningham, R. N., C. D. Simpson, and M. C. Keifer. 2012. "Hazards Faced by Informal Recyclers in the Squatter Communities of Asunción, Paraguay." *International Journal of Occupational and Environmental Health* 18 (3): 181–87.

da Costa, B. R., and E. R. Vieira. 2010. "Risk Factors for Work-Related Musculoskeletal Disorders: A Systematic Review of Recent Longitudinal Studies." *American Journal of Industrial Medicine* 53 (3): 285–323.

David, S., and K. Goel. 2001. "Knowledge, Attitude, and Practice of Sugarcane Crushers towards Hand Injury Prevention Strategies in India." *Injury Prevention* 7 (4): 329–30.

de Castro, A. B., K. Fujishiro, T. Rue, E. A. Tagalog, L. P. Samaco-Paquiz, and others. 2010. "Associations between Work Schedule Characteristics and Occupational Injury and Illness." *International Nursing Review* 57 (2): 188–94.

Dembe, A. E., R. Delbos, and J. B. Erickson. 2008. "The Effect of Occupation and Industry on the Injury Risks from Demanding Work Schedules." *Journal of Occupational and Environmental Medicine* 50 (10): 1185–94.

Dennerlein, J. T., K. Hopcia, G. Sembajwe, C. Kenwood, A. M. Stoddard, and others. 2012. "Ergonomic Practices within Patient Care Units Are Associated with Musculoskeletal Pain and Limitations." *American Journal of Industrial Medicine* 55 (2): 107–16.

Dianati, M., N. M. Ajorpaz, S. Heidari-Moghaddam, and M. Heidari. 2012. "Effect of a Face-to-Face Education Program Versus an Official-Imperative Method on Needle Disposal Behaviour of Nurses Working in Kashan, Iran." *Nursing and Midwifery Studies* 1 (1): 3–6.

Dorne, J. L., G. E. Kass, L. R. Bordajandi, B. Amzal, U. Bertelsen, and others. 2011. "Human Risk Assessment of Heavy Metals: Principles and Applications." *Metal Ions in Life Sciences* 8: 27–60.

Drebit, S., S. Shajari, H. Alamgir, S. Yu, and D. Keen. 2010. "Occupational and Environmental Risk Factors for Falls among Workers in the Healthcare Sector." *Ergonomics* 53 (4): 525–36.

Driessen, M. T., K. I. Proper, J. R. Anema, D. L. Knol, P. M. Bongers, and others. 2011. "The Effectiveness of Participatory Ergonomics to Prevent Low-Back and Neck Pain: Results of a Cluster Randomized Controlled Trial." *Scandinavian Journal of Work, Environment, and Health* 37 (5): 383–93.

Dunser, M. W., I. Baelani, and L. Ganbold. 2006. "A Review and Analysis of Intensive Care Medicine in the Least Developed Countries." *Critical Care Medicine* 34 (4): 1234–42.

Eakin, J. M., D. Champoux, and E. MacEachen. 2010. "Health and Safety in Small Workplaces: Refocusing Upstream." *Canadian Journal of Public Health* 101: S29–33.

Ecorys. 2012. "EU SMEs in 2012: At the Crossroads." Report prepared for the European Commission, Ecorys, Rotterdam, the Netherlands.

Ehnes, H. 2012. "Improvement of National Reporting, Data Collection, and Analysis of Occupational Accidents and Diseases." International Labour Organization, Geneva.

El Ghaziri, M., S. Zhu, J. Lipscomb, and B. A. Smith. 2014. "Work Schedule and Client Characteristics Associated with Workplace Violence Experience among Nurses and Midwives in Sub-Saharan Africa." *Journal of the Association of Nurses in AIDS Care* 25 (Suppl 1): S79–89.

Eltschinger, C. 2007. *Source Code China: The New Global Hub of IT Outsourcing.* Hoboken, NJ: John Wiley and Sons.

EU-OSHA (European Agency for Safety and Health at Work). n.d. "Case Studies: Driver Assistant System." EU-OSHA, Luxembourg. http://archive.beswic.be/data/case-studies/driver-assistant-system/Driver-assistant-system.pdf.

———. n.d. "Safeguarding Europe's Micro and Small Enterprises: The Development of the Online Interactive Risk Assessment Tool." EU-OSHA, Luxembourg. http://www.oiraproject.eu.

———. 2007. *Expert Forecast on Emerging Psychosocial Risks Related to Occupational Safety and Health.* Luxembourg: Office for Official Publications of the European Communities.

Eurofound. 2010. "European Working Conditions Survey (EWCS): 2010." European Foundation for the Improvement of Living and Working Conditions, Dublin.

Fabiano, B., F. Currò, and R. Pastorino. 2004. "A Study of the Relationship between Occupational Injuries and Firm Size and Type in the Italian Industry." *Safety Science* 42 (7): 587–600.

Farrow, A., and F. Reynolds. 2012. "Health and Safety of the Older Worker." *Occupational Medicine* 62 (1): 4–11.

Foley, M., Z. J. Fan, E. Rauser, and B. Silverstein. 2012. "The Impact of Regulatory Enforcement and Consultation Visits on Workers' Compensation Claims, Incidence Rates, and

Costs, 1999–2008." *American Journal of Industrial Medicine* 55 (11): 976–90.

Folkard, S., and T. Åkerstedt. 2004. "Trends in the Risk of Accidents and Injuries and Their Implications for Models of Fatigue and Performance." *Aviation, Space, and Environmental Medicine* 75 (3): A161–67.

Folkard, S., and D. A. Lombardi. 2006. "Modeling the Impact of the Components of Long Work Hours on Injuries and 'Accidents.'" *American Journal of Industrial Medicine* 49 (11): 953–63.

Folkard, S., and P. Tucker. 2003. "Shift Work, Safety, and Productivity." *Occupational Medicine* 53 (2): 95–101.

Frank, A. L., R. McKnight, S. R. Kirkhorn, and P. Gunderson. 2004. "Issues of Agricultural Safety and Health." *Annual Review of Public Health* 25 (1): 225–45.

Frenkel, S. J. 2001. "Globalization, Athletic Footwear Commodity Chains, and Employment Relations in China." *Organization Studies* 22 (4): 531–62.

Friedman, L. S., and L. Forst. 2007. "The Impact of OSHA Recordkeeping Regulation Changes on Occupational Injury and Illness Trends in the U.S.: A Time-Series Analysis." *Occupational and Environmental Medicine* 64 (7): 454–60.

Fu, C., M. Zhu, T. S. Yu, and Y. He. 2013. "Effectiveness of Participatory Training on Improving Occupational Health in Small and Medium Enterprises in China." *International Journal of Occupational and Environmental Health* 19 (2): 85–90.

Fujishiro, K., J. L. Weaver, C. A. Heaney, C. A. Hamrick, and W. S. Marras. 2005. "The Effect of Ergonomic Interventions in Healthcare Facilities on Musculoskeletal Disorders." *American Journal of Industrial Medicine* 48 (5): 338–47.

Gander, P., L. Hartley, D. Powell, P. Cabon, E. Hitchcock, and others. 2011. "Fatigue Risk Management: Organizational Factors at the Regulatory and Industry/Company Level." *Accident Analysis and Prevention* 43 (2): 573–90.

Gangwar, M., and P. Goodrum. 2005. "The Effect of Time on Safety Incentive Programs in the U.S. Construction Industry." *Construction Management and Economics* 23 (8): 851–59.

GAO (Government Accountability Office). 2012. "Workplace Safety and Health: Better Guidance Needed on Safety Incentive Programs." U.S. GAO, Washington, DC.

Gap. 2012. "Gap Inc. 2011 / 2012 Social and Environmental Responsibility Report." Gap Inc., San Francisco, CA.

Garg, A., and B. Owen. 1992. "Reducing Back Stress to Nursing Personnel: An Ergonomic Intervention in a Nursing Home." *Ergonomics* 35 (11): 1353–75.

Gervais, R. L., Z. Pawlowska, A. Kouvonen, M. Karanika-Murray, K. Van den Broek, and others. 2009. "Occupational Safety and Health and Economic Performance in Small and Medium-Sized Enterprises: A Review." Working Environment Information Working Paper, European Agency for Safety and Health at Work, Bilbao, Spain.

Ghaffari, M., A. Alipour, A. A. Farshad, I. Jensen, M. Josephson, and others. 2008. "Effect of Psychosocial Factors on Low Back Pain in Industrial Workers." *Occupational Medicine* 58 (5): 341–47.

Girard, S. A., M. Picard, A. C. Davis, M. Simard, R. Larocque, and others. 2009. "Multiple Work-Related Accidents: Tracing the Role of Hearing Status and Noise Exposure." *Occupational and Environmental Medicine* 66 (5): 319–24.

Glasscock, D. J., K. Rasmussen, O. Carstensen, and O. N. Hansen. 2006. "Psychosocial Factors and Safety Behaviour as Predictors of Accidental Work Injuries in Farming." *Work and Stress* 20 (2): 173–89.

Gonese, E., R. Matchaba-Hove, G. Chirimumba, Z. Hwalima, J. Chirenda, and others. 2006. "Occupational Injuries among Workers in the Cleansing Section of the City Council's Health Services Department: Bulawayo, Zimbabwe, 2001–2002." *Morbidity and Mortality Weekly Report* 55 (Suppl 1): 7–10.

Goosen, J., D. M. Bowley, E. Degiannis, and F. Plani. 2003. "Trauma Care Systems in South Africa." *Injury* 34 (9): 704–8.

Gray, W., and J. Mendeloff. 2002. "The Declining Effects of OSHA Inspections in Manufacturing, 1979–1998." Working Paper 9119, National Bureau of Economic Research, Cambridge, MA.

———. 2005. "The Declining Effects of OSHA Inspections of Manufacturing Injuries, 1979–1998." *Industrial and Labor Relations Review* 58 (4): 571–87.

Green, F. 2005. *Demanding Work.* Princeton, NJ: Princeton University Press.

Guimaraes, L. B., J. L. Ribeiro, and J. S. Renner. 2012. "Cost-Benefit Analysis of a Socio-Technical Intervention in a Brazilian Footwear Company." *Applied Ergonomics* 43 (5): 948–57.

Gyekye, S. A., and S. Salminen. 2007. "Workplace Safety Perceptions and Perceived Organizational Support: Do Supportive Perceptions Influence Safety Perceptions?" *International Journal of Occupational Safety and Ergonomics* 13 (2): 189–200.

Haig, A. J., J. Im, D. Adewole, V. Nelson, and B. Krabak. 2009. "The Practice of Physical and Rehabilitation Medicine in Sub-Saharan Africa and Antarctica: A White Paper or a Black Mark?" *Journal of Rehabilitation Medicine* 41 (6): 401–5.

Hale, A. R., F. W. Guldenmund, P. L. C. H. van Loenhout, and J. I. H. Oh. 2010. "Evaluating Safety Management and Culture Interventions to Improve Safety: Effective Intervention Strategies." *Safety Science* 48 (8): 1026–35.

Hämäläinen, P., J. Takala, and K. L. Saarela. 2006. "Global Estimates of Occupational Accidents." *Safety Science* 44 (2): 137–56.

Hämmig, O., M. Knecht, T. Läubli, and G. F. Bauer. 2011. "Work-Life Conflict and Musculoskeletal Disorders: A Cross-Sectional Study of an Unexplored Association." *BMC Musculoskeletal Disorders* 12 (1): 60–71.

Hanafi, M. I., A. M. Mohamed, M. S. Kassem, and M. Shawki. 2011. "Needlestick Injuries among Health Care Workers of University of Alexandria Hospitals." *Eastern Mediterranean Health Journal* 17 (1): 26–35.

Hasle, P., and H. J. Limborg. 2006. "A Review of the Literature on Preventive Occupational Health and Safety Activities in Small Enterprises." *Industrial Health* 44 (1): 6–12.

Haviland, A., R. Burns, W. Gray, T. Ruder, and J. Mendeloff. 2010. "What Kinds of Injuries Do OSHA Inspections Prevent?" *Journal of Safety Research* 41 (4): 339–45.

Hayter, S., and V. Stoevska. 2011. "Social Dialogue Indicators: International Statistical Inquiry 2008–09; Technical Brief." International Labour Organization, Geneva.

Headd, B. 2000. "The Characteristics of Small Business Enterprises." *Monthly Labor Review* 123 (4): 13–18.

HSE (Health and Safety Executive). 2014a. "Health and Safety in Construction in Great Britain, 2014." HSE, London.

———. 2014b. "Health and Safety in Manufacturing in Great Britain, 2014." HSE, London.

Hu, S. C., C. C. Lee, J. S. Shiao, and Y. L. Guo. 1998. "Employers' Awareness and Compliance with Occupational Health and Safety Regulations in Taiwan." *Occupational Medicine (London)* 48 (1): 17–22.

Huang, Y.-H., S. K. Verma, W.-R. Chang, T. K. Courtney, D. A. Lombardi, and others. 2012. "Management Commitment to Safety vs. Employee Perceived Safety Training and Association with Future Injury." *Accident Analysis and Prevention* 47: 94–101.

ILO (International Labour Organization). 2002. "Women and Men in the Informal Economy: A Statistical Picture." ILO, Geneva.

———. 2003. "Code of Practice on Workplace Violence in Services Sectors and Measures to Combat the Phenomenon." ILO, Geneva.

———. 2011a. "Children in Hazardous Work: What We Know, What We Need to Do." ILO, International Programme on the Elimination of Child Labour, Geneva.

———. 2011b. "Promoting Decent Employment for Rural Migrant Workers." ILO, Geneva.

———. 2012a. "Decent Work Country Profile: Zambia." ILO, Geneva.

———. 2012b. "Decent Work Indicators in Africa: A First Assessment Based on National Sources." ILO, Geneva.

———. 2012c. "Global Employment Trends 2012: World Faces a 600 Million Jobs Challenge, Warns ILO." ILO, Geneva.

———. 2012d. "Practices with Good Potential: Towards the Elimination of Hazardous Child Labour." International Programme on the Elimination of Child Labour (IPEC), ILO, Geneva.

———. 2013a. "ILO Calls for Urgent Global Action to Fight Occupational Diseases." ILO, Geneva.

———. 2013b. "Marking Progress against Child Labour: Global Estimates and Trends 2000–2012." IPEC, ILO, Geneva.

———. 2013c. "Rural-Urban Migrants Employed in Domestic Work: Issues and Challenges." Paper prepared for ILO forum "Making Decent Work a Reality for Domestic Workers in Africa: A Regional Knowledge Sharing Forum," 1–5. International Labor Office, Dar es Salaam, May 28–30.

———. 2014a. "ILO-ACTRAV Symposium: Role of Trade Unions in the Promotion of OSH in Asia-Pacific." ILO, Geneva.

———. 2014b. "Safety and Health in the Construction Sector: Overcoming the Challenges." Webinar, ILO, Geneva, November 7. http://www.ilo.org/empent/Eventsandmeetings/WCMS_310993/lang--en/index.htm.

ISSA (International Social Security Association). 2014. "Towards a Global Culture of Prevention: Working Conditions Have a Major and Direct Impact on the Health and Well-Being of Workers." ISSA, Geneva. http://www.issa.int/topics/occupational-risks/introduction.

Jaishankar, M., T. Tseten, N. Anbalagan, B. B. Mathew, and K. N. Beeregowda. 2014. "Toxicity, Mechanism, and Health Effects of Some Heavy Metals." *Interdisciplinary Toxicology* 7 (2): 60–72.

Jansen, N. W. H., D. C. L. Mohren, L. G. P. M. van Amelsvoort, N. Janssen, and I. Kant. 2010. "Changes in Working Time Arrangements over Time as a Consequence of Work-Family Conflict." *Chronobiology International* 27 (5): 1045–61.

Jun, M., W. Jingjing, M. Collins, W. Malei, S. Orlins, and others. 2012. "Sustainable Apparel's Critical Blind Spot." Friends of Nature, Institute of Public and Environmental Affairs, Green Beagle, Envirofriends, and Nanjing Green Stone, Beijing.

Kamchuchat, C., V. Chongsuvivatwong, S. Oncheunjit, T. W. Yip, and R. Sangthong. 2008. "Workplace Violence Directed at Nursing Staff at a General Hospital in Southern Thailand." *Journal of Occupational Health* 50 (2): 201–7.

Kauppinen, T., S. Uuksulainen, A. Saalo, and I. Mäkinen. 2013. "Trends of Occupational Exposure to Chemical Agents in Finland in 1950–2020." *Annals of Occupational Hygiene* 57 (5): 593–609.

Kawakami, T. 2007. "Participatory Approaches to Improving Safety, Health, and Working Conditions in Informal Economy Workplaces: Experiences of Cambodia, Thailand, and Vietnam." Subregional Office for East Asia, International Labour Organization, Bangkok.

Kawakami, T., L. Tong, Y. Kannitha, and T. Sophorn. 2011. "Participatory Approach to Improving Safety, Health, and Working Conditions in Informal Economy Workplaces in Cambodia." *Work* 38 (3): 235–40.

Kelsh, M. A., and J. D. Sahl. 1996. "Sex Differences in Work-Related Injury Rates among Electric Utility Workers." *American Journal of Epidemiology* 143 (10): 1050–58.

Kim, H.-C., J.-Y. Min, K.-B. Min, and S.-G. Park. 2009. "Job Strain and the Risk for Occupational Injury in Small- to Medium-Sized Manufacturing Enterprises: A Prospective Study of 1,209 Korean Employees." *American Journal of Industrial Medicine* 52 (4): 322–30.

Knight, E. B., D. N. Castillo, and L. A. Layne. 1995. "A Detailed Analysis of Work-Related Injury among Youth Treated in Emergency Departments." *American Journal of Industrial Medicine* 27 (6): 793–805.

Kraemer, B. 2010. "Impact of Economic Crisis on Occupational Health and Safety Management." Institute of Economic and Social Research (WSI), Dusseldorf.

Kubo, J,. M. R. Cullen, L. Cantley, M. Slade, B. Tessier-Sherman, and others. 2013. "Piecewise Exponential Models to Assess the Influence of Job-Specific Experience on the Hazard of Acute Injury for Hourly Factory Workers." *BMC Medical Research and Methodology* 13: 89.

Kubo, J., B. A. Goldstein, L. F. Cantley, B. Tessier-Sherman, D. Galusha, and others. 2014. "Contribution of Health Status and Prevalent Chronic Disease to Individual Risk for Workplace Injury in the Manufacturing Environment." *Occupational and Environmental Medicine* 71 (3): 159–66.

Lahiri, S., J. Gold, and C. Levenstein. 2005. "Net-Cost Model for Workplace Interventions." *Journal of Safety Research* 36 (3): 241–55.

Lambert, D. M., and M. C. Cooper. 2000. "Issues in Supply Chain Management." *Industrial Marketing Management* 29: 65–83.

Lapointe, J. M., C. E. P. Dionne, C. P. Brisson, and S. P. Montreuil. 2009. "Interaction between Postural Risk Factors and Job Strain on Self-Reported Musculoskeletal Symptoms among Users of Video Display Units: A Three-Year Prospective Study." *Scandinavian Journal of Work, Environment, and Health* 35 (2): 134–44.

Lauver, K. J., and S. W. Lester. 2007. "Get Safety Problems to the Surface: Using Human Resource Practices to Improve Injury Reporting." *Journal of Leadership and Organizational Studies* 14 (2): 168–79.

Lavack, A. M., S. L. Magnuson, S. Deshpande, D. Z. Basil, M. D. Basil, and others. 2008. "Enhancing Occupational Health and Safety in Young Workers: The Role of Social Marketing." *International Journal of Nonprofit and Voluntary Sector Marketing* 13 (3): 193–204.

Lehtola, M. M., R. H. Rautiainen, L. M. Day, E. Schonstein, J. Suutarinen, and others. 2008. "Effectiveness of Interventions in Preventing Injuries in Agriculture: A Systematic Review and Meta-Analysis." *Scandinavian Journal of Work, Environment, and Health* 34 (5): 327–36.

Leigh, J. P., and J. P. Marcin. 2012. "Workers' Compensation Benefits and Shifting Costs for Occupational Injury and Illness." *Journal of Occupational and Environmental Medicine* 54 (4): 445–50.

Levine, D. I., M. W. Toffel, and M. S. Johnson. 2012. "Randomized Government Safety Inspections Reduce Worker Injuries with No Detectable Job Loss." *Science* 336 (6083): 907–11.

Lin, Y.-H., C.-Y. Chen, and J.-L. Luo. 2008. "Gender and Age Distribution of Occupational Fatalities in Taiwan." *Accident Analysis and Prevention* 40 (4): 1604–10.

———. 2011. "Statistical Analysis of Fatalities in Construction Workers." *Journal of Occupational Safety and Health* 19: 75–85.

Lippel, K. 2005. "Precarious Employment and Occupational Health and Safety Regulation in Quebec." In *Precarious Employment: Understanding Labour Market Insecurity in Canada*, edited by L. F. Vosko, 241–55. Montreal: McGill-Queen's University Press.

Lipscomb, H. J., J. Nolan, D. Patterson, V. Sticca, and D. J. Myers. 2013. "Safety, Incentives, and the Reporting of Work-Related Injuries among Union Carpenters: 'You're Pretty Much Screwed If You Get Hurt at Work.'" *American Journal of Industrial Medicine* 56 (4): 389–99.

Locke, R. M. 2013. *The Promise and Limits of Private Power: Promoting Labor Standards in a Global Economy.* New York: Cambridge University Press.

Locke, R. M., and M. Romis. 2007. "Improving Work Conditions in a Global Supply Chain." *MIT Sloan Management Review* 48 (Winter): 54–62.

Loewenson, R. H. 1998. "Health Impact of Occupational Risks in the Informal Sector in Zimbabwe." *International Journal of Occupational and Environmental Health* 4 (4): 264–74.

Lombardi, D. A., S. Folkard, J. L. Willetts, and G. S. Smith. 2010. "Daily Sleep, Weekly Working Hours, and Risk of Work-Related Injury: U.S. National Health Interview Survey (2004–2008)." *Chronobiology International* 27 (5): 1013–30.

Lundqvist, P., and C. A. Svennefelt. 2012. "Health and Safety Strategy in Swedish Agriculture." *Work* 41 (Suppl 1): 5304–7.

———. 2014. "Swedish Strategies for Health and Safety in Agriculture: A Coordinated Multiagency Approach." *Work* 49 (1): 33–37.

Magnavita, N., M. Elovainio, I. De Nardis, T. Heponiemi, and A. Bergamaschi. 2011. "Environmental Discomfort and Musculoskeletal Disorders." *Occupational Medicine* 61 (3): 196–201.

Manothum, A., and J. Rukijkanpanich. 2010. "A Participatory Approach to Health Promotion for Informal Sector Workers in Thailand." *Journal of Injury and Violence Research* 2 (2): 111–20.

Manothum, A., J. Rukijkanpanich, D. Thawesaengskulthai, B. Thampitakkul, C. Chaikittiporn, and others. 2009. "A Participatory Model for Improving Occupational Health and Safety: Improving Informal Sector Working Conditions in Thailand." *International Journal of Occupational and Environmental Health* 15 (3): 305–14.

Marilda, M., and C. Maciel. 2014. "Strikes in Sugarcane Mills: The Forms of Resistance of Migrant Workers in Brazil." Paper prepared for the Fourth RUFORUM Biennial Regional Conference, Maputo, Mozambique, July 19–24.

Marras, W. S., W. G. Allread, D. L. Burr, and F. A. Fathallah. 2000. "Prospective Validation of a Low-Back Disorder Risk Model and Assessment of Ergonomic Interventions Associated with Manual Materials Handling Tasks." *Ergonomics* 43 (11): 1866–86.

Marucci-Wellman, H., T. B. Leamon, J. L. Willetts, T. T. Binh, N. B. Diep, and others. 2011. "Occupational Injuries in a Commune in Rural Vietnam Transitioning from Agriculture to New Industries." *American Journal of Public Health* 101 (5): 854–60.

Marucci-Wellman, H., D. H. Wegman, T. B. Leamon, T. T. Binh, N. B. Diep, and others. 2013. "Work-Related Injury Surveillance in Vietnam: A National Reporting System Model." *American Journal of Public Health* 103 (11): 1989–96.

Mayhew, C., and M. Quinlan. 1999. "The Effects of Outsourcing on Occupational Health and Safety: A Comparative Study of Factory-Based Workers and Outworkers in the Australian Clothing Industry." *International Journal of Health Services* 29 (1): 83–107.

Mbaisi, E. M., Z. Ng'ang'a, P. Wanzala, and J. Omolo. 2013. "Prevalence and Factors Associated with Percutaneous Injuries and Splash Exposures among Health-Care Workers in a Provincial Hospital, Kenya, 2010." *Pan African Medical Journal* 14: 10.

McKay, S., M. Craw, and D. Chopra. 2006. *Migrant Workers in England and Wales: An Assessment of Migrant Worker Health and Safety Risks.* London: Health and Safety Executive.

McSweeney, K. P., B. N. Craig, J. J. Congleton, and D. Miller. 2002. "Ergonomic Program Effectiveness: Ergonomic and

Medical Intervention." *International Journal of Occupational and Safety Ergonomics* 8 (4): 433–49.

Mendeloff, J., and W. B. Gray. 2005. "Inside the Black Box: How Do OSHA Inspections Lead to Reductions in Workplace Injuries?" *Law and Policy* 27 (2): 219–37.

Mendeloff, J., and L. Staetsky. 2014. "Occupational Fatality Risks in the United States and the United Kingdom." *American Journal of Industrial Medicine* 57 (1): 4–14.

Mischke, C., J. H. Verbeek, J. C. Job, T. C. Morata, A. Alvesalo-Kuusi, and others. 2013. "Occupational Safety and Health Enforcement Tools for Preventing Occupational Diseases and Injuries." *Cochrane Database of Systematic Reviews* 8: CD010183.

Mohan, D., and R. Patel. 1992. "Design of Safer Agricultural Equipment: Application of Ergonomics and Epidemiology." *International Journal of Industrial Ergonomics* 10 (4): 301–9.

Monaghan, P. F., C. A. Bryant, J. A. Baldwin, Y. Zhu, B. Ibrahimou, and others. 2008. "Using Community-Based Prevention Marketing to Improve Farm Worker Safety." *Social Marketing Quarterly* 14 (4): 71–87.

Mora, A. M., M. G. Mora-Mora, T. Partanen, and C. Wesseling. 2011. "Registration of Fatal Occupational Injuries in Costa Rica, 2005–2006." *International Journal of Occupational and Environmental Health* 17 (3): 243–50.

Morassaei, S., F. C. Breslin, M. Shen, and P. M. Smith. 2013. "Examining Job Tenure and Lost-Time Claim Rates in Ontario, Canada, over a 10-Year Period, 1999–2008." *Occupational and Environmental Medicine* 70 (3): 171–78.

Mou, J., S. M. Griffiths, H. Fong, and M. G. Dawes. 2013. "Health of China's Rural-Urban Migrants and Their Families: A Review of Literature from 2000 to 2012." *British Medical Bulletin* 106 (1): 19–43.

Muntaner, C., O. Solar, C. Vanroelen, J. M. Martinez, M. Vergara, and others. 2010. "Unemployment, Informal Work, Precarious Employment, Child Labor, Slavery, and Health Inequalities: Pathways and Mechanisms." *International Journal of Health Services* 40 (2): 281–95.

Murad, M. K., S. Larsen, and H. Husum. 2012. "Prehospital Trauma Care Reduces Mortality: Ten-Year Results from a Time-Cohort and Trauma Audit Study in Iraq." *Scandinavian Journal of Trauma, Resuscitation, and Emergency Medicine* 20: 13.

Murdoch, H., and D. Gould. 2004. "Corporate Social Responsibility in China: Mapping the Environment." Report prepared for the Global Alliance for Workers and Communities, Baltimore, MD.

Murray, C. J. L., K. F. Ortblad, C. Guinovart, S. S. Lim, T. M. Wolock, and others. 2014. "Global, Regional, and National Incidence and Mortality for HIV, Tuberculosis, and Malaria during 1990–2013: A Systematic Analysis for the Global Burden of Disease Study 2013." *The Lancet* 384 (9947): 1005–70.

Mustard, C. 2007. "Can Social Marketing Campaigns Prevent Workplace Injury and Illness?" *At Work* 49 (Summer): 3.

Nakata, A., T. Ikeda, M. Takahashi, T. Haratani, M. Hojou, and others. 2006. "Impact of Psychosocial Job Stress on Non-Fatal Occupational Injuries in Small and Medium-Sized Manufacturing Enterprises." *American Journal of Industrial Medicine* 49 (8): 658–69.

Nasrullah, M., and S. Awan. 2012. "Burns and Use of Mirror to Prevent These Injuries among Young and Adult Workers at Hot Clay Ovens, Tandoors: An Innovative, Cost-Effective Solution in a Low-Income Setting." *Burns* 38 (7): 1089–90.

NFIB (National Federation of Independent Business). 2002. "National Small Business Poll." *Workplace Safety* 2 (1).

Ngai, P., and J. Chan. 2012. "Global Capital, the State, and Chinese Workers: The Foxconn Experience." *Modern China* 38 (4): 383–410.

NIOSH (National Institute for Occupational Safety and Health). 2002. "The Changing Organization of Work and the Safety and Health of Working People: Knowledge Gaps and Research Directions." NIOSH, Cincinnati, OH.

———. 2008. "NORA AgFF Sector Council National Agriculture, Forestry, and Fishing Agenda." NIOSH, Washington, DC.

———. 2007. "Use of Blunt-Tip Suture Needles to Decrease Percutaneous Injuries to Surgical Personnel." NIOSH, Cincinatti, OH.

Niskanen, T., J. Lehtelä, R. Ketola, and E. Nykyri. 2010. "Results of Finnish National Survey on EU Legislation Concerning Computer Work." *Applied Ergonomics* 41 (4): 542–48.

Niu, S. 2010. "Ergonomics and Occupational Safety and Health: An ILO Perspective." *Applied Ergonomics* 41 (6): 744–53.

Noe, R., J. Rocha, C. Clavel-Arcas, C. Aleman, M. E. Gonzales, and others. 2004. "Occupational Injuries Identified by an Emergency Department–Based Injury Surveillance System in Nicaragua." *Injury Prevention* 10 (4): 227–32.

Nordander, C., K. Ohlsson, I. Balogh, G.-Å. Hansson, A. Axmon, and others. 2008. "Gender Differences in Workers with Identical Repetitive Industrial Tasks: Exposure and Musculoskeletal Disorders." *International Archives of Occupational and Environmental Health* 81 (8): 939–47.

Nossar, I., R. Johnstone, and M. Quinlan. 2003. "Regulating Supply-Chains to Address the Occupational Health and Safety Problems Associated with Precarious Employment: The Case of Home-Based Clothing Workers in Australia." Working Paper 21, Australian National University, Canberra.

Noy, Y. I., W. J. Horrey, S. M. Popkin, S. Folkard, H. D. Howarth, and others. 2011. "Future Directions in Fatigue and Safety Research." *Accident Analysis and Prevention* 43 (2): 495–97.

Nsubuga, F. M., and M. S. Jaakkola. 2005. "Needle Stick Injuries among Nurses in Sub-Saharan Africa." *Tropical Medicine and International Health* 10 (8): 773–81.

Ntow, W. J., H. J. Gijzen, P. Kelderman, and P. Drechsel. 2006. "Farmer Perceptions and Pesticide Use Practices in Vegetable Production in Ghana." *Pest Management Science* 62 (4): 356–65.

Pai, H. C., and S. Lee. 2011. "Risk Factors for Workplace Violence in Clinical Registered Nurses in Taiwan." *Journal of Clinical Nursing* 20 (9–10): 1405–12.

Palácios, M., M. L. dos Santos, M. B. do Val, M. Medina, M. de Abreu, and others. 2003. "Workplace Violence in the Health Sector: Country Case Study, Brazil." World Health Organization, Geneva.

Palmer, K. T., E. C. Harris, and D. Coggon. 2008. "Chronic Health Problems and Risk of Accidental Injury in the

Workplace: A Systematic Literature Review." *Occupational and Environmental Medicine* 65 (11): 757–64.

Palmer, K. T., E. C. Harris, C. Linaker, M. Barker, W. Lawrence, and others. 2012. "Effectiveness of Community- and Workplace-Based Interventions to Manage Musculoskeletal-Related Sickness Absence and Job Loss: A Systematic Review." *Rheumatology* 51 (2): 230–42.

Pehkonen, I., E.-P. Takala, R. Ketola, E. Viikari-Juntura, P. Leino-Arjas, and others. 2009. "Evaluation of a Participatory Ergonomic Intervention Process in Kitchen Work." *Applied Ergonomics* 40 (1): 115–23.

Pfortmueller, C. A., D. Kradolfer, M. Kunz, B. Lehmann, G. Lindner, and others. 2013. "Injuries in Agriculture: Injury Severity and Mortality." *Swiss Medical Weekly* 143: w13846.

Phung, D. T., H. T. Nguyen, C. Mock, and M. Keifer. 2008. "Occupational Injuries Reported in a Population-Based Injury Survey in Vietnam." *International Journal of Occupational and Environmental Health* 14 (1): 35–44.

Powers, J. R. Jr., D. E. Anmons, and I. Brand. 2009. "Machine Safety." *Professional Safety* 54 (11): 28–31.

Pransky, G. S., P. Loisel, and J. R. Anema. 2011. "Work Disability Prevention Research: Current and Future Prospects." *Journal of Occupational Rehabilitation* 21 (3): 287–92.

Premji, S., P. Duguay, K. Messing, and K. Lippel. 2010. "Are Immigrants, Ethnic and Linguistic Minorities Over-Represented in Jobs with a High Level of Compensated Risk? Results from a Montréal, Canada Study Using Census and Workers' Compensation Data." *American Journal of Industrial Medicine* 53 (9): 875–85.

Premji, S., K. Lippel, and K. Messing. 2008. "'We Work by the Second!' Piecework Remuneration and Occupational Health and Safety from an Ethnicity- and Gender-Sensitive Perspective." *Pistes* 10 (1): 1–22.

Pringle, T. E., and S. D. Frost. 2003. "The Absence of Rigor and the Failure of Implementation: Occupational Health and Safety in China." *International Journal of Occupational and Environmental Health* 9 (4): 309–16.

ProcureITfair. 2008. "The Dark Side of Cyberspace." World Economy, Ecology, and Development and Students and Scholars against Corporate Misbehaviour, Berlin. http://www2.weed-online.org/uploads/press_release_dark_side_of_cyberspace.pdf.

Pueyo, V., C. Toupin, and S. Volkoff. 2011. "The Role of Experience in Night Work: Lessons from Two Ergonomic Studies." *Applied Ergonomics* 42 (2): 251–55.

Quinlan, M. 1999. "The Implications of Labour Market Restructuring in Industrialized Societies for Occupational Health and Safety." *Economic and Industrial Democracy* 20 (3): 427–60.

Quinlan, M., and P. Bohle. 2008. "Under Pressure, Out of Control, or Home Alone? Reviewing Research and Policy Debates on the Occupational Health and Safety Effects of Outsourcing and Home-Based Work." *International Journal of Health Services* 38 (3): 489–523.

Quinlan, M., C. Mayhew, and P. Bohle. 2001. "The Global Expansion of Precarious Employment, Work Disorganisation, and Occupational Health: A Review of Recent Research." *International Journal of Health Services* 31 (2): 335–414.

Rahman, S. 2004. "Global Shift: Bangladesh Garment Industry in Perspective." *Asian Affairs* 26 (1): 75–91.

Redinger, C. F., and S. P. Levine. 1998. "Development and Evaluation of the Michigan Occupational Health and Safety Management System Assessment Instrument: A Universal OHSMS Performance Measurement Tool." *American Industrial Hygiene Association Journal* 59 (8): 572–81.

Regoeng, K. 2003. "Safety and Health in the Informal Sector and Small-Scale Industries: The Experience of Botswana." *African Newsletter on Occupational Health and Safety* 13 (1): 10–12.

Rivoli, P. 2009. *The Travels of a T-Shirt in the Global Economy: An Economist Examines the Markets, Power, and Politics of World Trade.* Hoboken, NJ: John Wiley and Sons.

Robson, L. S., J. A. Clarke, K. Cullen, A. Bielecky, C. Severin, and others. 2007. "The Effectiveness of Occupational Health and Safety Management System Interventions: A Systematic Review." *Safety Science* 45 (3): 329–53.

Robson, L. S., C. M. Stephenson, P. A. Schulte, B. C. Amick III, E. L. Irvin, and others. 2012. "A Systematic Review of the Effectiveness of Occupational Health and Safety Training." *Scandinavian Journal of Work, Environment, and Health* 38 (3): 193 208.

Rosenstock, L., M. Cullen, C. A. Brodkin, and C. A. Redlich. 2005. *Textbook of Clinical Occupational and Environmental Medicine,* second edition. Philadelphia: Elsevier WB Saunders.

Ruff, T. 2010. "Innovative Safety Interventions." *IEEE Industry Applications Magazine* 16 (3): 45–49.

SafeWork. 2012. "Improvement of National Reporting, Data Collection, and Analysis of Occupational Accidents and Diseases." Programme on Safety and Health at Work and the Environment, International Labour Organization, Geneva.

Sandoval, M., and K. A. Bjurling. 2014. "Challenging Labor: Working Conditions in the Electronics Industry." In *Lessons for Social Change in the Global Economy: Voices from the Field,* edited by S. Garwood, S. Croeser, and C. Yakinthou, 99–124. Plymouth, U.K.: Lexington Books.

Schlick, C., M. Joachin, L. Briceno, D. Moraga, and K. Radon. 2014. "Occupational Injuries among Children and Adolescents in Cusco Province: A Cross-Sectional Study." *BMC Public Health* 14: 766.

Schulte, P. A., S. Pandalai, V. Wulsin, and H. Chun. 2012. "Interaction of Occupational and Personal Risk Factors in Workforce Health and Safety." *American Journal of Public Health* 102 (3): 434–48.

Shiao, J. S., M. L. McLaws, M. H. Lin, J. Jagger, and C. J. Chen. 2009. "Chinese EPINet and Recall Rates for Percutaneous Injuries: An Epidemic Proportion of Underreporting in the Taiwan Healthcare System." *Journal of Occupational Health* 51 (2): 132–36.

Siddiqi, F., and H. A. Patrinos. 1995. "Child Labor: Issues, Causes, and Interventions." Human Capital Development and Operations Policy Working Paper 56, World Bank, Washington, DC.

Silverstein, M. 2008. "Meeting the Challenges of an Aging Workforce." *American Journal of Industrial Medicine* 51 (4): 269–80.

Sinclair, R. C., T. R. Cunningham, and P. A. Schulte. 2013. "A Model for Occupational Safety and Health Intervention Diffusion to Small Businesses." *American Journal of Industrial Medicine* 56 (12): 1442–51.

Smith, P., A. Bielecky, M. Koehoorn, D. Beaton, S. Ibrahim, and others. 2014. "Are Age-Related Differences in the Consequence of Work Injury Greater When Occupational Physical Demands Are High?" *American Journal of Industrial Medicine* 57 (4): 438–44.

Smith, T., D. A. Sonnenfeld, and D. N. Pellow. 2006. *Challenging the Chip: Labor Rights and Environmental Justice in the Global Electronics Industry*. Philadelphia: Temple University Press.

Smith, W. A. 2006. "Social Marketing: An Overview of Approach and Effects." *Injury Prevention* 12 (Suppl 1): i38–43.

Soares, M. M., K. Jacobs, K. Olsen, S. Legg, and P. Hasle. 2012. "How to Use Programme Theory to Evaluate the Effectiveness of Schemes Designed to Improve the Work Environment in Small Businesses." *Work* 41 (Suppl 1): 5999–6006.

Sorensen, G., P. Landsbergis, L. Hammer, B. C. Amick III, L. Linnan, and others. 2011. "Preventing Chronic Disease in the Workplace: A Workshop Report and Recommendations." *American Journal of Public Health* 101 (Suppl 1): S196–207.

Sørensen, O. H., P. Hasle, and E. Bach. 2007. "Working in Small Enterprises: Is There a Special Risk?" *Safety Science* 45 (10): 1044–59.

Sripichyakan, K., P. Thungpunkum, and B. Supavititpatana. 2003. "Workplace Violence in the Health Sector: A Case Study in Thailand." International Labour Organization, Geneva.

Steege, A. L., S. L. Baron, S. M. Marsh, C. C. Menéndez, and J. R. Myers. 2014. "Examining Occupational Health and Safety Disparities Using National Data: A Cause for Continuing Concern." *American Journal of Industrial Medicine* 57 (5): 527–38.

Steinman, S. 2003. "Workplace Violence in the Health Sector: Country Case Study in South Africa." World Health Organization, Geneva.

Stocks, S. J., R. McNamee, H. F. van der Molen, C. Paris, P. Urban, and others. 2015. "Trends in Incidence of Occupational Asthma, Contact Dermatitis, Noise-Induced Hearing Loss, Carpal Tunnel Syndrome, and Upper-Limb Musculoskeletal Disorders in European Countries from 2000 to 2012." *Occupational and Environmental Medicine* 72 (4): 294–303.

Strong, L. L., and F. J. Zimmerman. 2005. "Occupational Injury and Absence from Work among African American, Hispanic, and Non-Hispanic White Workers in the National Longitudinal Survey of Youth." *American Journal of Public Health* 95 (7): 1226–32.

Symanski, E., L. L. Kupper, and S. M. Rappaport. 1998. "Comprehensive Evaluation of Long-Term Trends in Occupational Exposure: Part 1. Description of the Database." *Occupational and Environmental Medicine* 55 (5): 300–309.

Taiwo, O. A., L. F. Cantley, M. D. Slade, K. M. Pollack, S. Vegso, and others. 2009. "Sex Differences in Injury Patterns among Workers in Heavy Manufacturing." *American Journal of Epidemiology* 169 (2): 161–66.

Tak, S., and G. M. Calvert. 2011. "The Estimated National Burden of Physical Ergonomic Hazards among U.S. Workers." *American Journal of Industrial Medicine* 54 (5): 395–404.

Takala, J., and P. Hämäläinen. 2009. "Globalization of Risks." *African Newsletter on Occupational Health and Safety* 19 (3): 70–73.

Targoutzidi, A., T. Koukoulaki, E. Schmitz-Felten, K. Kuhl, K. M. O. Hengel, and others. 2013. "The Business Case for Safety and Health at Work: Cost-Benefit Analyses of Interventions in Small and Medium-Sized Enterprises." European Agency for Safety and Health at Work, Luxembourg.

Taswell, K., and P. Wingfield-Digby. 2008. *Occupational Injury Statistics from Household Surveys and Establishment Surveys: An ILO Manual on Methods*. Geneva: International Labour Organization.

Tawatsupa, B., V. Yiengprugsawan, T. Kjellstrom, J. Berecki-Gisolf, S. A. Seubsman, and others. 2013. "Association between Heat Stress and Occupational Injury among Thai Workers: Findings of the Thai Cohort Study." *Industrial Health* 51 (1): 34–46.

Tessier-Sherman, B., L. F. Cantley, D. Galusha, M. D. Slade, O. A. Taiwo, and others. 2014. "Occupational Injury Risk by Sex in a Manufacturing Cohort." *Occupational and Environmental Medicine* 71 (9): 605–10.

Texido, E., and E. Warn. 2013. "Migrant Well-Being and Development: South America." Working Paper for the World Migration Report 2013, International Organization for Migration, Geneva.

Tinney, M. J., A. Chiodo, A. Haig, and E. Wiredu. 2007. "Medical Rehabilitation in Ghana." *Disability and Rehabilitation* 29 (11–12): 921–27.

Tompa, E., R. Dolinschi, C. de Oliveira, B. C. Amick III, and E. Irvin. 2010. "A Systematic Review of Workplace Ergonomic Interventions with Economic Analyses." *Journal of Occupational Rehabilitation* 20 (2): 220–34.

Tompa, E., R. Dolinschi, C. de Oliveira, and E. Irvin. 2009. "A Systematic Review of Occupational Health and Safety Interventions with Economic Analyses." *Journal of Occupational and Environmental Medicine* 51 (9): 1004–23.

Tompa, E., R. Dolinschi, and A. Laing. 2009. "An Economic Evaluation of a Participatory Ergonomics Process in an Auto Parts Manufacturer." *Journal of Safety Research* 40 (1): 41–47.

Tompa, E., R. Dolinschi, and J. Natale. 2013. "Economic Evaluation of a Participatory Ergonomics Intervention in a Textile Plant." *Applied Ergonomics* 44 (3): 480–87.

Tompa, E., S. Trevithick, and C. McLeod. 2007. "Systematic Review of the Prevention Incentives of Insurance and Regulatory Mechanisms for Occupational Health and Safety." *Scandinavian Journal of Work and Environmental Health* 33 (2): 85–95.

Törnström, L., J. Amprazis, M. Christmansson, and J. Eklund. 2008. "A Corporate Workplace Model for Ergonomic Assessments and Improvements." *Applied Ergonomics* 39 (2): 219–28.

Turgoose, C., L. Hall, A. Carter, and C. Stride. 2006. "Encouraging an Increase in the Employment of Women

Returners in Areas of Skill Shortage in Traditionally Male Industries." Institute of Work Psychology, University of Sheffield, Sheffield, U.K.

UN DESA (United Nations Department of Economic and Social Affairs). 2010. *The World's Women 2010: Trends and Statistics.* New York: UN DESA.

Ustailieva, E., L. Eeckelaery, and I. Nunes. 2012. *Promoting Occupational Safety and Health through the Supply Chain Literature Review.* Luxembourg: European Agency for Safety and Health at Work.

Valcour, M. 2007. "Work-Based Resources as Moderators of the Relationship between Work Hours and Satisfaction with Work-Family Balance." *Journal of Applied Psychology* 92 (6): 1512–23.

Vandergrift, J. L., J. E. Gold, A. Hanlon, and L. Punnett. 2012. "Physical and Psychosocial Ergonomic Risk Factors for Low Back Pain in Automobile Manufacturing Workers." *Occupational and Environmental Medicine* 69 (1): 29–34.

van der Molen, H. F., J. K. Sluiter, C. T. J. Hulshof, P. Vink, and M. H. W. Frings-Dresen. 2005. "Effectiveness of Measures and Implementation Strategies in Reducing Physical Work Demands due to Manual Handling at Work." *Scandinavian Journal of Work, Environment, and Health* 31 (Suppl 2): 75–87.

Van Dongen, H. P. A., J. A. Caldwell Jr., and J. L. Caldwell. 2011. "Individual Differences in Cognitive Vulnerability to Fatigue in the Laboratory and in the Workplace." In *Progress in Brain Research*, edited by A. K. Gerard, 145–53. Amsterdam: Elsevier.

van Stolk, C., L. Staetsky, E. Hassan, and C. W. Kim. 2012. "Management of Psychosocial Risks at Work: An Analysis of the Findings of the European Survey of Enterprises on New and Emerging Risks (ESENER)." European Agency for Safety and Health at Work, Luxembourg.

Verbeek, J., and I. Ivanov. 2013. "Essential Occupational Safety and Health Interventions for Low- and Middle-Income Countries: An Overview of the Evidence." *Safety and Health at Work* 4 (2): 77–83.

Verbeek, J., M. Pulliainen, and E. Kankaanpää. 2009. "A Systematic Review of Occupational Safety and Health Business Cases." *Scandinavian Journal of Work, Environment, and Health* 35 (6): 403–12.

Vigneswaran, D. 2007. "Special Report: Fact or Fiction? Examining Zimbabwean Cross-Border Migration to South Africa." Forced Migration Studies Programme and Musina Legal Advice Office, Johannesburg.

Vijayvergiya, S. C., A. K. Bohra, and P. Jhanwar. 2012. "Pattern of Agriculture-Related Injuries Presented in a Tertiary Care Hospital of South-Eastern Rajasthan." *Journal of Pharmaceutical and Biomedical Sciences* 17 (17).

Vink, P., E. A. P. Koningsveld, and J. F. Molenbroek. 2006. "Positive Outcomes of Participatory Ergonomics in Terms of Greater Comfort and Higher Productivity." *Applied Ergonomics* 37 (4): 537–46.

Virtanen, P., U. Janlert, and A. Hammarström. 2011. "Exposure to Temporary Employment and Job Insecurity: A Longitudinal Study of the Health Effects." *Occupational and Environmental Medicine* 68 (8): 570–74.

Wang, D. 2008. *Rural-Urban Migration and Policy Responses in China: Challenges and Options.* Bangkok: ILO Asian Regional Programming on Governance of Labour Migration, International Labour Office.

Wang, H., K. Fennie, G. He, J. Burgess, and A. B. Williams. 2003. "A Training Programme for Prevention of Occupational Exposure to Bloodborne Pathogens: Impact on Knowledge, Behaviour, and Incidence of Needle Stick Injuries among Student Nurses in Changsha, People's Republic of China." *Journal of Advanced Nursing* 41 (2): 187–94.

Wang, X., S. Wu, Q. Song, L.-A. Tse, I. T. S. Yu, and others. 2011. "Occupational Health and Safety Challenges in China: Focusing on Township-Village Enterprises." *Archives of Environmental and Occupational Health* 66 (1): 3–11.

Welford, R., and S. Frost. 2006. "Corporate Social Responsibility in Asian Supply Chains." *Corporate Social Responsibility and Environmental Management* 13 (3): 166–76.

WHO (World Health Organization). 2001. *Occupational Health: A Manual for Primary Health Care Workers.* Geneva: WHO.

———. 2004. *Guidelines on the Prevention of Toxic Exposures: Education and Public Awareness Activities.* Geneva: International Programme on Chemical Safety, WHO.

———. 2006a. "Managing Exits from the Workforce." In *The World Health Report 2006: Working Together for Health*, 97–118. Geneva: WHO.

———. 2006b. *Safer Access to Pesticides: Community Interventions.* Geneva: International Association for Suicide Prevention, WHO.

———. 2011. "Safe Injection Global Network: Summaries of Injection Safety Country Success Stories." WHO, Geneva.

———. 2012. "Connecting Health and Labour: Bringing Together Occupational Health and Primary Care to Improve the Health of Working People." Executive Summary of the WHO Global Conference "Connecting Health and Labour: What Role for Occupational Health in Primary Health Care," The Hague, November 29–December 1, 2011.

Williamson, A., D. A. Lombardi, S. Folkard, J. Stutts, T. K. Courtney, and others. 2011. "The Link between Fatigue and Safety." *Accident Analysis and Prevention* 43 (2): 498–515.

Wirtz, A., F. Nachreiner, and K. Rolfes. 2011. "Working on Sundays: Effects on Safety, Health, and Work-Life Balance." *Chronobiology International* 28 (4): 361–70.

World Bank. 2014. *World Development Indicators: Children at Work.* Washington, DC: World Bank. http://wdi.worldbank.org/tables.

WTO (World Trade Organization). 2013. *International Trade Statistics 2013.* Geneva: WTO.

Xia, Q. H., Y. Jiang, N. Yin, J. Hu, and C. J. Niu. 2012. "Injury among Migrant Workers in Changning District, Shanghai, China." *International Journal of Injury Control and Safety Promotion* 19 (1): 81–85.

Yang, Y. H., S. H. Liou, C. J. Chen, C. Y. Yang, C. L. Wang, and others. 2007. "The Effectiveness of a Training Program on Reducing Needlestick Injuries/Sharp Object Injuries among Soon Graduate Vocational Nursing School Students in Southern Taiwan." *Journal of Occupational Health* 49 (5): 424–29.

Yessuf Serkalem, S., G. Moges Haimanot, and N. Ahmed Ansha. 2014. "Determinants of Occupational Injury in Kombolcha Textile Factory, North-East Ethiopia." *International Journal of Occupational and Environmental Medicine* 5 (2): 84–93.

Yu, W., I. T. Yu, Z. Li, X. Wang, T. Sun, and others. 2012. "Work-Related Injuries and Musculoskeletal Disorders among Factory Workers in a Major City of China." *Accident Analysis and Prevention* 48 (September): 457–63.

Yu, X. 2007. "Impacts of Corporate Code of Conduct on Labor Standards: A Case Study of Reebok's Athletic Footwear Supplier Factory in China." *Journal of Business Ethics* 81 (3): 513–29.

Zawilla, N. H., and D. Ahmed. 2013. "Sharps Injuries among Health Care Workers in Cairo University Hospitals." *International Journal of Risk and Safety in Medicine* 25 (2): 79–92.

Zhuang, Z., T. J. Stobbe, J. W. Collins, H. Hongwei, and G. R. Hobbs. 2000. "Psychophysical Assessment of Assistive Devices for Transferring Patients/Residents." *Applied Ergonomics* 31 (1): 35–44.

Zink, K. J., U. Steimle, and D. Schröder. 2008. "Comprehensive Change Management Concepts: Development of a Participatory Approach." *Applied Ergonomics* 39 (4): 527–38.

# Chapter 7

# Household Air Pollution from Solid Cookfuels and Its Effects on Health

Kirk R. Smith and Ajay Pillarisetti

## INTRODUCTION

Since the earliest human times, humans have used wood as fuel for fires to cook their food. Indeed, learning to control fire is considered the defining moment between the pre-human and human condition (Wrangham 2009). With the agricultural revolution some 10,000 years ago, agricultural residues (including animal dung) were brought to the hearth as well. Around 1,000 years ago, coal became used in areas where it was mined easily—for example, the British Isles and China (Smil 1994). These three fuels—wood, agricultural residues, and coal—constitute the solid cooking fuels used by about 40 percent of humanity today (Bonjour and others 2013). Typically burned in simple cookstoves, these fuels produce smoke that is now understood to cause a large burden of disease (Smith and others 2014).

Cleaner fuels (coal gas, natural gas, liquefied petroleum gas [LPG], and electricity) began to make inroads only in the late nineteenth century. Although today 60 percent of the world's population uses these modern fuels (which are relatively clean in household use, even in simple cookstoves), growth in their use has never kept up with global population growth, primarily because of the persistence of biomass use among the poor. Today, almost 3 billion people use solid cookfuels, which probably is more than at any time in world history (Bonjour and others 2013) and more than the entire world population before 1960.

Household air pollution (HAP) is now understood to be a major risk factor for health. According to the 2013 Global Burden of Disease Study (GBD), HAP is ranked as the single most significant environmental health risk factor globally. In poor countries where many households rely on biomass for cooking (such as in Sub-Saharan Africa), HAP is ranked among the top risk factors examined in the GBD assessments. Depending on which set of estimates is used, some 3 million to 4 million premature deaths are thought to be caused annually by HAP. Between 3 and 5 percent of the GBD in terms of disability-adjusted life years (DALYs) is attributed to it, about one-third in children younger than age five years and the rest divided between adult men and women (for background on DALYs, see Salomon 2014).

This chapter relies on two major reviews published in recent years. One was done as part of the Comparative Risk Assessment (CRA) of the GBD project (Lim and others 2012; Lozano and others 2012; Smith and others 2014), and the other was done as background documentation for the World Health Organization's (WHO) Indoor Air Quality Guidelines (IAQGs) (WHO 2014b). This chapter summarizes what is known about effective and cost-effective interventions to reduce the health effects of exposure to HAP from solid cooking fuels[1] and then explores some of the issues regarding framing, interactions, and viable interventions. The discussion follows the classic environmental health pathway described in box 7.1.

Corresponding author: Kirk R. Smith, School of Public Health, University of California, Berkeley, California, United States; krksmith@berkeley.edu.

**Box 7.1**

## The Environmental Health Pathway

This chapter relies loosely on the classic environmental health pathway for describing and understanding pollution risks (figure B7.1.1), which starts with sources and emissions of pollution, moves to environmental levels, then to human exposures, then to doses within the body, and finally to health impacts (Smith 1987). In the case of household air pollution, a source could be any type of biomass combustion, but we focus here primarily on biomass combustion used in cooking. Different kinds of evidence come to bear at each stage of the pathway, and each stage offers different avenues for control. Because some of the terminology in the pathway is discipline specific, we must briefly clarify what we mean by emissions, concentration, exposure, biomarkers of exposure, and biomarkers of effect.

*Emissions* refer to the rate of release of a pollutant per unit of time or per unit of fuel (the "source" in figure B7.1.1). Measurements of emissions require sampling directly from the source of combustion. Emissions samples often are taken during a cooking cycle—either actual or simulated—and rarely are captured for the entire day. Experience shows that lab measurements or simulated measurements in homes usually underestimate actual emissions in the field (Johnson and others 2008; Johnson and others 2011).

*Concentrations* (generally measured in mass of pollutant per volume of air) are a function of emissions, conditions in the room of interest (such as the room's ventilation rate), and processes like deposition and exfiltration of pollutants through openings. Concentrations are not necessarily equivalent to exposures; for example, a monitor that measures pollution in a kitchen (defined here as the built environment around the cooking area, whether indoors or outdoors) for 24 hours does not reflect a person's exposure to that pollution unless he or she, too, is in the kitchen for 24 hours.

*Exposures* are a result of the spatiotemporal relationship between individuals and the pollution in their immediate surroundings. An individual's daily exposure is affected by the number, type, and duration of contact with all sources he or she comes into contact with, either directly (for example, one's own household cooking fire) or indirectly (for example, local traffic sources or a neighbor's household cooking fire). Exposure can be assessed either through personal measurement, in which an individual wears a monitor, or through exposure reconstruction, in which time-activity information (for example, a diary of time spent in various locations and time spent in proximity to potential sources) is coupled with area monitors measuring concentration in various microenvironments. Personal exposure typically is assessed for 24 or 48 hours.

*Biomarkers* of exposure are measurable metabolites or products of an interaction between an external agent and a target molecule, cell, or organ. Biomarkers of effect are chemical, biological, or physical alterations resulting from an exposure that can be associated with a health endpoint or disease (WHO 1993).

**Figure B7.1.1** Classic Environmental Health Pathway

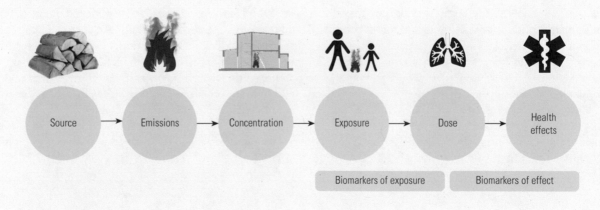

Most of the older literature and even some modern studies refer to the problem as one of indoor air pollution, but the CRA (Lim and others 2012) carefully redefined it as HAP for several reasons (Smith and others 2014):

- Much of the health-relevant exposure to air pollution from cooking fuel occurs in the environment around households, not just indoors.
- Solid cooking fuel is sufficiently polluting to affect widespread ambient (outdoor) air pollution levels appreciably and, thus, to cause ill health far from the source.
- The term *indoor* implies that an effective chimney or other venting would solve the problem entirely, when the basic problem is dirty combustion near people.
- In some parts of the world, incompletely combusted solid fuels are commonly used for space heating or lighting, as well as for cooking, thus confusing the attribution of risk and assessment of appropriate interventions unless the household uses being considered are specified.
- The term *indoor air pollution* overlaps with much research on indoor pollution from other sources (for example, from household furnishings and consumer products). For example, the CRA now separately includes risks from indoor exposure to radon.

This chapter focuses on the evidence base for health effects, because the causality between HAP and ill health is only now being firmly established. This is unlike contaminated water and poor sanitation, for which the connection to ill health was established in the nineteenth century. The causality and scale of the effects from HAP have only recently received recognition in health effects studies, which are now appearing in large numbers. This recent appearance perhaps explains why there are relatively few evaluations of large-scale interventions to date. Initiatives presently under way provide excellent opportunities to do so.

## SOURCES AND EMISSIONS

Burning biomass completely in simple stoves is extremely difficult. Even though wood and most other types of biomass have few intrinsic contaminants (unlike coal), substantial fractions of the fuel carbon are not completely oxidized to carbon dioxide; instead, they are converted to a vast range of products of incomplete combustion (PIC). As much as 20 percent of the fuel carbon can be diverted into these products, although more typical levels are 5–10 percent (Naeher and others 2007; Zhang and others 2000). By mass, the largest PIC component by far is carbon monoxide (CO), but thousands of other compounds have been measured in wood smoke, including nontrivial levels of dozens of well-known toxic chemical species, such as polycyclic aromatic hydrocarbons, benzene, formaldehyde, and even dioxin (Naeher and others 2007; Northcross and others 2012). In broad terms, the mixture is similar to the PIC produced from combustion of the most well-studied form of biomass: tobacco. Indeed, despite their differences, exposures to these two forms of smoke have many similar health effects.

As with tobacco smoke, the risks of different diseases resulting from exposure to HAP probably depend in different ways on the landscape of components. However, insufficient evidence exists to pin specific diseases on particular components of wood smoke. Indeed, given the many decades, more controlled conditions, and extensive resources devoted to studying tobacco smoke, still without being able to distinguish differences in detail, the issue of wood smoke mixtures is unlikely to be resolved in the foreseeable future. Therefore, like tobacco researchers, HAP researchers rely on two main indicator pollutants for measurement and risk assessment: $PM_{2.5}$ (particulate matter with an aerodynamic diameter of less than 2.5 micrometers, called tar in tobacco smoke, the most well-studied component of air pollution correlated with adverse health risk) and CO. Unlike tobacco smoke, smoke from other types of biomass does not contain measurable nicotine. However, smoke resulting from biomass combustion contains a vast range of other components for which $PM_{2.5}$ and CO are just indicators.[2]

In terms of $PM_{2.5}$, a typical wood fuel cookstove used by a single family for cooking household meals produces substantial pollution by any comparison. In laboratory simulations, the wood-fired three-stone stove (the most common stove used worldwide) produces some 6 grams or about 400 cigarettes worth of $PM_{2.5}$ per hour (figure 7.1) (Jetter and others 2002; Jetter and others 2012). To put it into another context, one year of cooking on a three-stone stove emits particles equivalent to the emissions of 20 diesel trucks driving 50,000 kilometers a year and meeting Euro 6 standards, the standard planned for India in 2020. Considering that 170 million households in India use biomass cooking fuel today, the emissions are roughly equivalent to those of a mixed fleet of 400 million diesel trucks meeting 2010 standards (Euro 4), far more emissions than are expected in India. In practice, field-based measurements of both biomass stoves and diesel trucks likely record even more pollution than is indicated by these numbers (which are based on laboratory evidence).

**Figure 7.1** Emissions of PM$_{2.5}$ in Grams per Hour for Common Types of Stoves Showing Range of Reported Lab Measurements

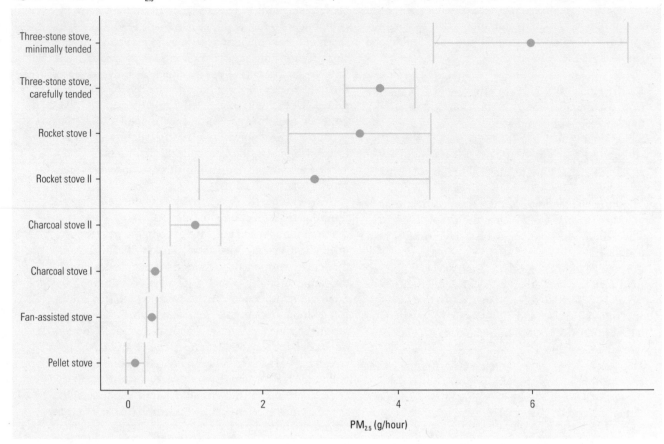

*Source:* Adapted from the comprehensive stove performance database in Jetter and others 2012; adapted with permission from Jetter, Zhao, Smith, Khan, Yelverton, Decarlo, and Hays. "Pollutant Emissions and Energy Efficiency under Controlled Conditions for Household Biomass Cookstoves and Implications for Metrics Useful in Setting International Test Standards." *Environmental Science and Technology* 46 (19): 10827–34. Copyright 2012. American Chemical Society.
*Note:* Data displayed are for dry fuel during hot start tests. g/hour = grams per hour; PM$_{2.5}$ = particulate matter with an aerodynamic diameter of less than 2.5 micrometers.

Toxicology studies of biomass particulates find some effects on cells and animals to be stronger than those produced by typical ambient air pollution or diesel particles and some to be weaker, with no clear trends (Naeher and others 2007; Zelikoff and others 2002). Growing epidemiological evidence suggests that diesel particles are likely to be more hazardous than average ambient particles or wood smoke particles, but all major assessments to date—for example, those of the WHO (2014b) and the U.S. Environmental Protection Agency—conclude that, at present, insufficient evidence exists to treat PM$_{2.5}$ of different origins differently with regard to control priorities.[3]

## CONCENTRATIONS

In indoor kitchens, PM$_{2.5}$ concentrations can become extremely high when cooking with solid fuels (Balakrishnan and others 2011), often reaching many thousands of micrograms per cubic meter of PM$_{2.5}$ and causing much eye and throat irritation, particularly in persons unaccustomed to such levels (Diaz and others 2007).[4] The iconic blackening of walls and ceilings in village kitchens using such fuels is testimony to these levels.

Although few systematic survey data are available, including those from the Demographic and Health Survey, the World Health Organization (WHO 2014a), and the World Bank, worldwide only a small fraction of households using biomass for cooking have working chimneys. The exception is China, where most rural kitchens have chimney stoves, partly because of the success of the largest stove dissemination program in history, the National Improved Stove Program (NISP), which operated from the early 1980s to the mid-1990s (Edwards and others 2007; Smith and others 2014; Zhang and Smith 2007). Unlike India's National Program on Improved Chulhas, which operated during roughly the same period (Venkataraman and others 2010), all stoves disseminated under the NISP had chimneys.

Good chimney stoves lower peak levels of indoor pollution, but they lower long-term average exposures only by a factor of two, at most, because even good chimney stoves do not intrinsically reduce emissions; they merely move emissions out of the immediate room and into the surrounding household and village environment, where people also spend time. They further require regular maintenance and proper use to function correctly.

Of course, a chimney does nothing to decrease outdoor air pollution, which is now understood to be heavily influenced by household sources in some countries. In India, for example, an estimated 25–50 percent of population-weighted outdoor $PM_{2.5}$ exposure results from emissions of primary particles from cookstoves (Chafe and others 2014; Guttikunda 2016; Lelieveld and others 2015). Outdoor $PM_{2.5}$ levels also include secondary particles from gaseous precursors, such as sulfur oxide, nitrogen oxide, and semivolatile compounds; though not yet well quantified, these compounds also are emitted from households, as well as from vehicles, power plants, and other more traditional sources of outdoor air pollution. If one considers primary particle emissions alone, household cooking is responsible for an estimated 370,000 premature deaths globally from its contribution to general outdoor air pollution on top of the mortality produced from exposure in the household environment itself (Chafe and others 2014).

## EXPOSURE

Household cooking is nearly universally done by women, who often also are responsible for the care of young children. These two groups generally have the highest HAP exposure, because they tend to be near the stove during combustion. As cooking fire smoke permeates the household environment, men and older children also may have significant exposure. However, studies have not characterized these exposures nearly as well. The importance of focusing on exposure (as opposed to just indoor air pollution) is illustrated by the fairly high exposure of women cooking on open fires outdoors.

Because monitors placed in a kitchen or living area cannot capture actual human exposure from a single location (particularly for different family members), the growing practice in epidemiological and other health-oriented research on HAP is to measure personal exposures. This is generally done by asking participants to wear portable monitoring devices for a day or in 24-hour increments for several days (Baumgartner and others 2011; Ni and others 2016; Smith and others 2010; Van Vliet and others 2013), an expensive and somewhat intrusive exercise given the available technology. Early studies commonly measured exposure only during periods of cooking, when exposure rates often are highest. These levels are hard to interpret, because relative risks and exposure-response relationships typically exist for annual average exposures, not for exposures only during cooking, heating, or other activities.

Evaluation of exposure is made more difficult by high within- and between-household variability (McCracken and others 2009; Pillarisetti and others 2016). Several parameters can influence both concentration and exposure, including (1) the cooking location, with some households cooking indoors, while others cook outdoors, in an open area, or in a separate cooking house; (2) cooking habits and type of cuisine, with some cuisines requiring constant attention during cooking, while others can be left unattended; and (3) the use of multiple fires for cooking. Each of these parameters influences exposure and complicates exposure assessment.

In the past, researchers generally assumed that as long as measurement days were typical of patterns throughout the year, then one or a few days of measurements would provide reasonable estimates of long-term averages. In recent years, however, because of high intrinsic intrahousehold variability, researchers have demonstrated that reliable estimates of long-term averages can be achieved only with multiple days of measurement (McCracken and others 2009; Pillarisetti and others 2016). Although studies have detected effects even with one or a few measurements, investigators risk not being able to do so even when effects exist because of the high degree of exposure misclassification that occurs.

Additional methods of measuring exposure involve measurements of "surrogate" pollutants, such as CO, or reconstruction of exposures using area measurements in multiple microenvironments and time-activity diaries. Exposure surrogates may be chosen because they facilitate more rapid or less difficult measurement of a specific pollutant. However, the decision to measure a surrogate in place of the pollutant of interest requires local, field-based validation of the surrogate as a proxy for the pollutant. Exposure reconstruction using microenvironmental models relies on area measurements of pollutant concentrations in multiple environments in which people spend time (for instance, kitchens, the outdoors, and living quarters), as well as recall or sensor-based data on the time spent in each location. Individual exposures are then estimated by estimating time-weighted average pollutant concentrations (see Balakrishnan and others [2011] for a database of HAP studies using proxy measures and time-activity methods).

## BIOMARKERS AND OTHER SIGNS OF HAP EFFECT

Recent reviews (Smith and others 2014; Tolunay and Chockalingam 2012; WHO 2014b) discuss studies that have found biomarkers of HAP exposure (CO breath, carboxyhemoglobin, urinary metabolites, DNA [deoxyribonucleic acid] adducts) and biomarkers of HAP effect (eye opacity, lung function, blood pressure, electrocardiogram ST-segment). These findings are consistent with the disease endpoints documented for HAP and provide support for interpolating between ambient air pollution and smoking exposures for cardiovascular outcomes.

## HEALTH IMPACTS

The health impacts of air pollution exposures of various sorts, including from household fuels, are based on two general categories of evidence:

- Direct epidemiological studies of health impacts in populations exposed to differing categories of exposure
- Interpolation of risks taken from integrated exposure-response (IER) functions derived by combining the results of epidemiological studies of a wide range of air pollution exposures in different situations.

Relying heavily on recent major reviews, this section summarizes the results of both kinds of evidence as they relate to HAP and discusses their relative merits and remaining gaps and uncertainties. The focus is on outcomes ranked as Class I, indicating multiple high-quality epidemiological studies from households in low- and middle-income countries (LMICs), with consistent results and particle exposures at both higher and lower exposures, and using exposure-response data across several particle exposure settings. See Table 7.1, where Class I is defined.

### Direct Epidemiological Studies of HAP Exposures

Most health studies of HAP published to date have relied on simple binary indicators of exposure, such as whether a household's primary cooking fuel is clean versus dirty fuel. Although simplistic, these indicators are more stable over a year than a single measurement of personal exposure or area of concentration. Most of the evaluated studies are cross-sectional in design, which poses the risk of bias by unmeasured confounders (such as socioeconomic status, smoking, and fuel/stove stacking). Many dozens of studies done by different investigators have

found similar ranges of effects for each of various health outcomes in different populations, providing considerable confidence that a degree of effect likely is real. A brief description of each category of disease for which there is epidemiological evidence follows. For a detailed literature review, see Smith and others (2014).

### Acute Lower Respiratory Infection in Children

Acute lower respiratory infection (ALRI) is a leading killer of children younger than age five years (GBD Risk Factors Collaborators 2015). Smith and others (2014) identified 24 studies that met their inclusion criteria during a systematic review and meta-analysis. Very few of the studies directly measured exposure to HAP, and many used poor-quality proxies of exposure. Furthermore, the case definitions of pneumonia varied among studies. All studies save one randomized control trial (RCT) were observational. The pooled odds ratio (OR) from their study was 1.78 (1.45, 2.18).

Although several trials are near completion, results from just one RCT have been published to date: the RESPIRE study of child ALRI in Guatemala, which compared a wood-fired cookstove with a chimney to the traditional open wood-fired cookstove (Smith and others 2010; Smith and others 2011). Results (summarized in figure 7.2) show a significant effect for severe forms of ALRI, but only marginally significant effects for all cases of ALRI. Of relevance is that the pilot studies justifying the conclusion that this stove would be an effective intervention focused on indoor air quality in the kitchen and not on personal exposures. In the RCT, kitchen concentrations dropped 90 percent, similar to the pilot results, but the actual exposure experienced by women and young children dropped only 50 percent, which was below the power of the study. This is because babies and mothers do not spend all day in the kitchen, and the locations where people spend time during the rest of the day were not appreciably affected by the intervention. The wood-fired cookstove with a chimney moved most of the smoke out of the kitchen and into the surrounding environment, where it still affected people and their exposures. The most important result of the RCT was the exposure-response analysis, enabled by the development of a means to measure infant exposures directly and facilitated by a validated relationship between CO and $PM_{2.5}$.

### Chronic Obstructive Pulmonary Disease

Chronic obstructive pulmonary disease (COPD), the fourth leading cause of death globally (GBD Risk Factors Collaborators 2015), is characterized by persistent airflow limitation associated with chronic inflammation of the airway and lungs in response to exposure to particles and gases (GOLD 2016). A previous systematic review and meta-analysis evaluating the risk of adult COPD from exposure to HAP identified 24 studies from 12 countries as suitable for inclusion (Smith and others 2014). The majority were cross-sectional (17), 6 were case-control studies, and 1 was a retrospective cohort. All but two studies had positive risk ratios. Stratifying by gender indicated a stronger effect in women (OR, 2.30; 1.73, 2.06) than in men (OR, 1.90; 1.15, 3.13); a subanalysis of duration of exposure indicated a stronger summary effect when comparing the longest to the shortest duration of exposure. All studies used proxy measures of exposure. The pooled OR reported was 1.94 (1.62, 2.33).

## Lung Cancer

Lung cancer (LC) is the seventh leading cause of death globally (IHME 2016). While the use of coal for heating and cooking is recognized as a group I carcinogen by the International Agency for Research on Cancer, use of biomass for cooking is considered only a probable carcinogen because of weaker epidemiological evidence, even though several chemicals with group I status are found in wood smoke. Smith and others (2014) identified 14 studies, providing 13 individual estimates in a review of the relationship between biomass use for cooking and LC (Bruce and others 2015). Ten studies were focused in Asia, with the remaining four spread across Canada, Europe, and the United States. Exposure assessment relied on survey-based recall of the type of fuel used for cooking or heating, along with the duration and period of life for which biomass was used in a subset. The overall OR was 1.17 (1.01, 1.37) for biomass used for cooking or heating and 1.15 (0.97, 1.37) for cooking only. ORs were 1.21 (1.05, 1.39) and 1.95 (1.16, 3.27) for men and women, respectively, for studies with adequate adjustment and a reference category.

## Cataracts

Cataracts (the clouding of the lens of the eye, preventing the passage of light) are a leading cause of blindness globally and account for approximately 0.12 percent of all DALYs (GBD Risk Factors Collaborators 2015). Toxicological evidence from animal models and epidemiological evidence from smokers indicated a potential relationship between cooking with solid fuels and cataracts. Smith and others (2014) identified seven eligible studies providing eight estimates for review, all from India and Nepal. The pooled OR was 2.64 (1.74, 3.50); however, evidence for men was deemed insufficient for cataracts to be listed as a class I outcome. Therefore, only the estimate for women of 2.47 (1.61, 3.73) was deemed reliable. Table 7.1 summarizes the ORs for primary disease outcomes.

Although not RCTs, a set of retrospective studies of a "natural experiment" in China in which coal stoves with

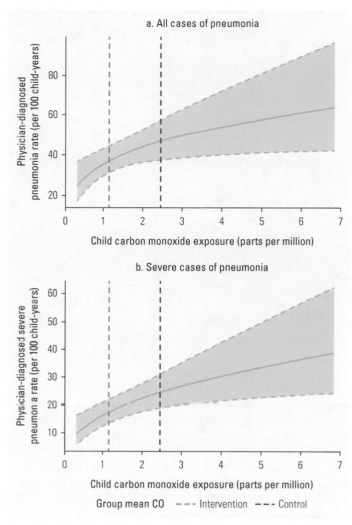

**Figure 7.2** Relationships between Carbon Monoxide Exposure in Children and Pneumonia and Severe Pneumonia from the RESPIRE Trial in Guatemala

*Source:* Adapted from Smith and others 2011; reprinted from *The Lancet*, Vol. 378, Smith, McCracken, Weber, Hubbard, Jenny, Thompson, Balmes, Diaz, Arana, and Bruce, "Effect of Reduction in Household Air Pollution on Childhood Pneumonia in Guatemala (RESPIRE): A Randomised Controlled Trial." 1717–26, 2011, with permission from Elsevier.
*Note:* CO = carbon monoxide. Shaded areas represent 95% confidence bounds. During the RESPIRE trial, CO was validated for this study population as a surrogate for particulate matter exposure, which is thought to be the best metric of hazard. The dashed lines represent the mean exposure levels.

chimneys were introduced rapidly in areas with no chimneys and in one county starting around 1980 also are an important part of the evidence base (Chapman and others 2005; Seow and others 2014; Shen and others 2009). As they relate to coal smoke, however, their direct relevance to the much more prevalent use of biomass fuel worldwide is not clear, although they do show significant reductions in LC as well as COPD and adult pneumonia. Unfortunately, too little exposure assessment was conducted to include these results in the development of IER functions.

**Table 7.1** Summary of Odds Ratio for Primary Outcomes Derived from the Systematic Review and Meta-Analysis Performed for the 2010 Comparative Risk Assessment of the Global Burden of Disease

| Outcome | Group studied[a] | 2010 systematic review and meta-analysis estimates | 2004 CRA estimates |
|---|---|---|---|
| Acute lower respiratory infection | Children | 1.78 (1.45, 2.18) | 2.3 (1.9, 2.7) |
| Chronic obstructive pulmonary disease | Females | 2.30 (1.73, 2.06) | 3.2 (2.3, 4.8) |
| | Males | 1.90 (1.15, 3.13) | 1.8 (1.0, 3.2) |
| *Lung cancer* | | | |
| Coal | Females | 1.98 (1.16, 3.36) | 1.94 (1.09, 3.47) |
| | Males | 1.31 (1.05, 1.76) | 1.51 (0.97, 2.46) |
| Biomass | Females | 1.95 (1.16, 3.27)[b] | — |
| | Males | 1.21 (1.05, 1.39)[b] | — |
| Cataracts | Females | 2.47 (1.63, 3.73) | — |

*Note:* — = not available; CRA = comparative risk assessment; OR = odds ratio.
a. Children younger than age five years; females and males ages 15 years and older.
b. ORs from Bruce and others 2015.

## Interpolation of Risks Using Integrated-Exposure Response Functions

IER functions were created spanning the range of global exposures to PM$_{2.5}$ by separately modeling the relationship between exposure from four sources (ambient air pollution, secondhand smoke, HAP, and active tobacco smoking) and five health endpoints (COPD, stroke, heart disease, LC in adults, and ALRI in children younger than age five years) (Burnett and others 2014; Pope and

others 2009). The complete list of data points used to create the model is in Burnett and others (2014, supplementary material table S1).

In using a wide range of concentrations from a variety of sources, the IERs assume that risk associated with these disparate sources is only a function of exposure, not smoke type, enabling the creation of a continuous response function that spans many orders of magnitude and is bounded on the low end by ambient exposure to PM$_{2.5}$ and on the high end by active tobacco smoking (Burnett and others 2014; Pope and others 2009). The modeled relative risks are thus a function of PM$_{2.5}$ exposures in terms of mass concentration; all PM$_{2.5}$ particles are considered equally damaging to health. The resulting functions are highly nonlinear for all outcomes except LC (figure 7.3).

Use of the IERs enabled estimation of the risk associated with exposures at levels common in households that use solid fuel for which there are no or very few HAP studies, but that have intermediate exposures between passive and active smoking. Additionally, it enabled use of the same idealized counterfactual level of approximately 7 micrograms per cubic meter for calculating the burden of disease attributable to HAP and ambient air pollution. Finally, it enabled comparison of IER-modeled risk estimates with estimates backed by evidence based on epidemiological studies (Smith and others 2014). A brief description of the modeled risk estimates for cardiovascular disease (CVD) (including stroke and heart disease) follows, along with a comparison of IER-modeled and epidemiological-study-based estimates for ALRI.

**Figure 7.3** Integrated-Exposure Response Curves Relating Exposure to PM$_{2.5}$ to Health Endpoints Associated with Exposure to Air Pollution

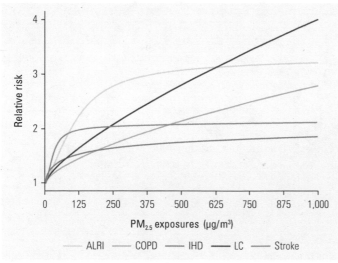

*Source:* Adapted from Burnett and others 2014.
*Note:* PM$_{2.5}$ = particulate matter with an aerodynamic diameter of less than 2.5 micrometers; μg/m³ = micrograms per cubic meter. Includes ischemic heart disease (IHD), stroke, chronic obstructive pulmonary disease (COPD), and lung cancer (LC) in adults and acute lower respiratory infection (ALRI) in children.

## Cardiovascular Disease

Although evidence exists linking exposure to HAP with biomarkers with known links to cardiovascular outcomes (including blood pressure and heart rate variability), few studies have specifically addressed CVD directly. The strong evidence of impacts at lower (ambient) and higher (active tobacco smoking) levels is good evidence for an effect at the intermediate levels of HAP exposure, however. Figure 7.4 indicates that, for both stroke and ischemic heart disease (IHD), risk flattens as exposure increases, although this effect is more pronounced for stroke.

## Acute Lower Respiratory Infection in Children

Unlike CVD outcomes, both exposure-response and many categorical analyses found that exposure to HAP was associated with child ALRI. The IER for ALRI was informed by studies of ambient air pollution, second-hand smoke, and HAP. Unlike other IERs, the one for ALRI contains directly measured risk and exposure data from RESPIRE, based on repeated measures of child personal exposure to CO, which were then converted to PM (McCracken and others 2013; Smith and others 2010).

Because children do not smoke, the upper bound of exposures in the IER for ALRI are from RESPIRE.

### Uncertainties and Emergent Issues

The health effects literature contains both uncertainties as well as new understandings with regard to exposure patterns that are influencing both research and intervention policies.

### Categories of Evidence: Exposure-Response

RCTs have substantial cachet in international health, and their results are beginning to inform the evidence base for HAP effects as well. However, RCTs are not as valuable or needed for HAP assessments as perhaps they are for other risk factors. Unlike the important risk factors in this volume that otherwise have many conceptual similarities—poor water, sanitation, and hygiene—HAP has a measurable exposure metric linked directly to health. Exposure units in, for example, micrograms per cubic meter annual levels, can thus be translated across populations and interventions. Indeed, this is the concept on which the IAQGs are based (WHO 2014b).

**Figure 7.4** Integrated-Exposure Response Curves for Cardiovascular Outcomes

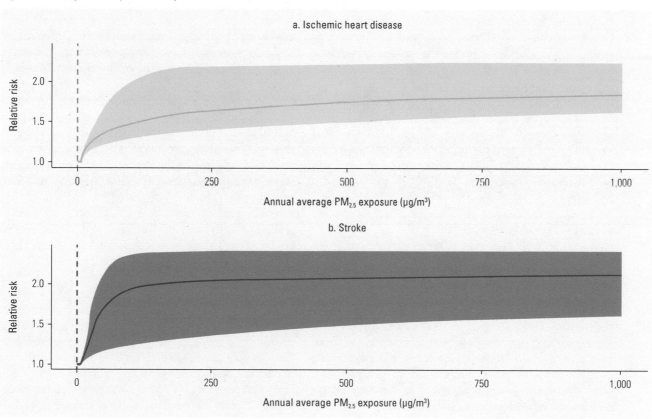

*Source:* Adapted from Burnett and others 2014.

*Note:* PM$_{2.5}$ = particulate matter with an aerodynamic diameter of less than 2.5 micrometers; μg/m$^3$ = micrograms per cubic meter. Shaded areas are model-based uncertainty bounds. Large uncertainties in areas approximating household air pollution exposures (300–1,000 micrograms per cubic meter) indicate a lack of evidence in those exposure ranges.

HAP RCTs alone, however, are idiosyncratic to the local situation and intervention and cannot meet the full requirements of an RCT, particularly the requirement to have placebo controls. Most important, unlike exposure-response relationships, the results do not translate easily to any other population—that is, they do not relate directly to exposure. This is one reason that exposure assessment is so fundamental to environmental health. No RCTs have been done or likely will be done for ambient air pollution, for example, but the effects are known and the benefits of interventions for a place that has never had a health study can be estimated with reasonable confidence if exposures are known. This is because multiple large-scale exposure-response results are available across the world. RCTs are most valuable for establishing causality if it is still in doubt, but they are rather poor at informing policy for HAP. What matters is how clean the fuel has to be to make a difference and how much the clean cooking technology displaces old, polluting technologies; that is, how much does exposure have to be reduced to achieve a meaningful health benefit, which is best informed by exposure-response analysis (Peel and others 2015).

RCTs can greatly improve exposure-response results, however. Although randomizing exposure itself in real populations is essentially impossible, randomizing one important cause of variability lessens the burden of potential confounders, increasing confidence in the results. In addition, the intervention spreads out the exposures more than occurs naturally and thus increases the chance of seeing effects. Exposure-response results have also been improved by the introduction of new means to measure the sources of high intrahousehold variability—in particular, the recent wide-scale introduction of stove use monitors (Pillarisetti and others 2014; Ruiz-Mercado, Canuz, and Smith 2012; Ruiz-Mercado and others 2013). These and other technical advances promise to reduce exposure misclassification further and to enhance the ability to detect effects.

An additional advantage of framing HAP effects in terms of exposure is the ability to combine effects across other major sources of air pollution into IERs. The same effects are found in a monotonically increasing trend with estimated exposure, and this provides a new class of evidence that supports results in all the other categories of exposure (ambient air pollution, secondhand tobacco smoke, and active tobacco smoking), but particularly HAP. Indeed, compared to ambient air pollution and active tobacco smoking, many fewer studies are available for all adult outcomes, and almost none are available for two important CVD outcomes—IHD and stroke. Interpolation along the IER function that is fixed by active tobacco smoking and ambient air pollution at the two

ends of the exposure spectrum and bolstered by results for environmental tobacco smoke thus seems justifiable. It is not credible that exposures that produce CVD effects at both higher and lower levels would not also produce CVD effects at the levels found for HAP. Extrapolation beyond the available data is fraught with potential problems, but a major reason to do graphs is to be able to do interpolation. Direct HAP studies of CVD risk factors, such as blood pressure and heart rate variability, further support the existence of CVD effects, but they do not themselves allow an estimate of the total CVD effect.

Although they are a major advance, the IERs include assumptions and show relationships that still need investigation. Three issues bear mention here. First, although three of the types of pollution are composed almost entirely of combustion particles, and although ambient air pollution typically is composed mostly of combustion particles, different types of combustion, fuels, and mixtures of other pollutants are involved with each. Diesel exhaust is different from tobacco smoke, for example, although both can be measured using $PM_{2.5}$. Second, the typical exposure patterns reflecting exposure to these different sources (both daily and over a lifetime) are quite different, even if they can be reduced to a common metric of an annual average. Third, studies use a different measure of exposure for each category of pollution. Ambient air pollution studies use ambient concentrations measured in central locations, such as on the roof of a building in a major metropolitan area. Measured changes of this type are found to reflect changes in actual exposures but are poor representations of absolute exposures. People do not live on top of buildings (where these central site monitors are located), but they do live near small sources that may not affect widespread ambient levels but that do affect individual exposures. Few studies of secondhand tobacco smoke and HAP in adults have measured personal exposure, but some have tried to estimate levels based on fixed monitors or models. Studies of active tobacco smoking use inhaled smoke levels or nominal dose (as measured by smoking machines) to estimate "exposure" per cigarette.

### Other Endpoints

Smith and others (2014) carefully assessed the evidence base for each outcome (disease) associated with HAP. As shown in table 7.2, three classes were established. Diseases in Class I were considered to have sufficient evidence to be included as formal outcomes in the CRA. Class II diseases had a sufficient number of epidemiological studies to conduct meta-analyses, which are found in Smith and others (2014), but the evidence was not considered consistent or otherwise convincing enough to be put forward as part of the formal burden

**Table 7.2** Evidence Classes

| Evidence class | Description | Criteria |
|---|---|---|
| Class IA | Quantified primary outcome, based on binary exposures in systematic reviews and meta-analyses | Multiple epidemiological studies of good quality in households in lower-income countries sufficient for meta-analyses; consistent results as well as significant and positive summary estimate; supporting epidemiological studies of other particle exposures, both at higher and lower exposures |
| Class IB | Quantified primary outcome, continued | Exposure-response data available from several particle exposure settings, allowing development of integrated exposure-response function covering (1) child ALRI, where studies have found that active tobacco smoking does not contribute, but studies have been conducted in the other three exposure settings (outdoor air pollution, secondhand smoke, and household air pollution); (2) CVD outcomes, where studies for outdoor air pollution, secondhand smoke, and active tobacco smoking exist, allowing estimates to be interpolated for HAP |
| Class II | Quantified secondary outcome | Multiple epidemiological studies in households in lower-income countries sufficient for meta-analyses; unconvincing adjustment for confounding or exposure assessment; inconsistent results or nonsignificant positive result; supporting epidemiological studies from other particle exposures |
| Class III | Nonquantified secondary outcome | Still thought likely to be causal; weak or insufficient epidemiological studies from households in lower-income countries for meta-analyses; some support from other particle exposure categories |

*Source:* Adapted from Smith and others 2014.

*Note:* ALRI = acute lower respiratory infection; CVD = cardiovascular disease; HAP = household air pollution. All evidence classes have plausible physiological mechanisms based on toxicology.

of HAP. These included adult ALRI; tuberculosis; nasopharyngeal carcinomas; tumors of the larynx, oropharynx, and hypopharynx; cervical cancer; and stillbirth. Diseases in Class III were considered to have suggestive, but insufficient, evidence for quantification. These diseases included asthma and preterm birth.

The CRA Expert Group found sufficient evidence to consider low birth weight as an outcome for HAP exposures, but the GBD project itself removed low birth weight as an outcome, focusing instead on preterm births. However, too few HAP studies had separated preterm birth from low birth weight for these outcomes to be included in the official CRA. (See Smith and others [2014] for a discussion of the available literature.)

A class of impacts not considered in the CRA consists of neurocognitive outcomes in children, although evidence of such effects has been growing, as has evidence of such effects with other pollution exposures (Smith and others 2014). This is an active area of HAP research.

All of the outcomes in Classes I, II, and III are firmly associated with tobacco smoking, a much more thoroughly studied source of exposure to biomass smoke. Thus, the fact that the same diseases that are associated with tobacco smoking have also been found to be associated with HAP exposures (albeit at lower risk levels) is not surprising. Indeed, the IERs provide quantitative evidence of the consistent relationship between HAP

and active smoking risks for the five main diseases associated with each.

## INTERVENTIONS

This section examines the traditional paradigms that have dominated thinking over the past half century regarding how to accelerate the transition to clean cooking technologies in poor populations. It then discusses more recent paradigms.[5]

### Old Paradigms

#### Let Development Take Care of It

Because the rich use clean fuels and the poor use dirty fuels (Bonjour and others 2013), one may be tempted simply to let development take care of the problem. Unfortunately, this has not worked. About the same number of people (almost 3 billion) are using dirty fuels today as 25 years ago, in spite of the considerable development that has occurred in that time. More people are using clean fuels (gas and electricity), but the absolute burden of exposure has not changed appreciably worldwide. However, the trends in the absolute numbers using solid fuels varies by region: going up in Sub-Saharan Africa, going down in East Asia (China), and remaining level in South Asia (Bonjour and others 2013).

## Make the Available Clean

Since the large national stove programs were initiated in China and India in the early 1980s, perhaps a dozen other national efforts and hundreds (if not thousands) of community and nongovernmental organization (NGO) programs, small and large, have been initiated worldwide to promote better stoves using the same local fuels (mainly different forms of biomass).[6] Although initially focused on fuel efficiency, many of these programs are also attempting to lower smoke levels—that is, to make the available fuels clean through better combustion, chimneys, and others approaches. As described in WHO (2014b), this improvement has been extremely elusive, and finding interventions that have reduced health-related exposures substantially and sustainably for a large population is difficult. Nevertheless, much progress has been made, and investments are needed to continue upgrading the engineering, business, and social marketing required to reach this goal.

One promising development is the parallel work of the International Standards Organization and the WHO to develop standards and guidelines for promoting only the cleanest devices in the future. Quantitative guidelines were made possible only by development of the IERs. Now a base of epidemiological evidence exists to support standards that quantify what emissions level is clean enough for good health (WHO 2014b). As mentioned, emissions reductions alone do not guarantee exposure reductions; rather, interventions must be adopted, maintained, and used regularly to achieve meaningful exposure reductions to protect health.

As part of the evidence review for the IAQGs (WHO 2014b), systematic reviews and meta-analyses were performed of the international literature on interventions (Dherani and others 2014). The methods and results are summarized in box 7.2. This review found that solid-fuel stoves with chimneys delivered the largest reductions in PM and CO concentrations, with CO levels often reaching WHO air quality guidelines. However, none achieved PM levels close to the guidelines. One key issue is the degree of heterogeneity between studies. For this reason, referring to the circumstances and results of individual stove and fuel evaluations is important for appropriate interpretation of these results. Continued efforts are needed to standardize the methods used for field evaluation.

---

**Box 7.2**

### Assessment of Improved Biomass Stove Interventions

To assess the potential health benefits that can be expected following the introduction of improved solid-fuel stoves, one must examine the reductions in HAP and personal exposure—and the absolute levels achieved—when these interventions are in everyday use. Although the results of laboratory emissions tests provide valuable information on the potential reductions in exposure, field evaluations provide a more realistic assessment of exposure when such interventions are adopted and used at scale. The key questions for the review were as follows:

- Are improved solid-fuel stoves in everyday use (compared to traditional solid-fuel stoves) effective for reducing average concentrations of, or exposure to, PM and CO in households in LMICs?
- By what amount (in absolute and relative terms) do the interventions reduce PM and CO, and how do postintervention (in-use) levels compare with the WHO air quality guidelines?

*Methods.* A search was conducted of electronic databases and specialist websites. Eligible studies included randomized trials, quasi-experimental and before-and-after studies, as well as observational designs and reported daily mean (24- or 48-hour) small PM (most reported $PM_{2.5}$, but two studies reported $PM_4$) or CO, with standard deviations or 95 percent confidence intervals. Interventions were categorized as standard combustion solid-fuel stoves with and without chimneys, advanced combustion solid-fuel stoves, clean fuels (LPG, biogas, ethanol, electricity, solar), and mixed interventions. Studies were selected, extracted, and assessed using standardized procedures and forms. Baseline and postintervention values, differences, and percentage changes from baseline were tabulated for each study, and weighted average values were calculated

*box continues next page*

**Box 7.2** (continued)

for all studies contributing data to each category of stove or fuel intervention. Subject to sufficient studies, meta-analysis of absolute changes in the two pollutants for each category of solid-fuel stove and clean fuel was carried out using the generic inverse-variance method, and publication bias was assessed. Narrative summaries were provided for intervention categories with very few eligible studies.

*Results*. A total of 38 eligible studies, some with multiple estimates, was included: 27 studies that provided data on kitchen PM, 3 on personal PM, 26 on kitchen CO, and 5 on personal CO. Only one or two studies were available for each intervention (LPG, electricity, charcoal, mixed). Baseline levels of PM and CO were variable, but all exceeded the annual WHO guideline for $PM_{2.5}$ of 35 micrograms per cubic meter by a factor of 10–100 times, and CO varied from just below to 6 times greater than the 24-hour air quality guideline for CO of 7 milligrams per cubic meter (5.68 parts per million). After intervention, reductions in pollutants were reported for almost all individual studies; when grouped, large reductions in the range of 38–82 percent were found for kitchen PM and CO levels, with the largest reductions for solid-fuel stoves with chimneys and the lowest for solid-fuel stoves without chimneys. Studies reporting impacts on personal exposure were identified only for solid-fuel chimney stoves, but reductions in the range of 47–76 percent were found.

Despite these large percentage reductions, post-intervention levels of PM remained well above the WHO guidelines for group-weighted means at around 400 micrograms per cubic meter, although the few personal exposure studies had a considerably lower weighted mean of 70 micrograms per cubic meter. In contrast, many interventions reduced CO to levels below the WHO 24-hour air quality guideline, with weighted mean values of 4–5 parts per million for stoves with chimneys, but almost 7 parts per million for stoves without chimneys. Postintervention personal exposure in the set of chimney-stove studies was 1.7 parts per million. Sensitivity analyses (conducted where the number of estimates was sufficient), including by study design, analytic approach (that is, comparing controls with only stoves in actual use or with all stoves allocated), and duration of use, did not find strong effects. Among the larger sets of studies, clear evidence of publication bias existed. Evidence from studies of improved wood stoves in high-income rural settings found, as expected, $PM_{2.5}$ levels much lower than those of improved wood stoves in developing countries (ranging from 13 to 54 micrograms per cubic meter) and an association between improved solid-fuel stoves (all of which were vented with some having advanced emissions control technology) and emissions reductions in a majority of households.

*Source:* Based directly on Dherani and others (2014), which also contains lengthy tables describing the published studies to date.

## New Paradigms

Based on the new evidence that exposures must be brought to low levels to achieve major health benefits, and the poor performance of "improved" biomass stoves to date, new paradigms are emerging in the field, although they have been operating on their own in the modern energy sector all along.

## Make the Clean Available

How one achieves clean cooking is no mystery. Gas and electricity are used by 60 percent of humanity, and these fuels cook every cuisine without problem (although with taste changes compared to traditional methods for some foods). Unlike typical biomass stoves, gas and electric stoves cannot be made dirty at the household level (even with nonoptimal use), and they do not require any special attention or training. They also are aspirational, with

attractive modern cooking appliances being an important sales advantage in most settings. They are not available to the populations using biomass, however, not only because of their cost but also because of unreliable or unavailable public and private infrastructure. Any kind of gas burns cleanly, including biogas and natural gas, but LPG is usually the first to reach rural areas. Rather than simply waiting passively for people to shift to clean fuels, there is clear need to find ways to promote these fuels to poor households in a more systematic and aggressive manner.

Several large and innovative initiatives for promoting LPG began in India in 2015. Although initiated by the Ministry of Petroleum and Natural Gas in collaboration with the three national oil companies that market LPG, these initiatives were driven by a desire to reduce the health impacts of solid fuel use for cooking. As of March 2016, more than US$1 billion had been committed to expand LPG to 50 million low-income households in three years, reaching perhaps 300 million people (Ministry of Finance 2016). This ambitious initiative has several innovative features designed to target LPG subsidies much more precisely to poor households and away from middle- and upper-class and commercial consumers. These features involve the use of modern digital technology, including bank accounts, cell phones, and biometric identification cards. In addition, widespread integrated use of formal and social media to promote the effort exists, including text messages, billboards, television and radio, Internet, and athletic events.

The most well-known of the programs is the Give It Up scheme, through which middle- and upper-income consumers are asked to give up their LPG subsidy to households below the poverty line. Households who give up their subsidy are listed on a Scroll of Honor on the website and can see which family benefited from their contribution.[7] Some 30,000 households a day were doing so at the height of the program. As a result, the government was able to focus new resources on providing the up-front costs (stove and cylinder) to enable poor households to take on LPG, and oil companies were incentivized to expand fuel access substantially and to improve the reliability of supply. In addition, new modes of distributing LPG are being tried, including promotion and sales by women's groups. Importantly, the government has specified that all new LPG connections since early 2016 are to be in the name of the woman of the house wherever possible, a significant movement toward improving gender engagement. Because shifting the subsidy from one income group to another does not entail additional government expenditure, the cost-effectiveness of this effort depends only on the additional expenditures for up-front costs.[8]

Another approach is to promote clean fuels that have not been widely adopted in high-income countries and thus have no established operational viability. The most prominent of these is biogas; although attractively clean and made renewably from animal dung, biogas is limited in scope by climate, capital cost, and the need for at least two large animals in each household. Second is ethanol, which burns cleanly and can be made renewably from several crops, including sugarcane and sorghum. Unknown, however, is whether large-scale production would trigger demand in other sectors (for example, as a petroleum enhancer or beverage) that would dominate its availability and price as a fuel.

The review described in box 7.2 also examined available studies for clean fuel interventions. It found none for electric cooking and too few for LPG or biogas to make an assessment. However, it found several for ethanol that indicated a reduction in overall exposure, but not enough to reach WHO air quality guidelines (WHO 2014b).

One major reason that clean fuel interventions do not show greater reductions is the remaining use of polluting fuels either in the same household or nearby, which has not been monitored well in past studies. More and better-designed studies are needed for all kinds of clean fuel interventions, as well as new intervention modes that promote usage and initial adoption.

### Embrace Leap-Frog Technologies

Highly advanced, electronic devices are now available for cooking. Depending on the task, electric induction stoves are 50 percent more efficient and 50 percent faster (as well as safer and longer-lived) than old-style electric stoves. They are so different as to provide a new entry into the cookstove landscape. Sales are booming in Asia, and prices are dropping, reaching as low as US$10 each in some markets. Most of the sales growth is occurring among customers now using gas, as cooking with induction stoves is sometimes cheaper than cooking with subsidized LPG. How far might induction stoves be pushed into rural areas when electricity supply becomes more reliable? Ecuador, for example, is replacing every stove in the country with an induction stove, and other countries with excess hydropower are considering taking such an approach. Could induction stoves be linked to local power made from renewable energy sources? This is an exciting prospect. Even when linked to coal power, induction stoves create substantially less pollution exposure and only minor increases in greenhouse gases (Smith 2014).

Synthetic liquid or gaseous fuels such as the bioethanol discussed earlier and synthetic LPG made from coal, which are clean at the household, also show promise but require additional study and evaluation of system requirements. Synthetic natural gas from coal is also being promoted in China and Mongolia but requires extensive pipeline infrastructure that makes it cost-prohibitive in most rural areas.

### Target the Community Level

Ongoing research and modeling show that, in many circumstances, changing one household in a village to clean fuels reduces exposure less than one might expect (Desai 2016; Smith 1987). This is because of a coverage or community effect—that is, even if you cook using LPG (or do not cook at all), you are affected by all of your neighbors who still cook on biomass stoves. Although varying by geography and meteorology, most of humanity lives in fairly close quarters, whether in cities or villages, and the community effect is common. For this reason, the most effective interventions are likely to occur at the community level. This has two other advantages: providing fuels, stoves, and service at the community scale usually is more efficient, lowering costs and increasing reliability, and it is possible to unleash social pressure to change social norms—for example, creating a smokeless village designation to encourage neighbors to work together (put pressure on each other) to avoid producing smoke in their village. Indeed, these other benefits of community interventions are likely to be the most critical.

The LPG initiatives in India are promoting "smokeless villages" designed to develop LPG connections by village rather than by household. As of mid-2016, at least 4,000 smokeless villages (defined as 100 percent of households being connected) had been certified, with thousands more being planned.

As with much of the rapid changes in the "make the clean available" agenda, however, evaluation of smokeless villages and other modes of LPG expansion have not yet been subjected to high-quality evaluation, something clearly needed.

## Recent Innovations

New ways of thinking have emerged from the literature but have not yet been well integrated into interventions. Among these is growing recognition of the following.

### Impact on Outdoor Pollution

A major reason that the field has moved away from the term *indoor* to *household* air pollution is the realization that, although pollution may start in the kitchen, it moves throughout the household, then into the community environment outside, where it adds to general ambient air pollution. The degree to which this matters depends on the situation; in India, for instance, as noted, an estimated 25–50 percent of primary ambient $PM_{2.5}$ comes from household cooking. Estimates are similar for China, although household use of solid fuel for heat is also seasonally important in much of the country (Liu and others 2016). Cleaning up household fuels clearly is a necessary step in dealing with outdoor pollution. Because outdoor air pollution has become a serious policy and public concern in many countries that still have significant household use of solid fuel, this connection provides a potential impetus for control programs and a framework for evaluation.

In late 2015, India's Ministry of Health and Family Welfare released a white paper proposing a pioneering approach to air pollution (Ministry of Health and Family Welfare 2015). It was the first ministry of health in the world to consider air pollution in the context of other health priorities, with the idea of using the health sector's unique assets to address it (air pollution generally has been handled by environmental agencies, which have a different agenda). India's Ministry of Health and Family Welfare is also the first government agency in the world to address household and ambient air pollution together by proposing a program to manage exposure, not concentrations, in particular locations (Sagar and others 2016). If implemented, this approach would focus more on pollution sources that are in close proximity to people (stoves and vehicles) and less on sources that are far from people (power plants and industries).

### Household Air Pollution as a Health Problem

Part of the poor progress of previous attempts to reduce HAP may be due to their origins in the technology sector rather than the health sector and the heavy emphasis the technology sector places on simple local technologies and community groups or NGOs. In contrast, the health sector taps the very best advanced scientific, technological, and manufacturing techniques to develop effective vaccines, antibiotics, and surgery tools; then, after those techniques have been proved worthwhile in highly structured field trials, the health sector makes them available through prepurchase, royalty agreements, and mass manufacture to reduce the cost. It then uses NGOs and other community groups to bring the vaccines to vulnerable populations. Unlike the technology sector, the health sector treats everyone the same; it does not promote less effective antibiotics in rural areas because the people there are poor. Unequal treatment may be satisfactory when addressing fuel efficiency or meeting local labor and materials goals, which are important issues in their own right. The technology sector is less effective at achieving health goals, and its priorities raise disquieting ethical issues.

One reason that often is given for continued cooking on open fires is the taste of the food, but the health sector would ask, is taste worth nearly one million lives a year in India? The health sector does not stop its programs because people like the taste of tobacco or dislike wearing seatbelts or dislike using condoms. It recognizes the importance of personal preferences, however, and brings social pressure to bear in an effort to change those tastes. The health sector has already recognized the importance of various kinds of "herd" effects—for example, with sanitation and mosquito protection. First is effectiveness on a large scale, which has often been promoted in biomass stove programs. Next is the household business model, which may come later. Finally, the health sector is not afraid of subsidies but provides the evidence needed to prove that expenditures on the health of the poor are cost-effective social investments.

### Common Challenges with Interventions

Although many relatively small-scale, low-cost interventions (such as the provision of better-burning biomass stoves) will continue, efforts to reach households at a large scale using existing infrastructure in the petroleum and power sectors are growing, but in ways that better focus on health. India is leading the way, but other countries have programs or are planning them.[9]

With LPG or electricity, little HAP concern exists, because the appliances that use these cooking fuels can stand up to variations in user behavior, and the appliances' performance is well known, with billions in use over many decades. Even with the most advanced biomass stoves, however, good field performance is difficult to maintain, even when the stoves are used regularly. Two common difficulties remain, however, with both approaches: cost and continued use of traditional polluting cookstoves.

### Cost and Subsidy

An advanced biomass stove with a chimney and blower (characteristics likely to be required for good health) is not cheap by low-income-country standards. The cost of the stove alone is likely to be more than US$100 and probably closer to US$200, as seen in successful chimney stove programs in China and Mexico, for example. The costs of dissemination, maintenance, repair, and replacement add to this. In addition, to date, only biomass pellet stoves are reliably clean enough to come close to the IAQGs for emissions. Pellet stoves require users to forfeit the greatest advantage of today's biomass fuel, which is that it can be gathered at no direct financial cost. Financing the stoves and pelletizing infrastructure in ways that are sustainable for poor populations is a major challenge.

The same is true of providing LPG or electric power reliably and sustainably. Electrification offers a way to spread costs, given its many social and other benefits in addition to health. Up-front costs are substantially lower than for nearly equivalently clean biomass stoves, but electricity entails recurring costs and access issues.

The very poor are unlikely to be able to afford any truly clean cooking technology. If significant progress is to occur, some form of public support likely will be needed for some years. This is not unusual: public support is accepted for many health-protective interventions for the poor, including vaccines, antenatal care, and basic antibiotics. The term *subsidy* often is applied to public support for fuels, usually in a pejorative way. However, subsidies for nuclear power, the coal industry, and the solar industry are not intended to target health protection for the poor, unlike support for HAP-reducing technologies such as LPG and advanced biomass stoves. Thus, if public expenditures can be shown to be as well targeted and effective as other expenditures on health-protective interventions, they may be considered social investments rather than subsidies, with a substantially different political and developmental connotation.

### Compliance and Stacking

The second issue is *stacking*, which refers to the common observation that people often do not switch to a new technology immediately, even if it is better in many ways and eventually takes over. In the case of cooking, people often continue to use their traditional fuel stove even if they also use an advanced biomass stove or LPG. It may take years, in the case of LPG, before they switch entirely, a process that has a generational component—young women often do not continue what their mothers find hard to give up.

As a result, with a new clean fuel alternative in the home, all of the HAP exposure is due to continued use of the traditional stove, and the exposure can be substantial. This is a familiar situation in health interventions: simply providing access and affordability does not guarantee high compliance (for example, in using bed nets, condoms, latrines, tuberculosis drugs, low-salt foods, and nicotine substitutes). In most of these examples, as with HAP, a high rate of compliance is needed to reduce risk adequately (seemingly more than 90 percent in the case of latrines and bed nets, for example). Accordingly, as with every other health intervention that must be accompanied by behavioral change, incentives must be found and implemented to enhance compliance (Fernald, Gertler, and Neufeld 2009; Fernald, Hou, and Gertler 2008; Lim and others 2010) or, in stove parlance, to reduce the degree and duration of stacking.

Additional research is needed to find ways to promote reduced use of the old and increased adoption and use of the new. Recent systematic reviews of adoption and barriers to adoption of clean stoves (Puzzolo and others 2016) and of clean fuels and electricity (Rehfuess and others 2014) highlight this need. They also challenge dissemination approaches that only market the new, as might be adequate for economic sustainability. Imagining a business model for eliminating the old polluting stove, however, is difficult, a phenomenon that is not uncommon with household or individual health interventions.

Approaches for triggering community pressure (for example, conditional cash transfers and cell phone messaging) have been applied successfully in other situations and could successfully reduce HAP as well. In addition, some innovations show promise even if they have never been applied—for example, linking the use of HAP-reducing cooking technology, such as LPG, to national life insurance and rural employment schemes, as is being considered in India.

## CONCLUSIONS

The health impacts of HAP have been suspected for decades, beginning with a few isolated studies more than a half century ago (Padmavati and Pathak 1959); only recently, sufficient evidence has been marshaled to make a systematic case for HAP's ill health effects across a range of diseases. This evidence is substantiated best in the two detailed reviews used so extensively in this chapter (Smith and others 2014; WHO 2014b). The conceptual and empirical connection between active and passive tobacco smoking and ambient air pollution provided by the IERs gives rise to a completely different and in itself compelling set of arguments for HAP's ill health effects, in addition to the growing base of epidemiological and toxicological evidence. Although the evidence is insufficient to pin down a precise risk for all diseases now attributed to HAP exposures or to establish a firm base for diseases that have some, but insufficient, evidence to include on the list, it seems likely that HAP will remain on the list of severe health risks affecting the world's poorest populations.

HAP will continue to constitute a major risk factor as long as billions of households worldwide use solid fuels. However, simply believing it to be a major risk is not sufficient to bring solutions. As noted in the introduction, fecal matter in the household environment was confirmed as a major risk factor for ill health in the late 1800s, but it still kills millions today in spite of considerable efforts to reduce this health burden. Both of these risk factors share uncomfortable similarities: they are significant, operate in poor populations, and require behavioral and engineering innovations and interventions. They both also seem to be refractory to cheap solutions. How can we be sure then that HAP (which only passed the threshold of acceptability in 2010 or so, and even still perhaps not as completely as fecal contamination) is not still killing millions a century from now?

Although basic epidemiological, toxicological, and exposure research continues, HAP's threshold of acceptability has been passed, and serious research is needed to determine what works on a large scale. Regarding poor sanitation, the failure to move in this direction is perhaps partly responsible for the long delay between recognition of the problem and its solution. Considering the question of scale—at the household level and the institutional level, in terms of the agencies and organizations that can operate on a large scale and perform careful monitoring and evaluation of natural interventions—is another way to frame this effort. This mode of thinking is particularly salient for those efforts now under way with clean fuels (such as LPG and electricity) in India, Bhutan, Paraguay, Ecuador, and elsewhere. As HAP has the advantage of a measurable exposure metric, much of this research can proceed more quickly and with less cost because exposure outcomes can be used as endpoints. If, in parallel, exposure-response is emphasized in the health research, the two together can help to find ways to provide the world with clean household environments effectively and steadily.

Providing empirical evidence of the cost-effectiveness of alternative interventions is difficult, although there is movement in this direction (Newcombe and others 2016; Pillarisetti, Mehta, and Smith 2016). The long-term solution is clear: clean fuels (although they will not be available for the very poorest populations for some years). Until then, however, the evident popularity of such fuels could be a model for how improved biomass stoves are designed and disseminated.[10] Only now are we beginning to understand how to bring clean fuels to the poor (but not the poorest) populations much faster than development alone has brought, while simultaneously accelerating the movement away from traditional practices during the transition.

## NOTES

World Bank Income Classifications as of July 2014 are as follows, based on estimates of gross national income (GNI) per capita for 2013:

- Low-income countries (LICs) = US$1,045 or less
- Middle-income countries (MICs) are subdivided:
  a) lower-middle-income = US$1,046 to US$4,125
  b) upper-middle-income (UMICs) = US$4,126 to US$12,745
- High-income countries (HICs) = US$12,746 or more.

1. This chapter focuses almost entirely on wood fuel, which dominates world use and research. Agricultural residues, including animal dung, are far less consistent and less well characterized. Coal pollution is even more difficult to summarize because of wide variations in the quality of coal around the world, including the content of toxic species, such as sulfur, arsenic, lead, mercury, ash, and others. For a good discussion, see WHO (2014b).
2. Few studies have been conducted on the impact of chronic CO exposures on health, and CO in wood smoke rarely causes acutely toxic exposures because of the warning of extreme irritation from other wood smoke components. Therefore, this chapter does not explore CO exposure further, though we note observed links between exposure to CO during pregnancy and adverse outcomes. However, low-volatile solid fuels, particularly charcoal and some coals, can produce acutely hazardous CO exposures. Indeed, despite the dearth of systematic assessments, thousands of deaths likely occur globally each year (some even in high-income countries) as a result of CO exposure (for example, from charcoal grills used indoors).
3. Kerosene, another middle distillate like diesel, is still used for household cooking in some countries and is widely used for lighting in hundreds of millions of households

without adequate electricity. Growing evidence suggests that, by mass, $PM_{2.5}$ from kerosene combustion is more toxic than $PM_{2.5}$ from biomass combustion. To date, however, the WHO has been unable to do more than recommend that kerosene be discouraged as a household fuel. (See WHO 2014b.)

4. The WHO guideline for annual average $PM_{2.5}$ concentrations is 10 micrograms per cubic meter (WHO 2014b).

5. This section draws on Smith and Sagar (2014) and Smith (2015), as well as on WHO (2014b).

6. See http://cleancookstoves.org/.

7. See http://mylpg.in/.

8. In 2016, the Give It Up program was folded into an even larger program to promote a total of 50 million LPG connections in India in three years.

9. See http://www.cooking-for-life.org/.

10. IAQGs has a section on the needs of the very poor in the transition to clean fuels for all.

## REFERENCES

Balakrishnan, K., G. Thangavel, S. Ghosh, S. Sambandam, K. Mukhopadhyay, and others. 2011. *The Global Household Air Pollution Measurement Database*. Geneva: World Health Organization. http://www.who.int/indoorair/health_impacts/databases/en/.

Baumgartner, J., J. J. Schauer, M. Ezzati, L. Lu, C. Cheng, and others. 2011. "Patterns and Predictors of Personal Exposure to Indoor Air Pollution from Biomass Combustion among Women and Children in Rural China." *Indoor Air* 21 (6): 479–88.

Bonjour, S., H. Adair-Rohani, J. Wolf, N. G. Bruce, S. Mehta, and others. 2013. "Solid Fuel Use for Household Cooking: Country and Regional Estimates for 1980–2010." *Environmental Health Perspectives* 121 (7): 784–90.

Bruce, N., M. Dherani, R. Liu, H. D. Hosgood III, A. Sapkota, and others. 2015. "Does Household Use of Biomass Fuel Cause Lung Cancer? A Systematic Review and Evaluation of the Evidence for the GBD 2010 Study." *Thorax* 70 (5): 433–41.

Burnett, R. T., C. A. Pope III, M. Ezzati, C. Olives, S. S. Lim, and others. 2014. "An Integrated Risk Function for Estimating the Global Burden of Disease Attributable to Ambient Fine Particulate Matter Exposure." *Environmental Health Perspectives* 122 (4): 397–403.

Chafe, Z. A., M. Brauer, Z. Klimont, R. Van Dingenen, S. Mehta, and others. 2014. "Household Cooking with Solid Fuels Contributes to Ambient $PM_{2.5}$ Air Pollution and the Burden of Disease." *Environmental Health Perspectives* 122 (12): 1314–20.

Chapman, R. S., X. He, A. E. Blair, and Q. Lan. 2005. "Improvement in Household Stoves and Risk of Chronic Obstructive Pulmonary Disease in Xuanwei, China: Retrospective Cohort Study." *BMJ* 331 (7524): 1050.

Desai, M. A. 2016. "Model of Postulated Coverage Effect from Clean Cooking Interventions." In *Multiscale Drivers of Global Environmental Health*. Doctoral dissertation submitted to the Environmental Health Sciences Graduate Group, University of California, Berkeley, 88–147.

Dherani, M., K. Jagoe, L. P. Naeher, and C. Noonan. 2014. "Review 6: Impacts of Interventions on Household Air Pollution Concentrations and Personal Exposure." In *WHO Indoor Air Quality Guidelines: Household Fuel Combustion*, edited by E. Rehfuess, D. Pope, and N. Bruce. Geneva: World Health Organization.

Diaz, E., T. Smith-Sivertsen, D. Pope, R. T. Lie, A. Diaz, and others. 2007. "Eye Discomfort, Headache, and Back Pain among Mayan Guatemalan Women Taking Part in a Randomised Stove Intervention Trial." *Journal of Epidemiology and Community Health* 61 (1): 74–79.

Edwards, R. D., Y. Liu, G. He, Z. Yin, J. Sinton, and others. 2007. "Household CO and PM Measured as Part of a Review of China's National Improved Stove Program." *Indoor Air* 17 (3): 189–203.

Fernald, L. C., P. J. Gertler, and L. M. Neufeld. 2009. "10-Year Effect of Oportunidades, Mexico's Conditional Cash Transfer Programme, on Child Growth, Cognition, Language, and Behaviour: A Longitudinal Follow-Up Study." *The Lancet* 374 (9706): 1997–2005.

Fernald, L. C., X. Hou, and P. J. Gertler. 2008. "Oportunidades Program Participation and Body Mass Index, Blood Pressure, and Self-Reported Health in Mexican Adults." *Preventing Chronic Disease* 5 (3): A81.

GBD Risk Factors Collaborators. 2015. "Global, Regional, and National Comparative Risk Assessment of 79 Behavioural, Environmental, Occupational, and Metabolic Risks or Clusters of Risks in 188 Countries, 1990–2013: A Systematic Analysis for the Global Burden of Disease Study 2013." *The Lancet* 386 (10010): 2287–323.

GOLD (Global Initiative for Chronic Obstructive Lung Disease). 2016. *Global Strategy for the Diagnosis, Management and Prevention of COPD*. GOLD. http://www.goldcopd.org/.

Guttikunda, S. 2016. *Urban Emissions*. http://www.urbanemissions.info/.

IHME (Institute for Health Metrics and Evaluation). 2016. "GBD Compare Data Visualization." IHME, University of Washington, Seattle. http://vizhub.healthdata.org/gbd-comparevizhub.healthdata.org/gbd-compare.

Jetter, J. J., Z. Guo, J. A. McBrian, and M. R. Flynn. 2002. "Characterization of Emissions from Burning Incense." *Science of the Total Environment* 295 (1–3): 51–67.

Jetter, J., Y. Zhao, K. R. Smith, B. Khan, T. Yelverton, and others. 2012. "Pollutant Emissions and Energy Efficiency under Controlled Conditions for Household Biomass Cookstoves and Implications for Metrics Useful in Setting International Test Standards." *Environmental Science and Technology* 46 (19): 10827–34.

Johnson, M., T. Bond, N. Lam, C. Weyant, Y. Chen, and others. 2011. "In-Home Assessment of Greenhouse Gas and Aerosol Emissions from Biomass Cookstoves in Developing Countries." In *Greenhouse Gas Strategies in a Changing Climate Conference 2011*, 530–42. Pittsburgh: Air and Waste Management Association.

Johnson, M., R. Edwards, C. A. Frenk, and O. Masera. 2008. "In-Field Greenhouse Gas Emissions from Cookstoves in Rural Mexican Households." *Atmospheric Environment* 42 (6): 1206–22.

Lelieveld, J., J. S. Evans, M. Fnais, D. Giannadaki, and A. Pozzer. 2015. "The Contribution of Outdoor Air Pollution Sources to Premature Mortality on a Global Scale." *Nature* 525 (7569): 367–71.

Lim, S. S., L. Dandona, J. A. Hoisington, S. L. James, M. C. Hogan, and others. 2010. "India's Janani Suraksha Yojana, A Conditional Cash Transfer Programme to Increase Births in Health Facilities: An Impact Evaluation." *The Lancet* 375 (9730): 2009–23.

Lim, S. S., T. Vos, A. D. Flaxman, G. Danaei, K. Shibuya, and others. 2012. "A Comparative Risk Assessment of Burden of Disease and Injury Attributable to 67 Risk Factors and Risk Factor Clusters in 21 Regions, 1990–2010: A Systematic Analysis for the Global Burden of Disease Study 2010." *The Lancet* 380 (9859): 2224–60.

Liu, J., D. L. Mauzerall, Q. Chen, Q. Zhang, Y. Song, and others. 2016. "Air Pollutant Emissions from Chinese Households: A Major and Underappreciated Ambient Pollution Source." *Proceedings of the National Academy of Sciences* 113 (28): 7756–61. http://www.pnas.org/cgi/doi/10.1073/pnas.1604537113.

Lozano, R., M. Naghavi, K. Foreman, S. Lim, K. Shibuya, and others. 2012. "Global and Regional Mortality from 235 Causes of Death for 20 Age Groups in 1990 and 2010: A Systematic Analysis for the Global Burden of Disease Study 2010." *The Lancet* 380 (9859): 2095–128.

McCracken, J. P., J. Schwartz, N. Bruce, M. Mittleman, L. M. Ryan, and others. 2009. "Combining Individual- and Group-Level Exposure Information: Child Carbon Monoxide in the Guatemala Woodstove Randomized Control Trial." *Epidemiology* 20 (1): 127–36.

McCracken, J. P., J. Schwartz, A. Diaz, N. Bruce, and K. R. Smith. 2013. "Longitudinal Relationship between Personal CO and Personal $PM_{2.5}$ among Women Cooking with Woodfired Cookstoves in Guatemala." *PLoS One* 8 (2): e55670.

Ministry of Finance. 2016. *Union Budget 2016–2017.* New Delhi: Ministry of Finance, Government of India.

Ministry of Health and Family Welfare. 2015. *Report of the Steering Committee on Air Pollution and Health-Related Issues.* New Delhi: Ministry of Health and Family Welfare, Government of India.

Naeher, L. P., M. Brauer, M. Lipsett, J. T. Zelikoff, C. D. Simpson, and others. 2007. "Woodsmoke Health Effects: A Review." *Inhalation Toxicology* 19 (1): 67–106.

Newcombe, K., T. Ramanathan, N. Ramanathan, and E. Ross. 2016. "Innovations in Payments for Health Benefits of Improved Cookstoves." In *Broken Pumps and Promises: Incentivizing Impact in Environmental Health*, edited by E. A. Thomas, 171–79. Cham, Switzerland: Springer International Publishing AG.

Ni, K., E. Carter, J. J. Schauer, M. Ezzati, Y. Zhang, and others. 2016. "Seasonal Variation in Outdoor, Indoor, and Personal Air Pollution Exposures of Women Using Wood Stoves in the Tibetan Plateau: Baseline Assessment for an Energy Intervention Study." *Environment International* 94: 449–57. doi:10.1016/j.envint.2016.05.029.

Northcross, A. L., S. K. Hammond, E. Canuz, and K. R. Smith. 2012. "Dioxin Inhalation Doses from Wood Combustion in Indoor Cookfires." *Atmospheric Environment* 49 (March): 415–18.

Padmavati, S., and S. N. Pathak. 1959. "Chronic Cor Pulmonale in Delhi: A Study of 127 Cases." *Circulation* 20 (3): 343–52.

Peel, J. L., J. Baumgartner, G. A. Wellenius, M. L. Clark, and K. R. Smith. 2015. "Are Randomized Trials Necessary to Advance Epidemiologic Research on Household Air Pollution?" *Current Epidemiology Reports* 2 (4): 263–70.

Pillarisetti, A., L. W. H. Alnes, J. P. McCracken, E. Canuz, and K. R. Smith. 2016. "Long-Term $PM_{2.5}$ in Kitchens Cooking with Wood: Implications for Measurement Strategies." *Environmental Science and Technology* 48: 14525–533.

Pillarisetti, A., S. Mehta, and K. R. Smith. 2016. "HAPIT, the Household Air Pollution Intervention Tool, to Evaluate the Health Benefits and Cost-Effectiveness of Clean Cooking Interventions." In *Broken Pumps and Promises: Incentivizing Impact in Environmental Health*, edited by E. A. Thomas, 147–70. Cham, Switzerland: Springer International Publishing AG.

Pillarisetti, A., M. Vaswani, D. Jack, K. Balakrishnan, M. N. Bates, and others. 2014. "Patterns of Stove Usage after Introduction of an Advanced Cookstove: The Long-Term Application of Household Sensors." *Environmental Science and Technology* 48 (24): 14525–33.

Pope, C. A. III, R. T. Burnett, D. Krewski, M. Jerrett, Y. Shi, and others. 2009. "Cardiovascular Mortality and Exposure to Airborne Fine Particulate Matter and Cigarette Smoke: Shape of the Exposure-Response Relationship." *Circulation* 120 (11): 941–48.

Puzzolo, E., D. Pope, D. Stanistreet, E. Rehfuess, and N. G. Bruce. 2016. "Clean Fuels for Resource-Poor Settings: A Systematic Review of Barriers and Enablers to Adoption and Sustained Use." *Environmental Research* 146 (April): 218–34.

Rehfuess, E. A., E. Puzzolo, D. Stanistreet, D. Pope, and N. G. Bruce. 2014. "Enablers and Barriers to Large-Scale Uptake of Improved Solid Fuel Stoves: A Systematic Review." *Environmental Health Perspectives* 122 (2): 120–30.

Ruiz-Mercado, I., E. Canuz, and K. R. Smith. 2012. "Temperature Dataloggers as Stove Use Monitors (SUMs): Field Methods and Signal Analysis." *Biomass and Bioenergy* 47 (December): 459–68.

Ruiz-Mercado, I., E. Canuz, J. L. Walker, and K. R. Smith. 2013. "Quantitative Metrics of Stove Adoption Using Stove Use Monitors (SUMs)." *Biomass and Bioenergy* 57 (October): 136–48.

Sagar, A. D., K. Balakrishnan, S. Guttikunda, A. Roychowdhury, and K. R. Smith. 2016. "India Leads the Way: A Health-Centered Strategy for Air Pollution." *Environmental Health Perspectives* 124 (7): A116–17.

Salomon, J. 2014. "Disability Adjusted Life Years." In *Encyclopedia of Health Economics*, edited by A. J. Cuyler, 200–03. San Diego, CA: Elsevier.

Seow, W. J., W. Hu, R. Vermeulen, H. D. Hosgood III, G. S. Downward, and others. 2014. "Household Air Pollution and Lung Cancer in China: A Review of Studies in Xuanwei." *Chinese Journal of Cancer* 33 (10): 471–75.

Shen, M., R. S. Chapman, R. Vermeulen, L. Tian, T. Zheng, and others. 2009. "Coal Use, Stove Improvement, and Adult Pneumonia Mortality in Xuanwei, China: A Retrospective Cohort Study." *Environmental Health Perspectives* 117 (2): 261–66.

Smil, V. 1994. *Energy and World History.* Boulder, CO: Westview Press.

Smith, K. R. 1987. *Biofuels, Air Pollution, and Health: A Global Review.* New York: Plenum Publishing.

———. 2014. "In Praise of Power." *Science* 345 (6197): 603.

———. 2015. "Changing Paradigms in Clean Cooking." *EcoHealth* 12 (1): 196–99.

Smith, K. R., N. Bruce, K. Balakrishnan, H. Adair-Rohani, J. Balmes, and others. 2014. "Millions Dead: How Do We Know and What Does It Mean? Methods Used in the Comparative Risk Assessment of Household Air Pollution." *Annual Review of Public Health* 35: 185–206.

Smith, K. R., J. P. McCracken, L. Thompson, R. Edwards, K. N. Shields, and others. 2010. "Personal Child and Mother Carbon Monoxide Exposures and Kitchen Levels: Methods and Results from a Randomized Trial of Woodfired Chimney Cookstoves in Guatemala (RESPIRE)." *Journal of Exposure Science and Environmental Epidemiology* 20 (5): 406–16.

Smith, K. R., J. P. McCracken, M. W. Weber, A. Hubbard, A. Jenny, and others. 2011. "Effect of Reduction in Household Air Pollution on Childhood Pneumonia in Guatemala (RESPIRE): A Randomised Controlled Trial." *The Lancet* 378 (9804): 1717–26.

Smith, K. R., and A. Sagar. 2014. "Making the Clean Available: Escaping India's Chulha Trap." *Energy Policy* 75 (December): 410–14.

Tolunay, H. E., and A. Chockalingam. 2012. "Indoor and Outdoor Air Pollution and Cardiovascular Health." *Global Heart* 7 (2): 87–196.

Van Vliet, E. D. S., K. Asante, D. W. Jack, P. L. Kinney, R. M. Whyatt, and others. 2013. "Personal Exposures to Fine Particulate Matter and Black Carbon in Households Cooking with Biomass Fuels in Rural Ghana." *Environmental Research* 127 (November): 40–48.

Venkataraman, C., A. D. Sagar, G. Habib, N. Lam, and K. R. Smith. 2010. "The Indian National Initiative for Advanced Biomass Cookstoves: The Benefits of Clean Combustion." *Energy for Sustainable Development* 14 (2): 63–72.

WHO (World Health Organization). 1993. *Biomarkers and Risk Assessment: Concepts and Principles, Environmental Health Criteria.* Geneva: WHO, International Programme on Chemical Safety.

———. 2014a. Global Health Observatory (database): Population Using Solid Fuels, by Country. WHO, Geneva. http://apps .who.int/gho/data/node.main.135?lang=en.

———. 2014b. *WHO Indoor Air Quality Guidelines: Household Fuel Combustion.* Geneva: WHO

Wrangham, R. W. 2009. *Catching Fire: How Cooking Made Us Human.* New York: Basic Books.

Zelikoff, J. T., L. C. Chen, M. D. Cohen, and R. B. Schlesinger. 2002. "The Toxicology of Inhaled Woodsmoke." *Journal of Toxicology and Environmental Health, Part B: Critical Reviews* 5 (3): 269–82.

Zhang, J. J., and K. R. Smith. 2007. "Household Air Pollution from Coal and Biomass Fuels in China: Measurements, Health Impacts, and Interventions." *Environmental Health Perspectives* 115 (6): 848–55.

Zhang J. J., K. R. Smith, Y. Ma, F. Jiang, W. Qi, and others. 2000. "Greenhouse Gases and Other Airborne Pollutants from Household Stoves in China: A Database for Emission Factors." *Atmospheric Environment* 34 (26): 4537–49.

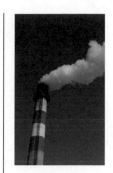

Chapter **8**

# Health Risks and Costs of Climate Variability and Change

Kristie L. Ebi, Jeremy J. Hess, and Paul Watkiss

## INTRODUCTION

The scientific community agrees that climate change is happening, is largely human induced, and will have serious consequences for human health (Field and others 2014). The health consequences of climate variability and change are diverse, potentially affecting the burden of a wide range of health outcomes. Changing weather patterns can affect the magnitude and pattern of morbidity and mortality from extreme weather and climate events, and from changing concentrations of ozone, particulate matter, and aeroallergens (Smith and others 2014). Changing weather patterns and climatic shifts may also create environmental conditions that facilitate alterations in the geographic range, seasonality, and incidence of some infectious diseases in some regions, such as the spread of malaria into highland areas in parts of Sub-Saharan Africa. Changes in water availability and agricultural productivity could affect undernutrition, particularly in some parts of Africa and Asia (Lloyd, Kovats, and Chalabi 2011). Although climate change will likely increase positive health outcomes in some regions, the overall balance will be detrimental for health and well-being, especially in low- and lower-middle-income countries that experience higher burdens of climate-sensitive health outcomes (Smith and others 2014).

The pathways between climate change and health outcomes are often complex and indirect, making attribution challenging. Climate change may not be the most important driver of climate-sensitive health outcomes over the next few decades but could be significant past

the middle of this century. Climate change is a stress multiplier, putting pressure on vulnerable systems, populations, and regions. For example, temperature is associated with the incidence of some food- and water-borne diseases that are significant sources of childhood mortality (Smith and others 2014). Reducing the burden of these diseases requires improved access to safe water and improved sanitation. Poverty is a primary driver underlying the health risks of climate change (Smith and others 2014). Poverty alleviation programs could improve the capacity of health systems to manage risks and reduce the overall costs of a changing climate.

Climate change entails other unique challenges:

- The magnitude, pattern, and rate of climate change over smaller spatial scales are inherently uncertain.
- Weather patterns will continue to change until mid-century, no matter to what extent greenhouse gas emissions (which drive climate change) are reduced in the short term.
- The magnitude and pattern of health risks past mid-century will be determined largely by the extent to which emissions are reduced in coming decades and the extent to which health systems are strengthened to manage current risks and prepare for projected ones in coming decades (Field and others 2014).

Significant reductions in greenhouse gas emissions (mitigation) in the next few years will be critical to preventing more severe climate change later in the century, but

Corresponding author: Kristie L. Ebi, Department of Global Health, University of Washington, Seattle, Washington, United States; krisebi@uw.edu.

they will have limited effects on weather patterns in the short term. In terms of costing, another complexity is that these policies and technologies are associated with short-term health benefits (Garcia-Menendez and others 2015).

Reducing and managing health risks over the next few decades will require modifying health systems to prepare for, cope with, and recover from the health consequences of climate variability and change; these changes are part of what is termed *adaptation*. Adaptation will be required across the century, with the extent of mitigation being a key determinant of health systems' ability to manage risks projected later in the century (Smith and others 2014). No matter the success of adaptation and mitigation, residual risks from climate change will burden health systems, particularly in low- and middle-income countries (LMICs).

Given these complexities, estimating the costs of managing the health risks of climate variability and change is not straightforward. The wide range of health outcomes potentially affected means counting (1) costs associated with increased health care and public health interventions for morbidity and mortality from a long list of climate-sensitive health outcomes; (2) costs associated with lost work days and lower productivity; and (3) costs associated with well-being. Costs could also accrue from repeated episodes of malaria, diarrhea, or other infectious diseases that affect childhood development and health in later life. Costs associated with actions taken in other sectors are also important for health, such as access to safe water and improved sanitation. A portion of the costs of managing the health risks associated with migrants and environmental refugees could be, but has not been, counted.

Further, costs and benefits will be displaced over time, with costs associated with increased health burdens occurring now because of past greenhouse gas emissions and benefits occurring later in the century because of mitigation implemented in the next few years. A few preliminary estimates have been made of the costs of adaptation. However, more work is needed to understand how climate variability and change could affect the ability of health systems to manage risks over long temporal scales.

This chapter reviews the health risks of climate variability and change, discusses key components of those risks, summarizes the attributes of climate-resilient health systems, provides an overview of the costs of increasing health resilience that arise from other sectors, reviews temporal and spatial scale issues, and summarizes key conclusions regarding the costs of the health risks of climate change.

## HEALTH RISKS OF CLIMATE VARIABILITY AND CHANGE

Climate change is affecting morbidity and mortality worldwide, with the risks projected to increase over coming decades (Smith and others 2014). Many health outcomes are affected by weather and climate, as shown in figure 8.1. The poor and vulnerable in LMICs, particularly children, are and will continue to be affected most. Until mid-century, the adverse health risks of climate change will mainly be exacerbations of current health problems, with the possibility that diseases (for example, vector-borne infections) may extend their geographic range into new areas. The largest risks will occur in populations that are currently most affected by climate-related health outcomes (Smith and others 2014).

Climate change affects health through various pathways:

- Changes in the frequency and intensity of extreme weather (including heat, windstorms, and heavy rain)
- Effects mediated through natural systems (for example, changes in the geographic range and incidence of infectious diseases, such as water-, food-, and vector-borne diseases, and health outcomes associated with poor air quality, such as high concentrations of ozone and aeroallergens)
- Effects heavily mediated by human systems (for example, occupational impacts, undernutrition, migration, and mental stress).

Climate change will affect mean weather variables (for example, temperature and precipitation); the frequency, intensity, and duration of some extreme weather and climate events; and sea level. Changes in the mean and variability of weather and climate can independently and jointly influence the burden of climate-sensitive health outcomes. For example, rising mean temperatures can create conditions conducive to the geographic spread of vector-borne diseases such as

**Figure 8.1** Impacts of Climate Change on Human Health

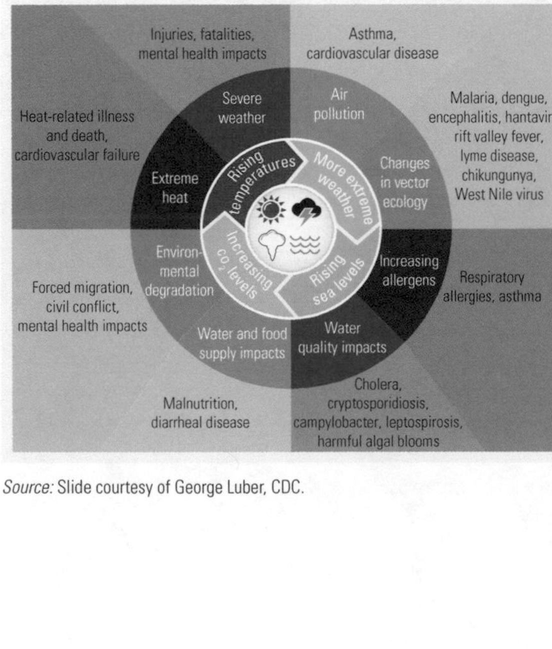

*Source:* Slide courtesy of George Luber, CDC.

malaria. At the same time, heavy precipitation events can wash away breeding grounds, resulting in short-term reductions in the number of *Anopheles* mosquitoes that can carry malaria. As changes continue over the century, thresholds may be crossed that could result in large increases or decreases in the incidence of climate-sensitive health outcomes.

Figure 8.2 shows the primary exposure pathways for the health risks of climate change. The figure shows that mediating factors, including environmental, social, and health factors, affect the burden of climate-sensitive health outcomes associated with changing weather patterns. The green arrows at the bottom indicate the possibility of positive or negative feedback mechanisms.

In the human health chapter of the Working Group II Contribution to the Intergovernmental Panel on Climate Change (IPCC) 5th Assessment Report, Smith and others (2014) conclude the following:

- The health of human populations is sensitive to shifts in weather patterns and other aspects of climate change. The effects occur directly, because of changes in temperature and precipitation and because of the occurrence of extreme weather and climate events (heatwaves, floods, droughts, and wildfires). Climate change can lead to ecological disruptions that indirectly affect health (for example, by reducing crop yields and altering the habitat of disease vectors). Social responses to climate change, such as migration, also can affect human health.

- Until mid-century, climate change mainly will exacerbate preexisting health problems. New health conditions may emerge, and diseases such as vector-borne infections may extend their geographic range into areas that currently are unaffected. The risks will be highest in populations most affected by climate-related health outcomes, such as in regions that currently are food insecure.

- Over the past few decades, climate change contributed to the burden of climate-sensitive health outcomes; however, the worldwide burden of ill health caused by climate change is relatively small compared with that caused by other stressors and is not well quantified.

- The major concerns with climate change include (1) morbidity and mortality from higher ambient temperatures and intense heatwaves; (2) higher risk of undernutrition from reduced food production in poor regions; (3) health consequences of lost work capacity and reduced labor productivity; and (4) higher risks of food-, water-, and vector-borne diseases.

**Figure 8.2 Conceptual Diagram of the Health Risks of Climate Change**

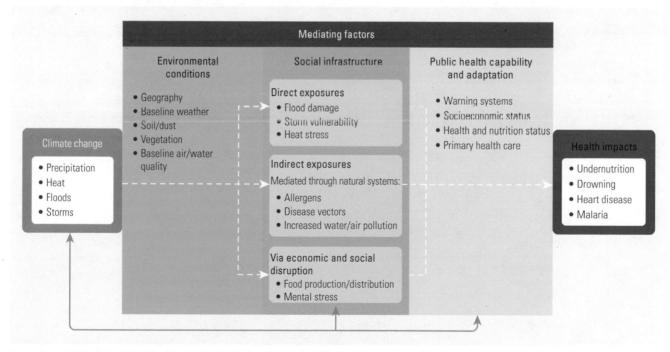

*Source:* Figure 11-1 from Smith, K. R., A. Woodward, D. Campbell-Lendrum, D. D. Chadee, Y. Honda, Q. Liu, J. M. Olwoch, B. Revich, and R. Sauerborn. 2014: "Human Health: Impacts, Adaptation, and Co-Benefits." In *Climate Change 2014: Impacts, Adaptation, and Vulnerability. Part A: Global and Sectoral Aspects.* Contribution of Working Group II to the Fifth Assessment Report of the Intergovernmental Panel on Climate Change [Field, C. B., V. R. Barros, D. J. Dokken, K. J. Mach, M. D. Mastrandrea, T. E. Bilir, M. Chatterjee, K. L. Ebi, Y. O. Estrada, R. C. Genova, B. Girma, E. S. Kissel, A. N. Levy, S. MacCracken, P. R. Mastrandrea, and L. L. White, eds.]. Cambridge University Press, Cambridge, United Kingdom, and New York, NY, United States.

- Impacts on health will be reduced, but not eliminated, in populations that benefit from rapid social and economic development, particularly among the poorest.
- The most effective measures to reduce vulnerability in the near term are programs that implement and improve basic health system measures, such as providing safe water, improving sanitation, securing essential health care, strengthening the capacity for disaster preparedness and response, and alleviating poverty.
- Important research gaps remain regarding the health risks of climate change, particularly in low-income countries (LICs).

The magnitude and pattern of risks in future decades will depend on actions taken to strengthen the resilience of health systems to prepare for, cope with, and recover from changing burdens of climate-sensitive health outcomes and on actions taken to reduce emissions of greenhouse gases that are driving climate change, sea-level rise, and ocean acidification.

## VULNERABILITY TO THE HEALTH RISKS OF CLIMATE VARIABILITY AND CHANGE

The magnitude and pattern of risks from climate change are due to the characteristics of the hazards created by changing weather patterns, the extent of exposure of human and natural systems to the hazard, the susceptibility of those systems to harm, and their ability to cope with and recover from exposure (Field and others 2012; Steinbruner, Stern, and Husbands 2013). Climate-related hazards can alter vulnerability to future events by changing the following (Field and others 2012; Steinbruner, Stern, and Husbands 2013):

- Extent of exposure (for example, reducing the presence or effectiveness of coastal barriers)
- Susceptibility of exposed human and natural systems (for example, making individuals and communities more or less susceptible by affecting their access to and the functioning of health care facilities or the proportion of the population vulnerable to an event)
- Ability of organizations and institutions to prepare for and manage events effectively and efficiently.

Understanding the magnitude and pattern of impacts and the factors that increase or decrease susceptibility and coping abilities is vital to modifying current policies and to implementing new policies and programs to increase resilience to climate change.

The wide range of factors that describe vulnerability to climate-related hazards can be divided into environmental, social, economic, health, and other dimensions (Cardona and others 2012; Field and others 2012). Environmental dimensions include physical variables (location-specific context for human-environment interactions); geography, location, and place; and settlement patterns and development trajectories. Social dimensions include demographic variables such as education and human health and well-being; cultural variables; and institutions and governance. Cross-cutting factors include relevant and accessible science and technology. In the health sector, important factors include the health of the population and the status of health systems (for example, the ability of health care facilities, laboratories, and other parts of the health system to manage an extreme event).

From the perspective of the health sector, vulnerability is the summation of all risk and protective factors that determine whether an individual or subpopulation experiences adverse health outcomes from exposure (Balbus and Malina 2009). Sensitivity to an event is a measure of the responsiveness of an individual or subpopulation to an event, often for biological reasons such as the presence of a chronic disease. A rich literature describes factors that increase vulnerability to extreme events. Individuals who are low on the socioeconomic scale, children, pregnant women, individuals with chronic medical conditions, and individuals with mobility or cognitive constraints are at higher risk of adverse health outcomes during an extreme event (Balbus and Malina 2009). In addition, the social determinants of health influence vulnerability. These determinants include access to health care services, access to and quality of education, availability of resources, transportation options, social capacity, and social norms and culture.

Figure 8.3 shows the framework used to explore the key drivers of vulnerability to extreme weather and climate events in the health sector (Ebi and Bowen 2016). Impacts can be categorized into those that affect environmental services, social and economic factors, or health status and health systems:

- Impacts on environmental services include availability of safe water (including quality and quantity), food security, and consequences that affect ecosystem services such as wildfires, coastal erosion, and saltwater intrusion into freshwater sources.
- Impacts on social and economic factors (such as community services, livelihoods, and social capital) include economic resources, infrastructure, access to services, and social capital.

**Figure 8.3** Key Drivers of Health Vulnerability to Extreme Weather and Climate Events

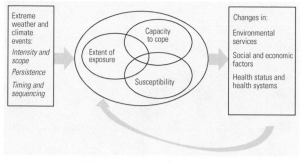

*Source:* Ebi and Bowen 2016.

- Impacts on health status and health systems include stress, mental illness as a consequence of the event or recovery, worsening chronic diseases, and undernutrition.

## CLIMATE-RESILIENT HEALTH SYSTEMS

Preparing for and managing the health risks of climate variability and change require strengthening the capacity of health systems to protect and improve population health in an unstable and changing climate (WHO 2015). To that end, the World Health Organization (WHO) defines a climate-resilient system as a system capable of anticipating, responding to, coping with, recovering from, and adapting to climate-related shocks and stresses to bring sustained improvements to the health of the population.

Health systems vary across and within countries, but all share common building blocks:

- Leadership and governance
- Health workforce
- Health information systems
- Essential medical products and technologies
- Service delivery
- Financing.

Figure 8.4 shows the 10 components for building climate-resilient health systems within these building blocks.

Within each component, specific characteristics or activities are needed to achieve resilience. For example, within leadership and governance, leadership and political will are needed to ensure collaboration across all relevant departments within a ministry, such as environmental health; vector control; water, sanitation, and hygiene; and disaster risk management. Also needed are policy prioritization and planning that explicitly incorporate the risks

of climate change; legal and regulatory systems that protect health; institutional mechanisms, capacities, and structures; accountability; and community participation. Indicators are needed to describe the current baseline and to measure progress as climate change is incorporated into policies and programs.

Costs are associated with implementing climate-resilient policies and programs within each component. Few efforts have been made to estimate these costs. Some costs will be limited, such as modifying five-year plans to incorporate climate change. Others will likely be significant, such as developing new products and technologies, ensuring adequate human and financial resources (particularly in LMICs), or improving infrastructure to ensure that health care facilities can withstand (and continue to function during) more frequent and intense floods and storm surges. Some costs will be ongoing, such as the need for regular reassessments of current and projected burdens of climate-sensitive health outcomes. Such assessments require ongoing research and development to project the magnitude and pattern of climate sensitive health outcomes as the climate continues to change, taking into account multiple drivers and adaptation options to reduce risks. Investments in surveillance, monitoring, and evaluation will be needed across the century to continue to prepare for and manage changing vulnerabilities and risks. New tools for mapping vulnerability, modeling future risks, developing scenarios, evaluating the effectiveness of public health prevention, and undertaking other activities are all components of the iterative management of climate change.

Other costs will be borne primarily by other sectors, such as developing and deploying new agricultural cultivars that are heat, drought, or salt tolerant. These activities will be critical for ensuring food security over coming decades. In the absence of these activities, the costs for health systems to manage risks will be considerably higher.

Table 8.1 lists some possible interventions within each of the six building blocks of health systems, providing an overview of the wide range of efforts needed to strengthen resilience. The costs associated with some of these activities, such as establishing and maintaining a malaria treatment program, are estimated in other chapters.

Limiting the magnitude of climate change risks past mid-century requires significant reductions in greenhouse gas emissions and deforestation, both now and in the years to come (Field and others 2014). Estimates of the costs of mitigation generally do not take into account the growing evidence that some mitigation options have extensive health co-benefits (Smith and others 2014). Mitigation policies and technologies (such as

**Figure 8.4** Components for Building Climate-Resilient Health Systems

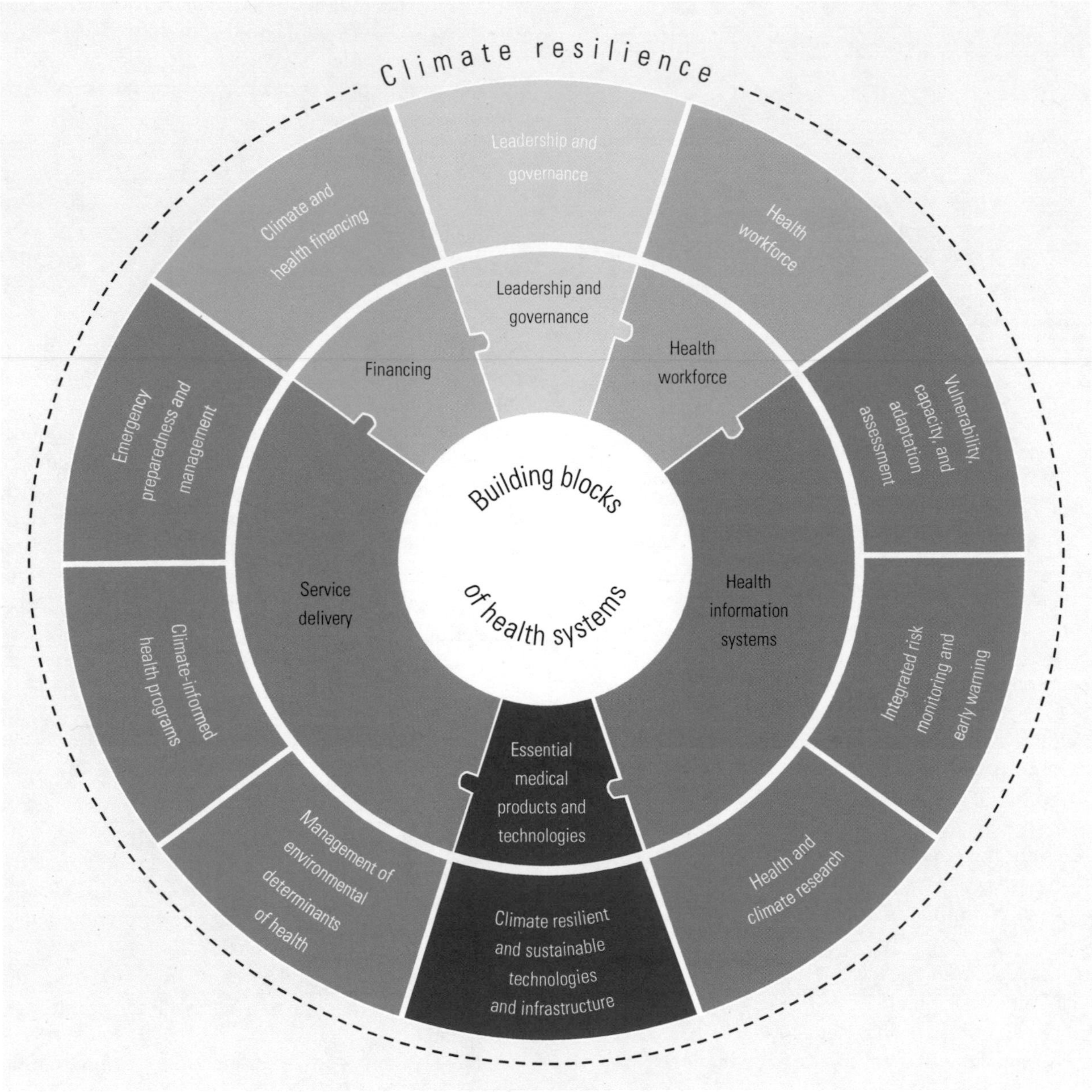

Climate resilience

Building blocks of health systems

- Leadership and governance
- Health workforce
- Vulnerability, capacity, and adaptation assessment
- Integrated risk monitoring and early warning
- Health and climate research
- Climate resilient and sustainable technologies and infrastructure
- Management of environmental determinants of health
- Climate-informed health programs
- Emergency preparedness and management
- Climate and health financing

Inner ring: Leadership and governance; Health workforce; Health information systems; Essential medical products and technologies; Service delivery; Financing

*Source:* WHO 2015.

transitioning energy generation to reduced use of fossil fuels; altering policies to increase mass transit and encourage active transportation such as walking and biking; and promoting dietary changes to reduce consumption of red meat) are associated with significant health benefits (termed *co-benefits*) that primarily will be local and will accrue well before the benefits of mitigation become evident, potentially making mitigation implementation more politically feasible.

Estimating the overall costs and benefits of mitigation to reduce health risks associated with climate change is an important research need.

## COSTS ARISING IN THE HEALTH SECTOR

The health effects of extreme weather and climate change will lead to potential costs. Important categories to consider when estimating impacts and subsequent

**Table 8.1** Examples of Climate-Informed Health Interventions

| Climate-related health risks and mechanisms | Examples of interventions |
|---|---|
| Extreme heat and thermal stress | • Establish occupational health exposure standards. |
| | • Improve health facility design, energy-efficient cooling and heating systems. |
| | • Ensure public education to promote behavior change (in relation to clothing and ventilation). |
| | • Develop heat-health action plans (including early warning, public communication, and response plans) such as cooling centers for high-risk populations. |
| Water- and food-borne diseases | • Enhance disease surveillance systems during high-risk seasons or periods. |
| | • Establish early warning systems to anticipate outbreaks associated with extreme weather and climate events. |
| | • Strengthen food and water quality control. |
| Zoonotic and vector-borne diseases | • Expand the scope of diseases monitored and conduct monitoring at the margins of current geographic distributions. |
| | • Establish early warning systems when data are sufficient and the association between environmental variables and health outcomes is robust. |
| | • Establish vector or pest surveillance and control programs. |
| | • Enhance diagnostic and treatment options in high-risk regions or periods. |
| | • Ensure adequate animal and human vaccination coverage. |
| Allergic diseases and cardiopulmonary health | • Develop exposure forecasts for air quality, allergens, and dust. |
| | • Enforce stricter air quality standards for pollution. |
| | • Establish programs to monitor pollen levels. |
| | • Establish allergen management. |
| | • Create plans for handling increased demand for treatment during high-risk seasons or weather conditions. |
| Nutrition | • Perform seasonal nutritional screening in high-risk communities. |
| | • Scale up integrated food security, nutrition, and health programming in fragile zones. |
| | • Promote public education and food hygiene. |
| Storms and floods | • Include climate risks in siting, designing, or retrofitting health infrastructure. |
| | • Establish early warning and early action systems, including education and community mobilization. |
| | • Assess and retrofit or construct public health infrastructure (health facilities in flood-prone areas) to be resilient to extreme weather conditions, warmer temperatures, and environmental changes. |
| Mental health and disability | • Address special needs of mental health patients (as well as patients with other disabilities) by developing emergency preparedness plans. |
| | • Address mental health needs of disaster- and trauma-exposed populations. |
| | • During extreme weather conditions, establish community watch for people with mental illness. |

*Source:* Adapted from WHO 2015.

responses include immediate health sector response costs (additional medicine and costs of treatment) when an extreme weather event occurs or an impact arises from changing weather trends. Other costs arise for those affected, including injuries, illnesses, and deaths and lost work time. Further effects relating to the impact on people's quality of life and well-being (or in economic terms, welfare) exist, even if these impacts are not captured by markets. Quantifying and valuing these effects is possible, expressing them in monetary terms to capture the economic, social, and environmental costs borne by society as a whole.

Estimating the full costs of climate variability and change includes three components: resource costs (medical treatment costs); opportunity costs (lost productivity); and welfare costs or disutility (pain or suffering, concern, and inconvenience to family and others). The magnitude of welfare costs usually is derived through elicitation techniques such as contingent valuation and stated preference. This valuation is somewhat controversial, but it is included because it is a way of comparing impacts using a common metric.

## Methods

A wide variety of methods have been used to estimate the costs of climate change effects on health. These methods capture different aspects of the resource, opportunity, and well-being costs and can use different approaches for valuation of these elements. Also, differences exist between the direct costs of the events and the indirect, wider costs for the economy.

Many studies focus on resource costs, although differences emerge even in the approach used for valuation. One set of studies explored the costs of adaptation to climate change using preventative costs. As an example, in the case of malaria, valuation includes estimating the number of malaria cases from climate change, then looking at the costs of adaptation (a proxy for impacts) based on the costs of programs and unit costs (per beneficiary) for insecticide-treated bed-nets plus case management and indoor residual insecticide spraying. These approaches have been widely used, particularly in studies in LMICs. Other approaches look at resource costs directly, for example, looking at the number of additional impacts, and then estimating the health care costs of treatment, that is, using estimates of the health care cost per patient and the number of hospital days spent on average for respiratory admissions. A variation on the resource cost method can be undertaken when working at aggregated scale, using investment and financial flow assessments. These look at existing expenditures and then apply a mark-up (an increase) to reflect rising impacts from climate change. One issue with all of these approaches is that they only cover one element of the total health costs.

One additional cost that arises from impacts is associated with the time or productivity lost from the illness—the opportunity costs. Some studies also estimate these, often using values based on loss, earnings, or, more appropriately, labor productivity. These costs are particularly relevant for studies that focus on outdoor worker productivity; the primary impact for these workers is associated with lost time, as worker output is reduced because of heat and humidity. However,

these opportunity costs also apply to other health impacts, and many studies estimate these in addition to resource costs.

Another set of studies takes the resource and opportunity costs estimated from these methods and inputs them into economy-wide economic models. This approach captures the impacts of costs on the wider economy, the linkages across sectors, and macroeconomic metrics such as gross domestic product (GDP).

Finally, in addition to estimating resource and opportunity costs, some studies derive values for the impacts on well-being (for example, the pain and suffering from illness). Techniques are available to capture this component, such as assessing the willingness to pay or the willingness to accept compensation for a particular health outcome. These are derived using survey-based stated preference methods and/or revealed preferences methods.

## Review of Studies

Altered weather patterns (particularly, extreme weather and climate events) could affect health sector costs initially through resource costs for diagnosis and treatment. As an example, six of the weather and climate events that struck the United States between 2000 and 2009 included higher concentrations of ground-level ozone, the 2002 outbreak of West Nile virus in Louisiana, the 2003 Southern California wildfires, the 2004 Florida hurricane season, the 2006 California heatwave, and the 2009 flooding of the Red River in North Dakota. In total, these events increased health care costs an estimated US$819 million, reflecting more than 760,000 encounters with the health care system (Knowlton and others 2011). The total health costs, including 1,689 lives lost prematurely (valued using nonmarket economic values), exceeded US$15.5 billion.

Health care facilities themselves can be damaged by extreme weather and climate events, including storm surges, floods, and wildfires, which compromise critical resources required to treat patients and repair or replace damaged or destroyed equipment and buildings (Carthey, Chandra, and Loosemore 2009). In 2011, 139.8 million people globally—57 percent of all disaster victims—were affected by hydrological disasters (floods and wet mass movements). These disasters were responsible for 20 percent of all people reportedly killed in disasters and 19 percent of total damages (Guha-Sapir and others 2012). Although the proportion of individuals seeking medical treatment during a disaster is typically a small subset of the total number of persons affected, the additional burden on health care facilities can be significant (Hess and others 2009). Floods and wildfires also can require the evacuation of critical care patients, with attendant risks.

When these extreme events are very large, they can affect the ability of health care systems to function properly and to care for patients with ongoing health issues that require medication or treatment. In cases where these events become significantly more frequent or intense, health facilities might need to add surge capacity to help them to manage such events without interrupting service (Banks, Shah, and Richards 2007; Hess and others 2009).

Climate change is projected to increase the burden of climate-sensitive health outcomes, leading to increased costs in the absence of mitigation and adaptation. As well as changing the patterns of extreme events, it will lead to shifts in climate variables that will affect health outcomes. This increase in health burdens will increase the demands on public health services (for example, surveillance and control programs) and the demands for health care and relevant supplies (for example, anti-malarials and oral rehydration). It also will increase opportunity and welfare costs. Studies use different methods and include different components, making inter-comparisons difficult.

Many earlier estimates of the additional costs of climate change typically focused on the health care costs associated with treating additional cases of disease, not the costs of providing additional health services (health system adaptation costs) or the wider societal costs. Therefore, they underestimated the total costs. Given these limitations, the global costs of treating future cases of adverse health outcomes from climate change from such studies are estimated at billions of U.S. dollars annually (Ebi 2008; Pandey 2010).

Ebi (2008) estimated the worldwide costs in 2030 of additional cases of malnutrition, diarrheal disease, and malaria due to climate change at US$5 billion to US$16 billion a year, for a high-emissions scenario, assuming no population or economic growth (undiscounted US$). This estimate was based on current costs of treatment and assumed no adaptation. The costs for additional infrastructure and health care workers were not included, nor were the costs of additional public health services, such as surveillance and monitoring. The estimated costs were distributed unevenly across regions. Markandya and Chiabai (2009) used these estimates to provide a regional breakdown of costs, finding the highest costs in Africa and South-East Asia.

Pandey (2010) estimated global health costs of climate change based on United Nations population projections, strong economic growth, updated projections of the current health burden of diarrheal diseases and malaria, two climate scenarios, and updated estimates of the costs of malaria treatment. In 2010, the average annual costs for treating diarrheal disease and malaria cases associated with climate change were estimated to be between US$4 billion and US$7 billion, with the costs expected to decline over time as basic health services improve. From 2010 to 2050, the average annual costs were estimated to be around US$3 billion, with most of the costs related to treating diarrheal disease; the largest burden was expected to be in Sub-Saharan Africa. Pandey's estimates differ from those of Ebi's primarily because of the assumption of a lower baseline burden of disease and lower costs for malaria treatment.

These studies considered only malnutrition, diarrheal disease, and malaria and therefore were underestimates. According to Parry and others (2009), the studies estimated only 30–50 percent of the extra health burden of climate change.

World Bank (2010) undertook a similar analysis of diarrheal disease and malaria and reported much lower estimates than these earlier studies. Whereas the earlier studies fixed the baseline incidence of disease, this study incorporated a future baseline based on the WHO Global Burden of Disease projections to 2030 (plus extensions through 2050). This led to a reduction in the baseline incidence of diarrheal disease and malaria, significantly reducing the additional cases due to climate change. The World Bank analysis also incorporated updated unit costs of prevention and treatment and risk factors. The resulting health adaptation costs in LMICs globally were estimated at between US$1.8 billion and US$2.4 billion a year in the period 2010–50, with most of these costs in Africa. Future health outcomes depend on multiple factors beyond the level of greenhouse gas emissions and resulting warming.

The recent Climate Impact Research and Response Coordination for a Larger Europe (CIRCLE) study used a combination of global models: a computable general equilibrium model to project effects to 2060 and the AD-RICE model to project effects beyond 2060 (OECD 2015).[1] It considered heat mortality in a stand-alone analysis, heat- and cold-related morbidity and mortality, and morbidity from infectious diseases such as malaria, schistosomiasis, dengue, diarrhea, cardiovascular disease, and respiratory disease. The changes in labor productivity from climate-sensitive diseases were taken from Bosello, Eboli, and Pierfederici (2012).

By 2060, the largest negative effects were projected to take place in Africa and the Middle East (−0.6 percent for South Africa, −0.5 percent for the Middle East and North Africa, and −0.4 percent for other African countries). Smaller impacts were projected for Brazil, Mexico, and LMICs in Asia (−0.3 percent), as well as for Indonesia, the United States, South-East Asia, and most of Latin America (−0.2 percent). Some regions were projected to experience positive impacts on labor productivity, the highest being the Russian Federation (+0.5 percent), Canada (+0.4 percent), and China (+0.2 percent). In other regions, the projected impacts were either very small or nonexistent. Changes in health care expenditures were also estimated. The costs of vector-borne diseases were based on prevention expenditures and treatment costs per person per month (Chima, Goodman, and Mills 2003).

Changes in health expenditure were small as a percentage of GDP. In 2060, they were projected to be highest in LMICs in Asia (0.5 percent), Brazil, and the Middle East and North Africa (0.3 percent). Additional demands for health services were projected to be very small in other regions and to be negative in Canada and large European Union economies, such as France and Germany (−0.1 percent).

Several regional and country studies support or extend these assessments:

- In India, Chiabai and others (2010) reported adaptation costs for malaria, diarrhea, and malnutrition. Using a similar prevention cost approach to the studies above, costs under different development scenarios were in the range of US$183 million to US$584 million with no mitigation and US$151 million to US$476 million with mitigation achieving stabilization at 550 parts per million.
- In Kenya, the Stockholm Environment Institute used a malaria risk model based on altitude to assess the national impact of future climate change (SEI 2009). The model projected that, by 2055, as a result of average climate warming of 4.3°F (2.3°C) across the projections, the population annually affected by malaria in rural areas above 1,000 meters (63 percent of the population) would increase as much as 74 percent (in the absence of adaptation). It also presented results for scenarios with average temperature increases of 2.2°F (1.2°C) and 5.6°F (3°C). The 10 model projections used a range of average climate warming increases from 36 to 89 percent. The additional economic burden of endemic malaria disease in the 2050s was estimated to be more than US$92 million annually (with a range of US$51 million to US$106 million annually across the temperature projections) based on the clinical and economic burden of malaria. The estimated welfare costs increased to a range of between US$154 million and US$197 million annually when disutility costs (discomfort, pain, and inconvenience measured by survey-based willingness-to-pay estimates) were taken into account.

- In 25 African countries, Egbendewe-Mondzozo and others (2011) used a semiparametric econometric model to estimate the climate change–related costs for inpatient and outpatient treatments for malaria at the end of the century (2080–100). Even marginal changes in temperature and precipitation were projected to affect the number of malaria cases, with most countries projected to see an increase and others a decrease. The end-of-century treatment costs as a proportion of year 2000 health expenditures per 1,000 people would be higher in the vast majority of countries, with increases of more than 20 percent in the costs of inpatient treatment in Burundi, Côte d'Ivoire, Malawi, Rwanda, and Sudan.
- In Tanzania, Traerup, Ortiz, and Markandya (2011) estimated the costs of cholera cases due to climate change in 2030 to be in the range of 0.32–1.4 percent of GDP.
- In India, Ramakrishnan (2011) estimated the costs of treating additional cases of diarrhea and malaria in 2030 to range between Rs 3,648 lakhs and Rs 7,787 lakhs, depending on the emissions scenario.[2]
- In Saint Lucia, the Economic Commission for Latin America and the Caribbean (ECLAC 2011) estimated the present value of treatment costs under two scenarios of greenhouse gas emissions in the period 2010–50 as US$634,000 for cardiorespiratory disease, US$33,000 for malaria, US$36,000 for dengue, and US$3.5 million for gastroenteritis, using a discount rate of 1 percent.
- In Paraguay, the United Nations Development Programme (UNDP 2011) applied an investment and financial flow assessment to health, estimating total costs to be US$160.5 million by 2030 (2005 US$).

Because adverse health outcomes are projected to occur predominantly in LICs, treatment costs will be borne primarily by families where governments provide limited health care (WHO 2004). Time off from work to care for sick children will have an adverse effect on productivity.

Estimates of the impact of climate change on outdoor worker productivity (primarily through heat stress) indicate that productivity has already declined during the hottest and most humid seasons in parts of Africa and Asia, with more than half of afternoon hours projected to be lost to the need for rest breaks in 2050 in South-East Asia and up to a 20 percent loss in global productivity in 2100 under a moderately low emission scenario (Representative Concentration Pathway 4.5) (Dunne, Stouffer, and John 2013; Kjellstrom and others 2009; Kjellstrom, Lemke, and Otto 2013). Trade-offs between worker health and productivity will be of particular concern for workers with limited control over work practices.

Kovats and others (2011) estimated the labor productivity losses for Europe at between US$321 million and US$792 million a year in the 2080s for a high-emissions scenario, falling to between US$64 million and US$160.5 million a year under a mitigation scenario, with impacts primarily in Southern Europe. For the loss of labor productivity, a value was derived from the GDP per labor force member. This represents the loss to society, differentiating it from a loss of earnings measure that reflects only the loss for the individual.

The CIRCLE project also considered these impacts and found that the highest impacts on labor productivity caused by occupational heat stress in 2060 likely would occur in regions with relatively large proportions of outdoor workers and warm climates (OECD 2015). The most severely affected regions were projected to experience productivity losses between 3 and 5 percent for outdoor activities for a 1.9°F (1°C) temperature increase in non–Organisation for Economic Co-operation and Development (OECD) countries, non–European Union European countries, Latin America (including Brazil and Chile), Mexico, China, LMICs in Asia, and South Africa. Most OECD countries, including Japan, the United States, and the OECD European Union countries, were projected to experience effects of less than 1 percent.

Nevertheless, some health impacts from climate change are likely to affect OECD countries, particularly mortality and morbidity from higher temperatures and heat extremes. Studies have assessed the impacts and full economic costs (including nonmarket valuation) in OECD countries. Watkiss and Hunt (2012) quantified and valued temperature-related mortality effects, salmonellosis, and coastal flooding–induced mental health impacts resulting from climate change in Europe in 2071–100, assessing the full welfare costs. The analysis found that the choice of valuation metric and inclusion or exclusion of acclimatization (autonomous adaptation)[3] had a major impact on the results, much more so than climate uncertainty.

In model runs without acclimatization, economic costs in current values were estimated at US$12.6 billion to US$31.6 billion a year by the 2020s using a value of statistical life metric, but US$1 billion to US$4.2 billion a year when acclimatization was included. By the 2080s, the annual values ranged from US$52.6 billion to US$189.5 billion (according to choice of function and climate model) without acclimatization, and US$8.4 billion to US$84.2 billion with acclimatization. The additional welfare costs for salmonellosis from climate change were estimated to be several hundred million dollars annually by 2071–100. They also found the potential reduction in cold-related mortality to be at least as large

as the increase in heat-related mortality, although recent literature (for example, Ebi and Mills 2013) has questioned whether these effects will be fully realized.

A similar analysis for Europe (Kovats and others 2011) estimated annual welfare costs for heat-related mortality at US$32.6 billion by the 2020s (2011–40), US$108.4 billion by the 2050s (2041–70), and US$154.8 billion by the 2080s (2071–100) under a high-emissions scenario. These values were more than an order of magnitude lower when using a different valuation approach. Under a mitigation scenario, broadly equivalent to the 3.7°F (2°C) target, these values fell significantly (after 2040), to US$84.2 billion a year by the 2050s (2041–70). Again, including (autonomous) acclimatization reduced these impacts significantly. As these studies highlight, choices regarding the response functions and valuation metrics, as well as autonomous adaptation, can have a very large impact on estimated overall health costs, leading to order of magnitude differences.

At the global level, OECD (2015) reported heat-related mortality under climate change in high income countries. Using a value of statistical life approach, they projected that the economic costs of heat-related deaths would increase from around US$100 billion today to US$320 billion in 2030 and US$670 billion in 2050, with the highest costs in Europe and North America.

## COSTS ARISING IN OTHER SECTORS

Adaptations in health systems and the health sector more generally are not the only climate change adaptations required to protect human health. Although determining the extent to which other sectors protect health can be challenging, certain sectors (such as electrical and water utilities) are clearly intimately tied to public health. These ties are complex. Some sectors provide health benefits via smooth and continuous operations, while the health sector, through regulation and other activities, minimizes the adverse health impacts imposed by other sectors. For example, electrification and a sustained, reliable power supply supports public health and health care delivery in numerous ways; power outages are associated with significant impacts on health. Yet, power generation, particularly based on fossil fuels, has serious adverse health consequences that regulations have only partially succeeded in limiting in most countries. Similarly, water treatment and distribution are fundamental to health, while certain water management decisions (such as dam construction) can have significant, if localized, adverse health consequences. Thus, in considering the costs associated with adaptation, costs also arise in sectors other than health whose activities are central to protecting health or whose adaptation choices may be maladaptive from a public health perspective.

Adaptation will vary by baseline status in these sectors and by location, with significant efforts needed to decrease exposure in a changing climate. In the water sector, several adaptations will likely be needed to address water scarcity, changes in water quality, and variability in precipitation. In the agriculture sector, adaptations will be needed to maintain an adequate supply of protein, energy, and micronutrients. In the forestry sector, adaptations will be needed to limit the incidence of forest fires and associated direct and pollution-driven health impacts, and to limit the socioeconomic impacts of disruptions to ecosystem services. In some settings, adaptations will be needed to enhance ongoing activities aimed at increasing resilience to worsening climate-sensitive health threats; in others, such as the water sector in the Arctic, fundamentally new approaches and infrastructure will be needed.

Other adaptations may fall outside of existing sectors. In anticipation of sea-level rise, widespread adaptation activities will be needed to protect infrastructure that is critical to public health (such as hospitals, clinics, and dialysis centers) and to prevent saltwater intrusion into groundwater sources (which can lead to hypertension, crop failure, and limitations on drinking water supply). Other adaptations will be needed to protect communities from extreme weather and climate events, such as flooding, severe storms, and extreme heat. Still others will be needed to manage population dislocation and resettlement, which can be a significant challenge to the health sector. In many cases, adaptation activities will entail managing risk, including risk reduction, risk sharing through insurance and other mechanisms, and enhanced recovery mechanisms.

Successful adaptation will require increased communication, coordination, and integration between health and other sectors. The public health sector has extensive experience collaborating with other sectors to achieve its goals and will need to build on this experience to facilitate intersectoral adaptation.

Some of this coordination will focus on highlighting the potential adverse consequences of adaptation activities in other sectors and, indeed, in the health sector itself. The appropriate balance between expenditures on activities that protect one population at one point in time but that potentially lead to some harm for other populations is not always clear. For instance, the widespread use of air conditioning to protect against extreme heat events is maladaptive to the extent that it has the potential not only to worsen the heat island effect locally in cities but also to affect climate change in the long term when power is generated by coal-fired power plants. Promoting health impact assessments of adaptation activities in other sectors is a powerful means for the health sector to highlight potential disbenefits of adaptation activities in other sectors.

## ISSUES RELATED TO SPATIAL AND TEMPORAL SCALE

Costs of preparing for, coping with, and recovering from the health risks of climate variability and change will vary across temporal and spatial scales.

### Spatial Scale

Poverty is a major driver of risk, which means that low- and lower-middle income countries generally will be at higher risk of adverse climate-sensitive health outcomes. Undernutrition, malaria, and diarrheal disease—among the largest health concerns related to climate change—are leading causes of morbidity and mortality in children younger than age five years (Liu and others 2015; Smith and others 2014). For example, despite recent progress, diarrhea kills 1,584 children every day, accounting for 9 percent of child deaths. Just 15 countries in Africa and Asia account for 71 percent of childhood mortality from diarrhea and pneumonia (IVAC 2014). These countries include low-income (Afghanistan, Chad, the Democratic Republic of Congo, Ethiopia, Niger, and Uganda), lower-middle-income (Bangladesh, India, Indonesia, Kenya, Nigeria, Pakistan, and Sudan), and upper-middle-income (Angola and China) countries.

The pathways leading to higher burdens of diarrheal diseases vary across countries, with lack of improved sanitation facilities a major risk; other drivers include food and water contaminated by humans or animals, improper food handling, and improper hand washing. Nine of these 15 countries are among the 10 countries that are home to two-thirds of the global population with limited access to improved drinking water sources: Bangladesh, China, the Democratic Republic of Congo, Ethiopia, India, Indonesia, Kenya, Nigeria, and Pakistan. Warmer temperatures mean faster replication of some pathogens associated with diarrheal diseases, and higher precipitation events can wash pathogens into water sources (Cann and others 2012; Kolstad and Johansson 2010). Without a significant improvement in access to safe water and improved sanitation, reducing the extent to which climate change could increase the burden of diarrheal disease will become increasingly challenging.

## Temporal Scale

Temporally, the rate of greenhouse gas emissions reductions will affect the magnitude and pattern of climate change past mid-century, with rapid and extensive reductions lowering adaptation needs later in this century (Smith and others 2014). Many policies and technologies to reduce greenhouse gas emissions are associated with health co-benefits; for example, reducing emissions from point sources such as coal-fired power plants and from mobile sources such as transportation could provide significant health benefits by reducing exposure to fine particulate matter (Balbus and others 2014).

Projecting how health costs could evolve as the climate continues to change also requires consideration of future development pathways (Ebi 2013). Five socioeconomic development pathways describe the evolution of demographic, political, social, cultural, institutional, economic, and technological trends through this century, along axes describing worlds with increasing socioeconomic and environmental challenges to adaptation and mitigation. Also considered are ecosystems and ecosystem services affected by human activities, such as air and water quality. Each development pathway has very different implications for the burdens of climate-sensitive health outcomes and health system capacities to prepare for and manage risks associated with climate variability and change. Using these pathways facilitates exploration of the possible impacts and costs associated with mitigating greenhouse gas emissions to a certain level and the extent of efforts required to adapt to that level.

One development pathway is a world aiming for sustainable development (Ebi 2013). This pathway includes the following features:

- Population health improves significantly, with increased emphasis on enhancing public health and health care functions.
- Coordinated, worldwide efforts through international institutions and nongovernmental organizations increase access to safe water, improved sanitation, medical care, education, and other factors in underserved populations.
- Life expectancies increase in LICs with decreasing burdens of key causes of childhood mortality (undernutrition, diarrheal diseases, and malaria).
- Funding increases for public health and health care organizations, and institutions enhance their capacities to prepare for, respond to, cope with, and recover from climate-related health risks.

Improvements in this development pathway will reduce the burden of climate-sensitive health outcomes even before considering any impacts of climate change. Meeting the challenges of climate change will be much easier in this pathway.

Another development pathway describes a world separated into regional blocks with little coordination between them (Ebi 2013). This world is failing to achieve global development goals, with regional blocks characterized by extreme poverty and pockets of moderate wealth and the bulk of countries struggling to maintain living standards for their rapidly growing populations. This pathway includes the following features:

- Mortality rates are high, with mortality from climate-related health outcomes (particularly undernutrition, diarrheal diseases, and malaria) increasing and life expectancy possibly falling in LMICs because of increased childhood mortality, although some sub-regions enjoy better health. All countries experience a double burden of climate-related infectious and chronic health outcomes.
- Large regions of the world are food and water insecure.
- Most urban growth in LMICs occurs in unplanned settlements and mostly fails to improve access to safe water and improved sanitation.
- Wealthier regions do not invest in research and development to help less well-off regions manage health risks. Further, governance and institutions are weak, international cooperation is limited, investments in public health and health care infrastructure are low, and the number of public health and health care personnel is too small to address health needs.

In this development pathway, the challenges to managing the health risks of climate variability and change increase over time, with rising and increasingly unaffordable costs in more vulnerable countries and regions.

The other three pathways explore a world that continues along its current trajectory, with health improving but at a slower rate than in the pathway aiming for sustainable development; a highly unequal world where adaptation is difficult, but technologies are developed and deployed to reduce greenhouse gas emissions; and a world with low challenges to adaptation, but where mitigation of greenhouse gas emissions is difficult for a range of technological and other reasons. Each has different implications for the health costs of climate variability and change.

## CHALLENGES RELATED TO ESTIMATING COSTS AND BENEFITS

Estimating the costs and benefits of climate change and adaptation to the associated risks presents many challenges. These include the unique nature of the threat of climate change to the incidence, geographic distribution, and seasonality of a wide range of health outcomes (with risks and uncertainty increasing over coming decades) and the temporal displacement between the causes of climate change (human activities leading to the release of greenhouse gases and natural climate variability) and the projected timing of health impacts. Further, the costs of proactive mitigation for managing health risks of climate change will be incurred years to decades before benefits in reducing climate change are evident. Precisely timing investments will not always be possible given inherent uncertainties about the magnitude, rate, and timing of climate change.

The hazards created by a changing climate will interact with the sensitivity of populations and regions and with their capacity to prepare for and cope with hazards as they arise. This creates complex relationships between climate change and health outcomes that will vary over temporal and spatial scales. Because LMICs have the highest sensitivity to climate-sensitive health outcomes and the least ability to adapt, they will be at highest risk (Smith and others 2014). All countries, however, will experience hazards, and all countries will need to adapt and mitigate. The differences across countries mean that the costs of adaptation will vary over time and space.

Given the limited capacity of health systems to manage current climate variability and change, the costs of adaptation are likely to be high in the longer-term, as health systems incorporate climate change into policies and programs. Once adaptive risk management processes are established and climate change mainstreamed into policies and programs, costs by mid-century will depend on the health impacts associated with the magnitude and pattern of climate change, which, in turn, will depend on the extent of mitigation over coming decades. Adding to these complexities are the costs associated with adaptation in other sectors.

It is not surprising that few costs of adaptation options have been estimated. Information on some adaptation options can be estimated from other chapters in this volume, such as the costs of surveillance and treatment for malaria or other vector-borne diseases. However, there are challenges in estimating what portion of the costs of extending current surveillance and health care systems to prepare for changes in the geographic range of malaria could be due to climate change versus other possible drivers of change, such as land use changes. Similar challenges present in estimating the benefits of interventions.

Other issues that arise when considering the costs of adaptation include how to limit double counting. For example, climate change is increasing the number of cases of undernutrition, malaria, and diarrheal disease in many regions (Smith and others 2014). However, these health outcomes are not independent; undernutrition increases a child's susceptibility to malaria and diarrheal disease. It is not clear how to count the costs of preventing and treating these health outcomes accurately.

Many researchers and modelers are estimating the costs of various mitigation options. Although health systems are a source of greenhouse gas emissions, the sector should reduce these emissions as quickly as possible. Lower emissions benefit everyone later in the century; unlike air pollutants, greenhouse gases do not remain local.

Interest in calculating the loss and damage due to climate change has been growing particularly in countries that are vulnerable to its adverse effects. Loss and damage refers to the impacts of climate-related stressors on human and natural systems that occur despite mitigation and adaptation efforts. Climate change that already is locked in because of the inertia in the climate system could adversely affect development in particularly vulnerable locations and populations. For example, saltwater intrusion from sea-level rise could mean that farmers can no longer grow crops or feed animals. The issue of loss and damage arose because most of the focus of the more than 20 years of negotiations under the United Nations Framework Convention on Climate Change has been on reducing greenhouse gas emissions, with less attention paid to ensuring that countries that are particularly vulnerable to climate change but who historically were responsible for only a tiny proportion of atmospheric greenhouse gases and who are experiencing adverse impacts have the financial resources to adapt. This issue has been contentious because some observers consider it to be synonymous with liability and compensation. This is an active area of research and negotiation.

## CONCLUSIONS

Climate variability and change present significant challenges for the health and well-being of individuals, communities, and nations. Preventing, preparing for, and managing climate-related risks to human and natural systems will be a recurring theme throughout the 21st century. Hallegatte and others (2016, xi) explored the intersection of climate change and poverty and offered the following conclusions:

> Without action, climate change would likely spark higher agricultural prices and could threaten food security in poorer regions such as Sub-Saharan Africa and South Asia. And in most countries where we have data, poor urban households are more exposed to floods than the average urban population. Climate change also will magnify many threats to health, as poor people are more susceptible to climate-related diseases such as malaria and diarrhea. . . . We need good, climate-informed development to reduce the impacts of climate change on the poor. This means, in part, providing poor people with social safety nets and universal health care. These efforts will need to be coupled with targeted climate resilience measures, such as the introduction of heat-resistant crops and disaster preparedness systems.

The report further concludes that, without climate-resilient development, climate change could force more than 100 million people into extreme poverty by 2030 (Hallegatte and others 2016). Rapid, inclusive development could avoid most of these impacts, and immediate reductions in emissions could avoid many of the projected risks later in the century.

Climate change underscores the urgency of strengthening basic public health infrastructure, particularly in poor and underserved areas. To be effective, health systems need to incorporate climate variability and change explicitly into all climate-sensitive policies and programs, including disaster risk management, air pollution control, infectious disease monitoring and surveillance, and water and food safety and security. Taking advantage of the growing body of knowledge about environmental drivers of climate-sensitive health outcomes can provide significant public health benefits. Continuing to take a business-as-usual approach to climate change will put lives and livelihoods at risk and result in higher health burdens that could have been prevented.

## NOTES

World Bank Income Classifications as of July 2014 are as follows, based on estimates of gross national income (GNI) per capita for 2013:

- Low-income countries (LICs) = US$1,045 or less
- Middle-income countries (MICs) are subdivided:
  a) lower-middle-income = US$1,046 to US$4,125
  b) upper-middle-income (UMICs) = US$4,126 to US$12,745
- High-income countries (HICs) = US$12,746 or more.

1. For information on the CIRCLE study, see http://www.circle-era.eu/np4/home.html.
2. A lakh is 100,000 rupees.
3. Future individuals will respond to higher temperatures through physiological and behavioral adjustments. Most studies ignore this effect and use impact functions derived from the current climate and apply these functions to the future. This overestimates impacts, because it assumes that no autonomous adaptation takes place (acclimatization). In reality, populations will adjust autonomously (that is, without planned adaptation) to climate change, and indeed, mortality rates today are fairly similar in countries with very different climates. Studies that build in acclimatization show much lower future health impacts. However, little information or evidence exists on which to base assumptions about the rate of future acclimatization. Estimating the rate of change of adaptation to climate change and the rate above which impacts might start to increase more sharply is difficult.

## REFERENCES

Balbus, J. M., J. B. Greenblatt, R. Chari, D. Millstein, and K. L. Ebi. 2014. "A Wedge-Based Approach to Estimating Health Co-Benefits of Climate Change Mitigation Activities in the United States." *Climatic Change* 127 (2): 199–210.

Balbus, J. M., and C. Malina. 2009. "Identifying Vulnerable Subpopulations for Climate Change Health Effects in the United States." *Journal of Occupational and Environmental Medicine* 51 (1): 33–37.

Banks, L. L., M. B. Shah, and M. E. Richards. 2007. "Effective Healthcare System Response to Consecutive Florida Hurricanes." *American Journal of Disaster Medicine* 2 (6): 285–95.

Bosello, F., F. Eboli, and R. Pierfederici. 2012. "Assessing the Economic Impacts of Climate Change: An Updated CGE Point of View." Working Paper 2, Research Paper 125, *Fondazione Eni Enrico Mattei, Euro-Mediterraneo per i Cambiamenti Climatici*, Venice.

Cann, K. F., D. R. Thomas, R. L. Salmon, A. P. Wyn-Jones, and D. Kay. 2012. "Extreme Water-Related Weather Events and Waterborne Disease." *Epidemiology and Infection* 141 (4): 671–86.

Cardona, O. D., M. G. Ordaz, E. Reinoso, L. Yamin, B. Barbat, and others. 2012. "CAPRA—Comprehensive Approach to Probabilistic Risk Assessment: International Initiative for Risk Management Effectiveness." Paper prepared for the 15th World Conference on Earthquake Engineering, Lisbon, September 24–28.

Carthey, J., V. Chandra, and M. Loosemore. 2009. "Adapting Australian Health Facilities to Cope with Climate-Related Extreme Weather Events." *Journal of Facilities Management* 7 (1): 36–51.

Chiabai, A., S. Balakrishnan, G. Sarangi, and S. Nischal. 2010. "Human Health." In *Costing Adaptation: Preparing for Climate Change in India*, edited by A. Markandya and A. Mishra. New Delhi: TERI Press.

Chima, R. I., C. A. Goodman, and A. Mills. 2003. "The Economic Impact of Malaria in Africa: A Critical Review of the Evidence." *Health Policy* 63: 17–36.

Dunne, J. P., R. J. Stouffer, and J. G. John. 2013. "Reductions in Labour Capacity from Heat Stress under Climate Warming." *Nature Climate Change* 3: 563–66.

Ebi, K. L. 2008. "Adaptation Costs for Climate Change–Related Cases of Diarrhoeal Disease, Malnutrition, and Malaria in 2030." *Globalization and Health* 4 (1): 9.

———. 2013. "Health in the New Scenarios for Climate Change Research." *International Journal of Environmental Research and Public Health* 11 (1): 30–46. doi:10.3390 /ijerph100x000x.

Ebi, K. L., and K. J. Bowen. 2016. "Extreme Events as Sources of Health Vulnerability: Drought as an Example." *Weather and Climate Extremes* 11: 95–102.

Ebi, K. L., and D. Mills. 2013. "Winter Mortality in a Warming Climate: A Reassessment." *WIREs Climate Change* 4 (3): 203–12.

ECLAC (Economic Commission for Latin America and the Caribbean). 2011. *An Assessment of the Economic Impact of Climate Change on the Health Sector in Saint Lucia.* Santiago: ECLAC.

Egbendewe-Mondzozo, A., M. Musumba, B. A. McCarl, and X. Wu. 2011. "Climate Change and Vector-borne Diseases: An Economic Impact Analysis of Malaria in Africa." *International Journal of Environmental Research and Public Health* 8 (12): 913–30.

Field, C. B., V. R. Barros, D. J. Dokken, K. J. Mach, M. D. Mastrandrea, and others, eds. 2014. *Impacts, Adaptation, and Vulnerability. Part A: Global and Sectoral Aspects. Contribution of Working Group II to the Fifth Assessment Report of the Intergovernmental Panel on Climate Change.* New York: Cambridge University Press.

Field, C. B., V. R. Barros, T. F. Stocker, D. Qin, D. J. Dokken, and others. 2012. *Managing the Risks of Extreme Events and Disasters to Advance Climate Change Adaptation, a Special Report of Working Groups I and II of the Intergovernmental Panel on Climate Change.* New York: Cambridge University Press.

Garcia-Menendez, F., R. K. Saari, E. Monier, and N. E. Selin. 2015. "U.S. Air Quality and Health Benefits from Avoided Climate Change under Greenhouse Gas Mitigation." *Environmental Science and Technology* 49: 7580–88.

Guha-Sapir, D., F. Vos, R. Below, and S. Ponserre. 2012. *Annual Disaster Statistical Review 2011: The Numbers and Trends.* Brussels: CRED.

Hallegatte, S., M. Bangalore, L. Bonzanigo, M. Fay, T. Kane, and others. 2016. *Shock Waves: Managing the Impacts of Climate Change on Poverty.* Washington, DC: World Bank.

Hess, J. J., K. L. Heilpern, T. E. Davis, and H. Frumkin. 2009. "Climate Change and Emergency Medicine: Impacts and Opportunities." *Academic Emergency Medicine* 16 (8): 782–94.

IVAC (International Vaccine Access Center). 2014. *Pneumonia and Diarrhea Progress Report.* Baltimore, MD: Johns Hopkins University.

Kjellstrom, T., R. S. Kovats, S. J. Lloyd, T. Holt, and R. S. J. Tol. 2009. "The Direct Impact of Climate Change on Regional Labor Productivity." *Archives of Environmental and Occupational Health* 64 (4): 217–27.

Kjellstrom, T., B. Lemke, and M. Otto. 2013. "Mapping Occupational Heat Exposure and Effects in South-East Asia: Ongoing Time Trends, 1980–2011 and Future Estimates to 2050." *Industrial Health* 51 (1): 56–67.

Knowlton, K., M. Rotkin-Ellman, L. Geballe, W. Max, and G. M. Solomon. 2011. "Six Climate Change-Related Events in the United States Accounted for about $14 Billion in Lost Lives and Health Costs." *Health Affairs* 30 (11): 2167–76.

Kolstad, E. W., and K. A. Johansson. 2010. "Uncertainties Associated with Quantifying Climate Change Impacts on Human Health: A Case Study for Diarrhea." *Environmental Health Perspectives* 119 (3): 299–305.

Kovats, S., S. Lloyd, A. Hunt, and P. Watkiss. 2011. "The Impacts and Economic Costs on Health in Europe and the Costs and Benefits of Adaptation, Results of the EC RTD ClimateCost Project." Technical Policy Briefing Note 8. In *The Climate Cost Project. Final Report. Volume 1: Europe,* edited by P. Watkiss. Stockholm: Stockholm Environment Institute.

Liu, J., H. Mooney, V. Hull, S. J. Davis, J. Gaskell, and others. 2015. "Systems Integration for Global Sustainability." *Science* 347 (6225): 1258832.

Lloyd, S. J., R. S. Kovats, and Z. Chalabi. 2011. "Climate Change, Crop Yields, and Undernutrition: Development of a Model to Quantify the Impact of Climate Scenarios on Child Undernutrition." *Environmental Health Perspectives* 119 (12): 1817–23.

Markandya, A., and A. Chiabai. 2009. "Valuing Climate Change Impacts on Human Health: Empirical Evidence from the Literature." *International Journal of Environmental Research and Public Health* 6 (2): 759–86.

OECD (Organisation for Economic Co-operation and Development). 2015. "Modelling the Economic Consequences of Climate Change." In *The Economic Consequences of Climate Change.* Paris: OECD.

Pandey, K. 2010. "Cost of Adapting to Climate Change for Human Health in Developing Countries." Discussion Paper 11, World Bank, Washington, DC.

Parry, M., N. Arnell, P. Berry, D. Dodman, S. Fankhauser, and others. 2009. "Assessing the Costs of Adaptation to Climate Change: A Review of the UNFCCC and Other Recent Estimates." International Institute for Environment and Development and Grantham Institute for Climate Change, London.

Ramakrishnan, S. 2011. "Adaptation Cost of Diarrhea and Malaria in 2030 for India." *Indian Journal of Occupational and Environmental Medicine* 15 (2): 64.

SEI (Stockholm Environment Institute). 2009. *The Economics of Climate Change in East Africa.* Final Report for DFID and DANIDA, SEI, Stockholm.

Smith, K. R., A. Woodward, D. Campbell-Lendrum, D. D. Chadee, Y. Honda, and others. 2014. "Human Health: Impacts, Adaptation, and Co-Benefits." In *Climate Change*

*2014: Impacts, Adaptation, and Vulnerability; Part A: Global and Sectoral Aspects.* Contribution of Working Group II to the Fifth Assessment Report of the Intergovernmental Panel on Climate Change, edited by C. B. Field, V. R. Barros, D. J. Dokken, K. J. Mach, M. D. Mastrandrea, and others, chapter 11, 709–54. New York: Cambridge University Press.

Steinbruner, J. D., P. C. Stern, and J. L. Husbands. 2013. *Climate and Social Stress: Implications for Security Analysis; National Climate Assessment.* Washington, DC: National Research Council.

Traerup, S. L. M., R. A. Ortiz, and A. Markandya. 2011. "The Costs of Climate Change: A Study of Cholera in Tanzania." *International Journal of Environmental Research and Public Health* 8 (12): 4386–405.

UNDP (United Nations Development Programme). 2011. "Assessment of Investment and Financial Flows to Address Climate Change (Capacity Development for Policy Makers to Address Climate Change): Country Summaries." UNDP, New York. http://www.undpcc.org/en/financial-analysis/results.

Watkiss, P., and A. Hunt. 2012. "Projection of Economic Impacts of Climate Change in Sectors of Europe Based on Bottom-Up Analysis: Human Health." *Climatic Change* 112 (1): 101–26.

WHO (World Health Organization). 2004. *World Health Report 2004: Changing History.* Geneva: WHO.

———. 2015. *Operational Framework for Building Climate Resilient Health Systems.* Geneva: WHO.

World Bank. 2010. *The Costs to Developing Countries of Adapting to Climate Change: New Methods and Estimates; the Global Report of the Economics of Adaptation to Climate Change Study.* Synthesis Report. Washington, DC: World Bank.

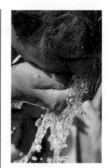

Chapter 9

# Water Supply, Sanitation, and Hygiene

Guy Hutton and Claire Chase

## INTRODUCTION

Safe drinking water, sanitation, and hygiene (WASH) are fundamental to improving standards of living for people. The improved standards made possible by WASH include, among others, better physical health, protection of the environment, better educational outcomes, convenience time savings, assurance of lives lived with dignity, and equal treatment for both men and women. Poor and vulnerable populations have lower access to improved WASH services and have poorer associated behaviors. Improved WASH is therefore central to reducing poverty, promoting equality, and supporting socioeconomic development. Drinking water and sanitation were targets in the Millennium Development Goals (MDGs) for 2015; under the Sustainable Development Goals (SDGs) for the post-2015 period, Member States of the United Nations (UN) aspire to achieve universal access to WASH by 2030. The Human Right to Safe Drinking Water and Sanitation (HRTWS) was adopted in 2010 under a UN resolution calling for safe, affordable, acceptable, available, and accessible drinking water and sanitation services for all.[1]

The scope of WASH services included in this chapter is shown in table 9.1. The focus is on services at the household and institutional level and on services for personal rather than productive uses.

This chapter summarizes global evidence on current WASH coverage and effects of intervention options, and it recommends areas for research and policy. Evidence comes from published synthesized evidence, such as systematic reviews and meta-analyses, evidence papers, and literature reviews. When those sources were not available, evidence was compiled from the next best sources of published research, thus using accepted criteria of the hierarchy of evidence for studies on health effectiveness. Unpublished and grey literature was used where no peer-reviewed published evidence exists.

This chapter is structured as follows:

- Progress in improving drinking water, sanitation, and hygiene coverage
- Impacts of poor WASH, thereby summarizing the evidence on the continued decline in mortality from diarrheal disease and the emerging evidence on the long-term developmental and cognitive effects of inadequate WASH on children
- Effectiveness of interventions, thereby examining the health effects of specific WASH interventions, the approaches to service delivery, and the key role of broader institutional policy in accelerating and sustaining progress
- Intervention costs, efficiency, and sustainability, thereby assessing the socioeconomic returns of improved WASH and considering the requirements for populations to have continued access to WASH services
- Challenges, opportunities, and recommendations.

This chapter uses the World Health Organization (WHO) classification of superregions as follows: Africa, the Americas, South-East Asia, Europe, Eastern Mediterranean, and Western Pacific.

Corresponding author: Guy Hutton, WASH Section, UNICEF. ghutton@unicef.org, formerly at the Water and Sanitation Program, World Bank.

**Table 9.1** Scope of Water, Sanitation, and Hygiene Services Included in This Chapter

| Service | Included | Excluded |
|---|---|---|
| **Water supply** | Water for drinking | Water for productive uses |
| | Other water uses in the home (cooking, hygiene, sanitation, cleaning, laundry) | |
| | Treatment, safe handling, and storage of water | |
| **Sanitation** | Toilets and onsite excreta management | Separate greywater management |
| | Management of septage (fecal sludge) | Industrial wastewater management |
| | Sewerage or combined sewer-drainage systems | Storm water drainage |
| | | Solid waste management |
| **Hygiene** | Handwashing and other personal hygiene practices | Food hygiene |
| | Menstrual hygiene management | Environmental hygiene and cleanliness measures |

## STATUS OF DRINKING WATER, SANITATION, AND HYGIENE

### Targets

The MDG targets called for halving the proportion of the population without sustainable access to safe drinking water and basic sanitation between 1990 and 2015. The targets were ambitious. In 1990, 76 percent of the global population used an improved drinking water source, and 54 percent had access to safe sanitation. The MDG's drinking water target was met in 2010; yet in 2015, the world remained 9 percentage points short of achieving the sanitation target. The SDGs for 2015–2030 have broadened from the MDG period to include (1) water-use efficiency across all sectors, sustainable withdrawals, and supply of freshwater to people suffering from water scarcity; (2) integrated water resource management, and (3) water-related ecosystems. The SDG also set ambitious WASH-related targets of universal access to safe water (target 6.1), adequate sanitation and hygiene, and the elimination of open defecation (target 6.2) as well as reduced untreated wastewater (target 6.3). In the overall aim of access for all, the SDG language and spirit emphasizes progressive reduction of inequalities and leaving no one behind, as well as providing inclusive, quality, and sustainable services—thereby ensuring access for women and for poor and vulnerable populations.

### Definitions

To understand the status of drinking water, sanitation, and hygiene, one must make a distinction between different levels of service access and population practices.

All populations meet water and sanitation needs in some way, but those ways are often not sufficient, reliable, safe, convenient, affordable, or dignified. To monitor the MDG water and sanitation target, the UN distinguished between improved and unimproved water and sanitation facilities at home. For the SDG targets, one indicator is proposed per target: (1) for target 6.1, the percentage of population using safely managed drinking water services and (2) for target 6.2, the percentage of population using safely managed sanitation services, including a handwashing facility with soap and water. Complementing these proposals is a broader set of indicators distinguishing basic and safely managed service levels (table 9.2) (WHO and UNICEF 2015a).

The indicators for global monitoring need to be kept simple for feasibility and cost. However, countries, organizations, and programs often monitor different aspects of service performance, such as quantity, quality, proximity, reliability, price, and affordability (Roaf, Khalfan, and Langford 2005). Some countries adopt more lenient definitions, and some adopt stricter definitions.

The definitions in existing monitoring systems have several limitations. Some limitations are partially addressed by the new indicators for higher-level services. The new indicators were informed by the five normative criteria, as stated in the HRTWS and shown in table 9.2: accessibility, acceptability, availability, affordability, and quality.[2]

- The Joint Monitoring Programme's (JMP) definition of improved facilities focuses on the technology type and is an imprecise proxy for the quality of services (Moriarty and others 2010; Onda, LoBuglio, and Bartram 2012; Potter and others 2010).

**Table 9.2** Proposed Service Level Definitions for Monitoring SDG 6 WASH Targets

| Service | Basic services | Safely managed services |
|---|---|---|
| **Water** | Percentage of population using an improved drinking water source with a total collection time of 30 minutes or less for a round trip, including queuing (termed "basic" water).[a] | Percentage of population using safely managed drinking water services. "Safely managed" refers to an improved[a] drinking water source that is located on premises, available when needed, and free from fecal (E. coli) and priority chemical (arsenic and flouride) contamination. |
| **Sanitation and hygiene** | Percentage of population not practicing open defecation. Percentage of population using an improved sanitation facility that is not shared with other households (basic sanitation).[b] Percentage of population with a handwashing facility with soap and water at home. | Percentage of population using safely managed sanitation services, including a handwashing facility with soap and water. "Safely managed" refers to an improved sanitation facility that is not shared with other households and where excreta are either safely disposed in situ or treated offsite. |

*Sources:* Definitions of improved, WHO and UNICEF 2006; definitions of indicators, WHO and UNICEF 2015a.

*Note:* The higher service level indicators are proposed for SDG monitoring. SDG = Sustainable Development Goal; WASH = drinking water, sanitation, and hygiene; WatSan = water and sanitation.

a. Same as improved water monitored as part of the MDG target 7c: piped water into dwelling, plot, or yard; public tap and standpipe; tubewell and borehole; protected dug well; protected spring; rainwater collection.

b. Same as improved sanitation monitored as part of the MDG target 7c: flush or pour-flush to piped sewer system, septic tank, pit latrine or ventilated improved pit latrine; pit latrine with slab and composting toilet.

- Self-reported responses of access by household members may be biased (Stanton and Clemens 1987).
- Statistics on household access provide no indication of variations in access and practices among different household members. For example, even in communities with high coverage rates for sanitation, children still commonly defecate in the open.[3]
- Indicators do not adequately reflect accountability and sustainability, which are key elements that cut across all the service levels.

The existing approach to measuring access does not provide a good indication of sustainability. The surveys use representative sampling and do not follow individual households over time. Effective monitoring of higher service levels requires regulatory data, but coverage is poor in low- and middle-income countries (LMICs), especially in rural areas.

## Coverage of Water Supply, Sanitation, and Hygiene

This section presents the coverage data at global and regional levels for drinking water and sanitation according to the JMP definitions used for monitoring MDG target 7c, thereby using the most recent update and MDG assessment report (WHO and UNICEF 2015b). Breakdowns are provided by rural and urban areas.[4]

### Water Supply

Globally, the use of improved drinking water sources increased from 76 percent in 1990 to 91 percent in 2015 (WHO and UNICEF 2015b). Regional breakdowns for progress between 1990 and 2015 are shown in figure 9.1. In its 2012 report presenting 2010 estimates, the UN showed that its MDG target of halving the proportion of the population without access to safe drinking water had been met (WHO and UNICEF 2012b); however, such global estimates mask regional disparities and inequities in access between urban and rural populations. As of 2015, 663 million people still used unimproved water sources, compared to 1.3 billion in 1990; 2.6 billion people have gained access to improved water since 1990. Rural dwellers remain unserved compared with urban dwellers (16 percent and 4 percent, respectively). In Sub-Saharan Africa, 44 percent of rural dwellers continue to use an unimproved water supply. Water hauling costs Sub-Saharan Africans, especially women, billions of hours each year. In 2008, more than 25 percent of the population in several Sub-Saharan African countries spent more than 30 minutes to make one round trip to collect water; 72 percent of the burden for collecting water fell on women (64 percent) and girls (8 percent), compared with men (24 percent) and boys (4 percent) (WHO and UNICEF 2010).

Urban areas enjoy a higher level of water service, as indicated by the use of piped water supply; in 2015,

**Figure 9.1** Drinking Water Coverage Trends, by Regions and World, Using the JMP Improved Water Definition, 1990–2015

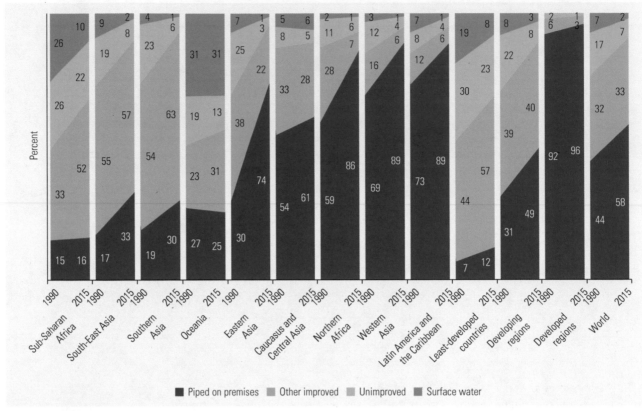

*Source:* WHO and UNICEF 2015b.
*Note:* JMP = Joint Monitoring Programme.

four of five people living in urban areas used piped water, compared to two of three in rural areas. Water sources classified as improved—even piped water—do not guarantee the safety or continuity of the water supply. Water quality surveys conducted in five countries showed that microbiological compliance with the WHO guidelines varied between water sources and countries (Onda, LoBuglio, and Bartram 2012). On average, compliance was close to 90 percent for piped water sources, and from 40 percent to 70 percent for other improved sources. Extrapolating to global estimates, the authors estimate that in 2010, 1.8 billion people (28 percent) used unsafe water, more than twice the population of 783 million (11 percent) that used an unimproved water supply.

**Sanitation**

The use of improved sanitation increased from 54 percent in 1990 to 68 percent in 2015, but those gains fell short of meeting the global MDG target (WHO and UNICEF 2015b). In 2015, 2.4 billion people still did not

have access to their own improved sanitation facility, a fact that, due to population growth, reflects no change in the unserved population of 1990. However, these numbers mask the fact that since 1990, 2.1 billion people have gained access to improved sanitation. Regional breakdowns in progress between 1990 and 2015 are shown in figure 9.2. Globally, the proportion of population practicing open defecation declined from 24 percent in 1990 to 13 percent in 2015. In South Asia, 34 percent still defecate in the open, compared to 23 percent in Sub-Saharan Africa. Globally, 638 million people (9 percent) share their sanitation facility with another family or families. Comparing rural and urban areas, 51 percent of rural dwellers have access to improved sanitation, compared with 82 percent of urban dwellers. Rates of improved sanitation do not reflect the amount of fecal waste that is not isolated, transported, or treated safely; a study of 12 cities in LMICs found that whereas 98 percent of households used toilets, only 29 percent of fecal waste was safely managed (Blackett, Hawkins, and Heymans 2014).

**Figure 9.2** Sanitation Coverage Trends, by Regions and World, Using the JMP Improved Sanitation Definition, 1990–2015

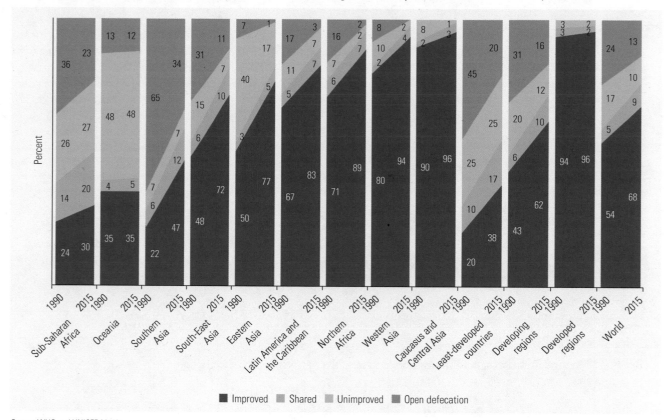

■ Improved ■ Shared ■ Unimproved ■ Open defecation

Source: WHO and UNICEF 2015b.
Note: JMP = Joint Monitoring Programme.

## Hygiene

Although the MDG target 7c does not provide a global indicator for hygiene, the data on the presence of a hand-washing facility with soap and water are increasingly collected as part of nationally representative surveys and will form the basis for efforts to monitor target 6.2 of the SDGs. Two main sources include nationally representative household surveys and a global review of published studies (Freeman and others 2014). Research studies suggest that the global prevalence of handwashing with soap after contact with excreta is 19 percent; rates are lower in Sub-Saharan Africa (14 percent) and South-East Asia (17 percent), where the most studies have been conducted (Freeman and others 2014). Proxy indicators for handwashing practice from nationally representative surveys are not reliable and tend to over report hygiene practices (Biran and others 2008).

## Distribution of Services

The JMP has reported the distribution of water supply and sanitation services by wealth status, breaking the population into five equal wealth quintiles using an asset index. In 35 Sub-Saharan African countries, households in the poorest wealth quintile are 6 times less likely to have water access compared with the richest quintile; the difference for sanitation is at least 2.5 times less likely (WHO and UNICEF 2013). Figure 9.3 illustrates the levels of disparity—between regions, between countries in a region, and at the country level—in the differences between rural and urban areas and between wealth quintiles. Limited datasets are available on the disparities between population subgroups—for example, slum populations, ethnic groups, women, the elderly, and persons who have physical impairments—as the sample size and sampling methodology in nationally representative surveys generally do not enable sufficiently robust comparisons.

Global reporting of institutional WASH has not yet been standardized as it has for household-level WASH; efforts are under way to build a global reporting system of WASH in schools and health facilities for SDG monitoring. The Demographic and Health Survey (DHS) Service

**Figure 9.3** Mozambique Example: How Average Values Mask Massive Disparities in Household Coverage

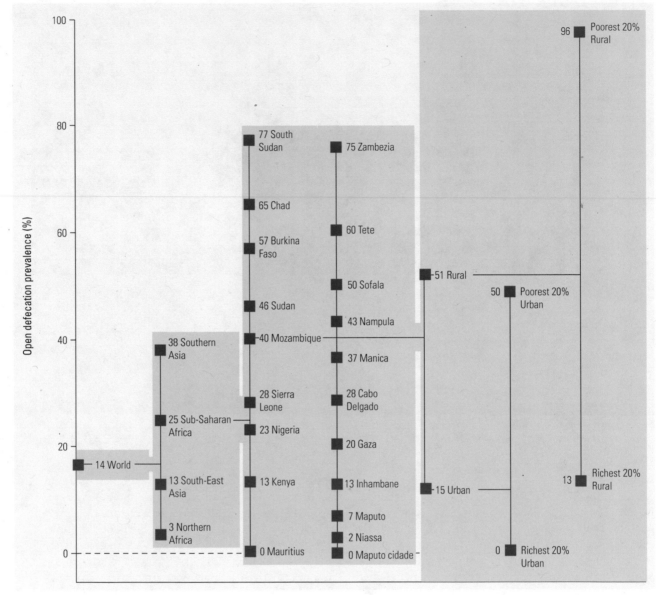

Source: WHO and UNICEF 2014.

Provision Assessment (SPA) monitors WASH in health facilities. WASH coverage in both primary schools and front-line health facilities is monitored and reported under the Service Delivery Indicators, currently for Sub-Saharan Africa. United Nations agencies collect data on WASH in schools (Education Management Information System operated by UNICEF), health facilities (Health Management Information System operated by the WHO), and refugee camps (UN High Commissioner for Refugees).

In addition to enhanced monitoring efforts by UN agencies, UN member countries need greater understanding of the challenges facing the world to meet the goal of universal access to institutional WASH within 15 years and to sustain that access beyond 2030. Unsustainable water extraction, along with competing demands, population growth and migration (including urbanization), and climate change and variability, puts significant pressure on water supply systems. In addition, new settlements require systematic, coordinated planning, and existing settlements require retrofitting to bring sustainable WASH services to citizens.

## IMPACTS OF INADEQUATE WASH

Understanding the nature and extent of the demonstrated negative effects of inadequate WASH on individuals, the environment, and societies is important for those designing interventions and assessing benefits and efficiency. Many benefits of WASH interventions are nonhealth in nature; including only health effects in impact evaluations can severely underestimate the intervention benefits (Loevensohn and others 2015).

### Health Consequences

Contaminated water and lack of sanitation lead to the transmission of pathogens through feces and, to a lesser extent, urine. The F-diagram explained here but not shown provides a basic understanding of these pathways by which pathogens from feces are ingested through transmission by fingers, flies, fluids, fields (soil), and food:

- Diseases transmitted by the fecal pathway include diarrheal disease, enteric infection, hepatitis A and E, poliomyelitis, helminths, trachoma, and adenoviruses (conjunctivitis) (Strickland 2000). Most of these diseases are transmitted through the fecal-oral pathway, but some are transmitted through the fecal-skin pathway (for example, schistosomiasis) and the fecal-eye pathway (for example, trachoma). These transmissions occur between humans, as well as between animals and humans.
- Pathogens carried through urine (for example, leptospirosis) mainly result from animal-to-human transmission.
- Poor personal hygiene causes fungal skin infections, such as ringworm (tinea) and scabies.
- Lack of handwashing is associated with respiratory infections (Rabie and Curtis 2006); inadequate hand hygiene during childbirth is linked to infection (Semmelweis 1983) and neonatal mortality (Blencowe and others 2011; Rhee and others 2008).

A systematic review and meta-analysis documented large and significant associations between poor water, sanitation, and maternal mortality (Benova, Cumming, and Campbell 2014). The precise mechanism has not been well established, but it is thought to be largely attributable to puerperal sepsis.

Children under age five years are especially vulnerable to infection. Regular exposure to environments with high fecal loads causes enteropathy[5]; compromises nutritional status; and leads to long-term consequences, such as stunting and retarded cognitive development (Humphrey 2009; Petri and others 2008).

The availability of water for drinking and household uses affects the quantity of water consumed and the time available to care for children in the household. Reducing the distance required to fetch water is associated with lower prevalence of diarrhea, improved nutrition, and lower mortality in children under age five years (Pickering and Davis 2012); these effects may be due to better hygiene practices (Curtis and Cairncross 2003; Esrey 1996; Esrey and others 1991), as well as to additional time available for child care or income-generating activities (Ilahi and Grimard 2000), thereby resulting in healthier children.

Inadequate quantities or consumption of water can also lead to dehydration, which has a number of adverse effects on physical and cognitive performance and bodily functions (Popkin, D'Anci, and Rosenberg 2010). Because there are no adequate biomarkers for measuring a population's hydration status, such an effect remains largely undocumented (Popkin, D'Anci, and Rosenberg 2010). Safe drinking water provides the basis for oral rehydration salts that save lives (Atia and Buchman 2009).

Exposure to harmful levels of arsenic in groundwater is estimated to affect 226 million people in more than 100 countries (Murcott 2012). Arsenic exposure causes skin lesions and long-term illnesses such as cancer, neurological disorders, cardiovascular diseases, diabetes, and cognitive deficits among children (Naujokas and others 2013).

Excess levels of water from heavy rainfall and inadequate drainage lead to flooding, thus causing injuries and death, as well as heightened risk of fecal-oral and skin diseases (Ahern and others 2005). Earthquakes, volcanic eruptions, tsunamis, and other natural disasters leave affected populations vulnerable to infection with waterborne diseases such as diarrhea, hepatitis A and E, and leptospirosis (Jafari and others 2011).

### Diarrheal Disease

The most recent study estimated 842,000 global deaths from diarrheal disease for 2012 (Prüss-Ustün and others 2014); 43 percent of these were children under age five years. An estimated 502,000 deaths were caused by inadequate drinking water, 280,000 by inadequate sanitation, and 297,000 by inadequate hand hygiene (table 9.3). The regional breakdowns indicate that the major share of global burden is in South-East Asia and Sub-Saharan Africa. Precise estimates remain elusive because of poor quality data on the cause of death; insufficient data on hygiene practices; and poor quality evidence on the effectiveness of some water and sanitation interventions, especially onsite sanitation. This paucity of reliable data has led to conflicting estimates of the burden of disease. The Institute for Health Metrics and

**Table 9.3** Diarrheal Disease Mortality Attributed to Poor Water Supply, Sanitation, and Hygiene in Low-and Middle-Income Countries, Regional and Risk Factor Breakdown

| Region | Water supply | Sanitation | Hygiene | WASH |
|---|---|---|---|---|
| Africa | 229,316 | 126,294 | 122,955 | 367,605 |
| The Americas | 6,441 | 2,370 | 5,026 | 11,519 |
| Eastern Mediterranean | 50,409 | 24,441 | 28,699 | 81,064 |
| Europe | 1,676 | 352 | 1,972 | 3,564 |
| South-East Asia | 207,773 | 123,279 | 131,519 | 363,904 |
| Western Pacific | 6,448 | 3,709 | 6,690 | 14,160 |
| **World** | **502,061** | **280,443** | **296,860** | **841,818** |

*Source:* Prüss-Ustün and others 2014.

*Note:* WASH = safe drinking water, sanitation, and hygiene. Totals may not be sum of rows because of rounding. Columns 2–4 do not sum to column 5 because of overlap in risk pathways.

Evaluation's Global Burden of Disease (GBD) study conducted a new meta-regression analysis of available experimental and quasi-experimental interventions. It found that poor water and sanitation account for 0.9 percent of global disability-adjusted life years (DALY) or 300,000 deaths per year (Lim and others 2012). The resulting difference between this study and the Prüss-Ustün and others (2014) study is 542,000 deaths, possibly because the studies included in the GBD study do not differentiate between different levels of quality of water supply and sanitation and between poor quality implementation and lack of effect.

Not all diarrheal diseases are caused by pathogens transmitted through inadequate WASH. Over time, different estimates have been made for the burden of diarrheal disease that can be attributed to fecal-oral transmission. Earlier estimates attribute 94 percent of diarrheal disease to poor WASH (Prüss-Ustün and Corvalan 2007); the more recent study attributes 58 percent (Prüss-Ustün and others 2014). This latter estimate is closely supported by a separate review of more than 200 studies that examined the causes of diarrhea in inpatients and found no pathogen present in 34 percent of cases (Lanata and others 2013). Importantly, deaths not easily preventable through WASH interventions (for example, rotavirus spread among young children and difficult to control) were excluded from the global burden of disease estimates for diarrheal disease shown in table 9.3. Thus, the data in table 9.3 provide a more realistic picture on how many deaths are considered preventable by WASH interventions.

Rising temperatures caused by climate change are expected to exacerbate the burden of diarrheal disease. The WHO estimates that an additional 48,000 deaths in children under age 15 years will be caused by climate change by 2030 and 33,000 deaths by 2050 (Hales and others 2014). These estimates may be conservative because they do not account for diarrheal deaths caused by other risk factors such as declining water availability and undernutrition.

Cholera is an endemic diarrheal disease, but it is strongly associated with natural disasters and civil conflict. An estimated 2.9 million cases of cholera cause 95,000 deaths each year in 69 endemic countries (Ali and others 2015). Cholera is transmitted through fecal contamination of water or food. Therefore, clean water and proper sanitation are critical to preventing its spread. However, good evidence is lacking as to which mix of interventions (including oral cholera vaccine, case management, and surveillance) is most cost-effective during outbreaks because few high-quality evaluation studies have been conducted (Taylor and others 2015).

Institutional settings—such as schools, health facilities, prisons, and other public settings such as refugee camps and public markets—can pose high risks if water and sanitation are not well managed. Studies have documented higher rates of diarrheal disease and gastrointestinal infection in schools that lack access to improved drinking water and sanitation facilities (Jasper, Le, and Bartram 2012). Improved hand hygiene is particularly important in institutional settings, given the ease with which infections spread in such environments.

**Helminth Infections**

Helminth infections are transmitted in water by fecal matter (schistosomiasis) and in soil by soil-transmitted helminths (STH). Although routine monitoring of infection rates is limited, the large number of prevalence surveys permits global estimates to be made.

One study of helminth prevalence data for 6,091 locations in 118 countries estimated that in 2010, 438.9 million people were infected with hookworm

(*Ancylostoma duodenale*), 819.0 million with roundworm (*A. lumbricoides*), and 464.6 million with whipworm (*T. trichiura*) (Pullan and others 2014). Of the 4.98 million years lived with disability (YLDs) attributable to STH, 65 percent of those were attributable to hookworm, 22 percent to *A. lumbricoides,* and 13 percent to *T. trichiura*. Most STH infections (67 percent) and YLDs (68 percent) occurred in Asia (Central, East, South, and South-East). A separate study estimated 89.9 million STH infections in school-age children in Sub-Saharan Africa (Brooker, Clements, and Bundy 2006). Annual global deaths are estimated at 2,700 for *A. lumbricoides* and 11,700 for schistosomiasis (Lozano and others 2010).

Helminth infections cause several adverse health outcomes, including anemia, malnutrition, growth stunting, and impaired physical and cognitive development; those outcomes result in low school attendance and educational deficits, thus leading to loss of future economic productivity (Victora and others 2008). The risk of STH infection is greatest for those in specific occupations and circumstances, such as people who work in agriculture, who live in slums, who are poor, who have poor sanitation, and who lack clean water (Hotez and others 2006).

## Undernutrition and Environmental Enteric Dysfunction

Undernutrition causes an estimated 45 percent of all child deaths (Black and others 2013) and is responsible for 11 percent of global disease burden (Black and others 2008). Inadequate dietary intake and disease are directly responsible for undernutrition; however, multiple indirect determinants exacerbate these direct causes, including food insecurity, inadequate child care practices, low maternal education, poor access to health services, lack of access to clean water and sanitation, and poor hygiene practices (UNICEF 1990). Political, cultural, social, and economic factors play a role as well. Stunting (height-for-age below minus two standard deviations from median height-for-age of reference population) and underweight (weight-for-age below minus two standard deviations from median weight-for-age of reference population) are forms of undernutrition associated with weakened immune systems and severe long-term consequences that include poor cognitive development, a lower rate of school attendance, a lower level of job attainment, and a potentially higher risk of chronic disease in adulthood (Victora and others 2008).

The links between diarrhea and child undernutrition (Fishman and others 2004; Prüss-Üstün and Corvalan 2006) and other enteric infections (Brown, Cairncross, and Ensink 2013; Checkley and others 2008; Guerrant and others 2008; Lin and others 2013) are well documented. An emerging body of evidence suggests

that a subclinical condition of the small intestine caused by chronic ingestion of pathogenic microorganisms results in nutrient malabsorption. This subclinical condition may be the primary causal pathway between poor WASH and child growth (Humphrey 2009).

The evidence on the etiology of diarrheal disease finds an association between levels of intestinal inflammation detected through fecal samples and subsequent growth deficits in infants. This evidence lends support to the environmental enteropathy hypothesis that stunting may be an outcome of frequent enteric infection and intestinal inflammation (Kotloff and others 2013). Because of the asymptomatic nature of environmental enteropathy, the extent and seriousness of the condition is not known; however, it appears to be nearly universal among those living in impoverished conditions (Salazar-Lindo and others 2004) and may be the cause of up to 43 percent of stunting (Guerrant and others 2013).

The risks of low birth weight and stunting are heightened in undernourished mothers (Özaltin, Hill, and Subramanian 2010), resulting in intergenerational consequences of undernutrition and related conditions.

## Social Welfare Consequences

Improved water supply and sanitation provide individuals with increased comfort, safety, dignity, status, and convenience, and also have broader effects on the living environment (Hutton and others 2014). The social welfare effects are difficult to quantify, given their subjective nature. Nevertheless, those benefits are consistently cited as among the most important for beneficiaries of water supply and sanitation (Cairncross 2004; Jenkins and Curtis 2005) and may be particularly relevant for women (Fisher 2006).

### In or Near Homes

Water supply in or adjacent to homes provides greater comfort to household members, notably women and girls tasked with fetching water; water sources closer to home, especially piped water, are associated with increased use (Howard and Bartram 2003; Olajuyigbe 2010).

Data from 18 countries indicate that women are five times more likely than men to have the responsibility for collecting household water (WHO and UNICEF 2012b). As the distance to the water source increases, the time that women could spend on income-generating activities, household chores, and child care decreases (Ilahi and Grimard 2000). A regular piped water supply can introduce the possibility of purchasing time- and labor-saving devices, such as washing machines and dishwashers. Although access to water infrastructure does not always translate into wage employment for women (Lokshin and Yemtsov 2005), one study finds that it can provide time savings in water collection, thus improving gender equality (Koolwal and Van de Walle 2013).

Individuals with access to on-plot sanitation benefit from greater privacy, comfort, and convenience. Accompanying a child to the toilet is more convenient if it is nearby and safe, and mothers can comfortably step away from household duties to practice hygiene. In Ghana, more than 50 percent of households considering adopting a toilet included convenience in their top three reasons for investing in sanitation (Jenkins and Scott 2007). In six countries of South-East Asia, the rural households that owned their own latrine saved from 4 to 20 minutes of travel time per trip (Hutton and others 2014). Privacy, comfort, and convenience benefits are magnified for vulnerable groups, such as the elderly or persons living with disabilities or debilitating chronic illness.

On-plot sanitation reduces the risk of theft or assault (including rape and sexual harassment), especially at night or in isolated locations. Improved pit latrines are safer, less likely to collapse, and easier for small children to use. On-plot water supply and sanitation help to avoid conflicts with neighbors, landowners, or others over the use of shared water resources and sanitation facilities and the use of fields or rivers for open defecation.

### Schools and Workplaces

Access to improved WASH services in schools and workplaces contributes to school attendance, school performance, and choice of where to work, especially for girls and women. Recent evidence from India shows that a national government program to build toilets in schools led to an 8 percent increase in enrollment among pubescent-age boys and girls and a 12 percent increase among younger children of both genders (Adukia 2014). The comparably large effect of school sanitation on primary school children and the robust effects for boys and girls at all ages suggest that at least some of the effect of school sanitation is related to health (Jasper, Le, and Bartram 2012). Research has seldom analyzed academic performance as an outcome; however, given the role that improved water and sanitation have on child health and school attendance rates, the current evidence lacks research into their role in academic performance.

### Menstrual Hygiene

Menstrual hygiene management (MHM) is a poorly understood and underresearched area of WASH services. This neglect has left women in many LMICs without access to appropriate products, facilities, and services (Sebastian, Hoffmann, and Adelman 2013). Lack of adequate MHM is frequently described as a hindrance to girls' education, but high-quality evidence is lacking (Sumpter and Torondel 2013). A randomized controlled trial in Nepal suggests that menses, and poor menstrual hygiene technology in particular, has no effect on absenteeism of girls; girls miss less than one school day a year on average because of menstruation (Oster and Thornton 2011). However, girls may avoid going to school while they are menstruating, not because they lack management methods but because they lack proper facilities for managing menses (Jasper, Le, and Bartram 2012).

### Environmental Consequences

Two major environmental consequences of poor WASH practices are (1) the excessive extraction of water to meet population needs and (2) the pollution caused by poorly managed human excreta.

The water supply for domestic use represents a small proportion of overall extraction, but the concept of virtual water trade[6] has led to a greater understanding of the implications of population consumption patterns for water use. Globally, the combined effects of socioeconomic growth and climate change indicate that, by 2050, the population at risk of exposure to at least a moderate level of water stress could reach 5 billion people (Schlosser and others 2014). A population of up to an estimated 3 billion in 2050 is nearly double the current estimate of 1.7 billion people who live in areas with a high degree of water stress. The projections are made on the basis of a risk metric of frequency of water shortage in reservoirs (Sadoff and others 2015). This metric combines hydrological variability and water usage trends, which may be mitigated by storage infrastructure. This class of water insecurity is most severe in South Asia and Northern China, although the risk of water shortage exists on all continents.

Overextraction of groundwater and pollution of local surface water bodies have led many large urban population centers to source municipal water supplies from reservoirs or rivers that are tens or hundreds of kilometers from the site of treatment or consumption. Such schemes cost tens of millions of dollars each in reservoir construction, pipeline, and pumping costs. Groundwater resources are under increasing stress from unsustainable agricultural practices resulting from crop choice and energy subsidies to enable farmers to pump groundwater. In India and Mexico, for example, subsidized electricity and kerosene for farmers have led to serious groundwater overdraft (Scott and Shah 2004).

Poorly managed human excreta have major environmental consequences; excreta pollute human settlements, groundwater, and surface water such as lakes, rivers, and oceans. The degree of pollution depends on wastewater, sludge, and sewage management practices; climatic factors; and the population size and density in relation to the volume of water. In highly populated river basins, municipal sewage and wastewater contribute a high proportion to overall biological oxygen demand (Corcoran and others 2011; Rabalais and Turner 2013).

Heavily polluted surface water has serious effects on ecosystems, food webs, and biodiversity (Turner and Rabalais 1991). Coastal areas that are near the discharge of large, polluted rivers have reported compromised fish catch, such as in Argentina (Dutto and others 2012). In the coastal areas of the Philippines, water pollution was estimated to cost US$26 million per year in lost fish catch and degraded coral reefs (World Bank 2009). Water pollution of recreational areas affects the tourism industry, thus lowering visit rates or causing gastrointestinal illness or both.

## Financial and Economic Consequences

Financial and economic studies convert the health, social, and environmental effects of poor WASH to a common money metric, thereby enabling aggregation as well as comparison across locations and over time. However, these estimates are often incomplete, using crude estimates of economic value or relying on the imprecise physical effects underlying the economic values.

Damage cost studies account for the broader welfare and productivity consequences of poor WASH beyond the health effects. A review of economic impacts of poor water and sanitation found estimates from more than 30 countries (see annex 9A), as well as global studies. Studies with economic impacts expressed as a percentage of gross domestic product (GDP) are shown in figure 9.4, disaggregated between health and nonhealth damages.

Although all the studies presented in figure 9.4 present effects in monetary units, the results are not directly comparable. They have different base years and different effects included; some include only sanitation, and others include water and sanitation. In East Asian and Pacific and Sub-Saharan African economies, the cost of poor sanitation exceeded 2 percent of total GDP; in South Asia, it exceeded 4 percent of GDP. A global study, including the health and time losses, valued the costs in LMICs at 1.5 percent of global domestic product (Hutton 2012). These significant economic effects raise awareness of the extent of the problem, but they do not indicate how to address the problem in a cost-effective manner.

## INTERVENTION OPTIONS AND EFFECTIVENESS

Three main categories of interventions to improve WASH are as follows:

- Technology options and WASH practices cover the type of hardware, equipment, and associated behaviors of WASH services. Not all water or sanitation technologies perform the same function, so they can be classified by the service level they provide.
- Service delivery models cover the components of WASH service implementation. Those components include (1) approaches to demand generation and WASH behavior change, (2) approaches to strengthen supply of water and sanitation goods and services, and (3) approaches to improve the effectiveness of WASH service delivery.
- Strengthening the enabling environment for WASH service delivery includes (1) measures to strengthen capacity, (2) legal framework, (3) policy and planning, (4) resource allocation, (5) monitoring and evaluation, and (6) other interventions to provide a stronger foundation for implementing the technology and service delivery models. The evidence is provided in annex 9B.

## Effectiveness of Technologies and Practices

Water technologies are designed to source, treat, distribute, and monitor the supply of water. Epidemiological studies evaluate the effectiveness of water interventions in terms of the quantity and (microbial) quality of water supplied (Waddington and others 2009). Increasing evidence enables the comparison of the incremental health benefits of different water interventions, such as improved community source, piped water, higher-quality piped water, and point-of-use treatment (chlorine, solar, and filter). Utility regulators, as well as regional and global initiatives, monitor water quality according to service standards, such as continuity, consumption, and number of complaints (IBNET 2014). In 2010, The International Benchmarking Network for Water and Sanitation Utilities (IBNET) of the World Bank reported that only 16 percent of utilities in low-income countries supply water continuously 24 hours per day, compared to 86 percent of utilities in middle-income countries (Van den Berg and Danilenko 2010). Even a few days of interrupted water supply can result in significant adverse health consequences if beneficiaries revert to using unimproved sources of water (Hunter, Zmirou-Navier, and Hartemann 2009).

**Figure 9.4** Economic Costs of Poor Water and Sanitation in Selected Countries, as a Percentage of GDP

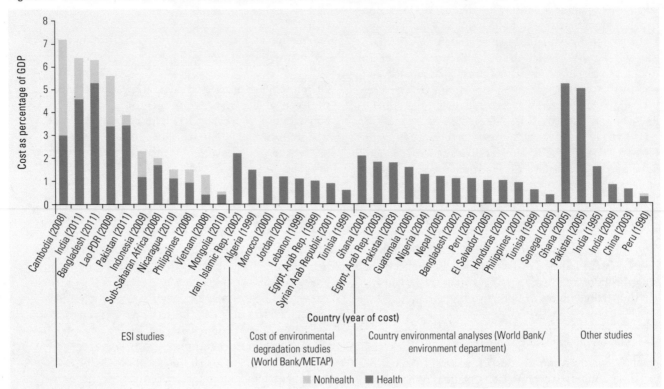

*Source:* See annex 9A for fuller datasets and references.

*Note:* GDP = gross domestic product. Economics of Sanitation Initiative (ESI) studies have been implemented by the World Bank's Water and Sanitation Program in 34 countries of Latin America and the Caribbean, East Asia and Pacific, South Asia, and Sub-Saharan Africa. These studies estimated the costs of poor sanitation, including health and nonhealth impacts (access time, costs of accessing safe water, tourism). The Mediterranean Environmental Technical Assistance Program (METAP) of the World Bank conducted studies on the costs of environmental degradation in eight Mediterranean countries from 1999 to 2002. Country environmental analyses conducted by the World Bank in more than 20 countries since 2003 have estimated the health costs of poor water and sanitation.

To increase safety, drinking water can be treated either at the source or at the point of use through a process of filtration or disinfection or both. The greatest health effects for improved water treatment technologies concern the piped water supply, with greater health benefits associated with higher-quality piped water (water that is safe and continuously available) (Wolf and others 2014). Among household-level studies, filter interventions that also provided safe storage (for example, ceramic filters) were associated with a large reduction in diarrheal disease (Wolf and others 2014). Neither chlorine treatment nor solar disinfection shows significant impact on diarrhea after meta-analysis adjusted for non-blinding of the intervention (Wolf and others 2014), although an earlier systematic review and meta-analysis of water quality interventions found household-level treatment to be more effective than source treatment (Clasen and others 2005). Blinding participants to the intervention and longer follow-up periods are recommended to better understand the impact of point-of-use water treatment interventions on diarrhea (Clasen and others 2005).

To reduce the transmission of pathogens, sanitation technologies isolate, transport, and treat fecal waste, and they also provide users with a dignified and comfortable experience when going to the toilet. Different rungs on the "sanitation ladder" confer different health impacts and user experiences; hence, utilization of different kinds of sanitation services or facilities can vary. For example, communal facilities may be poorly maintained, in which case they are less likely to be used by women, children, and individuals who are disabled or infirm. Distance also decreases usage of communal toilets (Biran and others 2011).

Hygiene technologies enable users to perform basic personal hygiene functions. Epidemiological studies have typically used the presence of a place for handwashing with soap and water as a proxy for handwashing practice; however, this has been shown to be only loosely correlated with observed handwashing behavior (Ram 2013).

One synthetic review and meta-analysis of health impact assessments of water and sanitation interventions includes 61 individual studies for water,

12 observations comparing unimproved and improved sanitation conditions, and only 2 observations comparing unimproved sanitation and sewer connections (Wolf and others 2014).

Table 9.4 shows relative risk reductions for different movements up the water supply and sanitation ladders. The summary risk ratio for all observations on diarrhea morbidity is 0.66 (95% confidence interval [CI]: 0.60–0.71) for water interventions and 0.72 (95% CI: 0.59–0.88) for sanitation interventions (Wolf and others 2014). An earlier review of 25 studies investigating the association between sewerage and diarrhea or other related outcomes estimated an average risk ratio of 0.70 (95% CI: 0.61–0.79), which increased to as much as 0.40 when starting sanitation conditions were very poor (Norman, Pedley, and Takkouche 2010).

A meta-analysis of hygiene interventions found an average risk ratio for diarrhea of 0.60 for promotion of handwashing with soap (95% CI: 0.53–0.68) and 0.76 for general hygiene education alone (95% CI: 0.67–0.86) (Freeman and others 2014). These results are summarized in table 9.4. An earlier systematic review found a relative risk compared to no handwashing of 0.84 (95% CI: 0.79–0.89) for respiratory infection (Rabie and Curtis 2006).

A meta-analysis that combined sanitation availability and use examined the impact of improved sanitation on soil-transmitted helminths. The meta-analysis reported the following overall odds ratios:[7] 0.51 (95% CI: 0.44–0.61) for the three soil-transmitted helminths combined, 0.54 (95% CI: 0.43–0.69) for *A. lumbricoides*, 0.58 (95% CI: 0.45–0.75) for *T. trichiura*, and 0.60 (95% CI: 0.48–0.75) for hookworm (Ziegelbauer and others 2012).

Access to sanitation has been associated with lower trachoma, as measured by the presence of trachomatous inflammation–follicular or trachomatous inflammation–intense with odds ratio 0.85 (95% CI: 0.75–0.95) and *C. trachomatis* infection with odds ratio 0.67 (95% CI: 0.55–0.78) (Stocks and others 2014).

A systematic review examined the impact of improved WASH on child nutritional status. Specifically, a meta-analysis of five randomized controlled trials found a mean difference of 0.08 in height-for-age z-scores of children under age five years (95% CI: 0.00–0.16) for solar disinfection of water, provision of soap, and improvements in water quality (Dangour and others 2013). However, the authors raised concerns about the low methodological quality of the included studies and the short follow-up periods; there was insufficient experimental evidence on water supply improvement and sanitation to include in the meta-analysis. Since publication of the Dangour and others (2013) review, several additional randomized controlled trials of household sanitation interventions have been completed (Briceno, Coville, and Martinez 2014; Cameron, Shah, and Olivia 2013; Clasen and others 2014; Hammer and Spears 2013; Patil and others 2014),

**Table 9.4** Meta-Regression Results for Water and Sanitation Interventions: Relative Risks Compared with No Improved Water, Sanitation, or Hygiene Practice

| Baseline | Outcome[a] | | | |
|---|---|---|---|---|
| *Baseline water* | *Outcome water* | | | |
| | *Improved community source* | *Piped water, noncontinuous* | *Piped water, high quality* | *Filter and safe storage in the household* |
| Unimproved source | 0.89 [0.78, 1.01] | 0.77 [0.64, 0.92] | 0.21 [0.08, 0.55] | 0.55 [0.38, 0.81] |
| Improved community source | | 0.86 [0.72, 1.03] | 0.23 [0.09, 0.62] | 0.62 [0.42, 0.93] |
| Basic piped water | | | 0.27 [0.10, 0.71] | 0.72 [0.47, 1.11] |
| *Baseline sanitation* | *Outcome sanitation* | | | |
| | *Improved sanitation, no sewer* | | *Sewer connection* | |
| Unimproved sanitation | 0.84 [0.77, 0.91] | | 0.31 [0.27, 0.36] | |
| Improved sanitation, no sewer | | | 0.37 [0.31, 0.44] | |
| *Baseline hygiene* | *Outcome hygiene* | | | |
| | *General hygiene education* | | *Handwashing with soap* | |
| No hygiene education or handwashing | 0.76 [0.67, 0.86] | | 0.60 [0.53, 0.68] | |

*Sources:* Water and sanitation: Wolf and others 2014; hygiene: Freeman and others 2014.
a. Brackets represent 95 percent confidence intervals.

most of them failing to find a significant relationship between the interventions and child health or growth outcomes. One exception is a study in rural Mali of Community-Led Total Sanitation (CLTS), which led to taller children on average (+0.18 height-for-age z-score, CI on z-score: 0.03–0.32). These children were 6 percentage points less likely to be stunted after the intervention (Pickering and others 2015). Econometric studies drawing on time series data establish links between open defecation and stunting (Spears 2013), between open defecation and childhood diarrhea in India (Andres and others 2014), and between open defecation and cognitive development in India (Spears and Lamba 2013). A source of regularly updated evidence reviews on WASH interventions with strict inclusion criteria is the Cochrane Library.[8]

## Effectiveness of Service Delivery Models

Effectiveness of service delivery models is measured by intervention uptake, change in risky behaviors, sustainability, and, to a lesser extent, health outcomes. Large-scale approaches that include demand raising and behavior change are needed to achieve universal access, but experience has shown these approaches result in lower average effectiveness.

### Approaches to Demand Generation and WASH Behavior Change

Demand-based approaches start from the premise that lasting change is brought about when individual and community behaviors are affected. CLTS and its school-based counterpart, School-Led Total Sanitation (SLTS), promote broader changes in sanitation and hygiene behaviors at the community level. Since its founding in 1999, the CLTS approach has rapidly expanded to more than 50 developing countries, where many thousand successful applications of the approach have been made; at least 16 national governments have adopted CLTS as national policy.[9] Rigorous evaluation of the CLTS approach has been limited, and the reliance on the emergence of natural leaders presents difficulties in testing the effectiveness of CLTS using conventional experimental methods. One exception comes from a recent example in rural Mali, in which CLTS was well implemented in a random set of villages and shown to almost double coverage of a private latrine (Pickering and others 2015).

Specific behaviors, such as household water treatment and storage (HWTS) and handwashing with soap, have been the subject of behavior change campaigns. HWTS combines marketing of low-cost water treatment (for example, boiling, filtration, disinfection using chemicals, solar and ultraviolet lamps, and flocculation) and safe storage technologies with communication- and behavior-change techniques (Peal, Evans, and van der Voorden 2010). Despite substantial evidence pointing to health benefits of HWTS, skepticism remains that the results may largely be the result of bias; concerns remain about the extent of uptake, use, and scalability of commercially marketed HWTS, particularly among poor populations most at risk of diarrheal disease (Schmidt and Cairncross 2009).

Handwashing promotion has been tested in formative research and has applied social cognitive models to determine what motivates and changes behavior. The promotion has used a variety of communication channels—such as television, radio, theater groups, community meetings, and face-to-face visits—to reach target groups who typically are mothers of young children or school-age children. A pre- and post-evaluation of the approach in Burkina Faso, which targeted the behavior of safe disposal of child feces and handwashing after contact, documented increases in handwashing (Curtis and others 2001). A similar approach to improve handwashing behavior was piloted on a large scale under the Water and Sanitation Program's Global Scaling Up Handwashing Projects in Peru, Senegal,[10] Tanzania, and Vietnam. Experimental evidence from Peru (Galiani and others 2015), Tanzania (Briceno, Coville, and Martinez 2014), and Vietnam (Chase and Do 2012) suggests the campaigns were only marginally successful. The Peru study did find large changes in behavior in a subset of communities with children who participated in a school-based handwashing promotion intervention. Effects on health were not observed in any of the countries, and the sustainability of handwashing was not measured. A key obstacle identified in both Tanzania and Vietnam was the difficult trade-off between scale and intensity of activities.

The Global Public-Private Partnership for Handwashing (PPPHW) combines the marketing expertise of the soap industry with government support and the enabling environment to trigger behavior change and reduce diarrhea. Whereas the PPPHW has expanded globally, the coalition has not yet been subject to rigorous effectiveness trials (Peal, Evans, and van der Voorden 2010). Evaluations of PPPHWs have been commissioned by private soap companies and involved providing free soap to households (Nicholson and others 2013), thus limiting their external validity.

### Approaches to Strengthening Supply of Water and Sanitation Goods and Services

Supply-side approaches to water and sanitation service delivery cover the full value chain from production and assembly of inputs, importation, sales, distribution, installation, and maintenance of water infrastructure and latrines. Services range from micro and small-scale independent water resellers; network operators; well and pit diggers; operators offering masonry, pit, and septic tank emptying; and public toilet operators to medium-scale sanitation markets—or sanimarts—offering a full range of sanitation goods and services. Small-scale operators can effectively serve rural markets, where the majority of people without access to piped water and sanitation live. However, the existing literature highlights several obstacles to growth and the ability of such providers to effectively serve these rural populations.

Rural operators often face higher per capita costs because they lack economies of scale enjoyed by larger utilities and therefore have lower revenue potential (Baker 2009). Investment financing needed for growth can be difficult to secure, and the lack of formalization in the sector can result in insecure operating environments (Sy, Warner, and Jamieson 2014). The availability of alternative sources of free or low-cost water makes rural areas less attractive to independent operators. Low or uneven demand has limited growth opportunities for small-scale onsite sanitation service providers. Despite these obstacles, small-scale service providers are increasingly recognized as a central part of the solution to close the gap in water and sanitation access, particularly among the poor.

Supply-side strengthening is predominant in the Community Approach to Total Sanitation (CATS) promoted by the United Nations Children's Fund and the Total Sanitation and Sanitation Marketing (TSSM) approach of the World Bank Water and Sanitation Program. Recent randomized control trial impact evaluations of TSSM in Madhya Pradesh, India (which included a hardware subsidy to households below the poverty line); East Java, Indonesia; and 10 rural districts of Tanzania found the approach varied widely in its effectiveness across the countries, with no increase in improved sanitation in Indonesia (Cameron, Shah, and Olivia 2013) and increases of 19 and 15.7 percent in Madhya Pradesh (Patil and others 2014) and Tanzania (Briceno, Coville, and Martinez 2014), respectively. Despite better sanitation coverage in Madhya Pradesh, large numbers of adults continued to practice open defecation.

### Approaches to Improve the Effectiveness of WASH Service Delivery

Addressing the supply- and demand-side constraints of WASH service delivery has led to large increases in access. But the persistence of regional and socioeconomic disparities in access suggests that current delivery models could be improved to enhance the quality of services as well as increase take-up of services, especially among the poorest populations.

Results-based approaches[11] to development that offer financial or nonmonetary rewards upon demonstration of measurable outputs or outcomes are used increasingly for achieving desirable outcomes. The specific details differ, but such approaches share a common aim of shifting the overall incentive structure from financing infrastructure to delivering services. Until recently, the experience using results-based approaches in water and sanitation was limited. A review by the World Bank in 2010 indicated that less than 5 percent of its output-based aid (OBA) portfolio was in water and sanitation (Mumssen, Johannes, and Kumar 2010). The use of OBA has increased under the Global Partnership on Output-Based Aid (GPOBA), which lists 22 projects in water supply and sanitation whose outputs include water, sewerage, or sanitation connections.[12] Multilateral and bilateral agencies such as the World Bank, Inter-American Development Bank, and Department for International Development (DfID) have shifted funding toward results-based approaches in water and sanitation. As of early 2016, the World Bank's Program-for-Results Financing (PforR) has six active operations in water supply, sanitation, and hygiene.

Microfinance or microcredit can help poor households facing liquidity constraints to invest in water supply and sanitation by (1) smoothing consumption over time, (2) encouraging households to be more willing to adopt improved services, and (3) giving those households an opportunity to purchase more durable, higher levels of service. Consumer credit has been applied successfully to increase the installation and use of household piped water connections (Devoto and others 2011), but experimental evidence of consumer lending for sanitation remains limited. However, emerging interest in the potential of microfinance for household sanitation and the results of small-scale pilots are promising. A randomized study in Cambodia found a fourfold increase in uptake when households were offered a 12-month low-interest loan to purchase a latrine (Shah 2013).

Finally, interest is emerging for using large-scale delivery platforms for social services and poverty reduction. These platforms can help improve the targeting of WASH services and will make use of the tools and mechanisms those programs have for improving livelihoods and outcomes for the poor. Examples include the following:

- Sanitation subsidies and financing can be targeted to conditional-cash transfer (CCT) participants, many of whom lack adequate sanitation. A more ambitious approach could make receipt of cash transfers conditional on a household's use of improved sanitation. These programs also provide outreach and counseling to reach target households with sanitation promotion messages that build awareness and help change behavior.

- Community-driven development (CDD) programs can be used as a platform to deliver CLTS and to follow up with participatory planning and budgeting to ensure that communities become free of open defecation.
- Safety-net programs that build skills and strengthen sources of livelihood can include sanitation businesses and services such as masonry, plumbing, and electrical skills among the list of profitable investments for beneficiaries.
- Many nutrition interventions already promote handwashing with soap, safe water, and sanitation. Handwashing demonstrations are often included in promotions for breastfeeding and interventions for feeding infants and young children, which also stress the use of safe water in food preparation.

More innovative integration approaches may use those same channels to discuss with the community sanitation product options and services that are available. Evidence is needed on the effectiveness and the cost of integrated approaches. Such information may highlight the need for more operational research and impact evaluations to inform policy and program design.

## INTERVENTION COSTS, EFFICIENCY, AND SUSTAINABILITY

Any intervention in the WASH sector requires an economic rationale, thus satisfying conditions of efficiency, affordability, and relevance. *Cost-benefit analysis* compares the intervention costs with the benefits, expressed in monetary units. *Cost-effectiveness analysis* compares the intervention costs with the benefits, expressed in some other common unit, such as lives gained or pollution load to the environment averted.

### Costs

The cost of interventions is one key piece of evidence for decision making, because it is relatively easy to obtain and is often cited as a constraint for an investment decision, whether by governments, private sectors, households, or individuals. Costs can be measured for the WASH technology (the hardware), the service delivery approach (the "software" or program management), and the enabling environment.

Despite its importance, cost information is not commonly tabulated in an appropriate format to support decision making. At the policy level, budgets and resource allocations are fragmented among subsectors, levels of government, and sector partners or financiers. Considerable differences exist between budget allocations and disbursements. WASH-BAT (bottleneck analysis tool), developed by UNICEF, helps consolidate the budgetary needs so that sector bottlenecks can be removed (see annex 9B) (UNICEF 2014). At the program or service delivery levels, implementers do not easily share information on their costs, and budgets may not be structured for simple breakdowns between software and hardware costs. Cost studies for WASH technologies are more abundant, and at the local level, the market or subsidized price is available. However, the price is rarely the same as the cost. The price commonly contains either a profit or a subsidy; because both are transfer payments, they should be excluded from economic analysis. However, to ease the research burden, it is common practice in economic analysis to use prices as a proxy for cost, adjusting for any known subsidy or profit.

Published cost evidence is available in aggregated and unit forms. Aggregated cost includes the expenditure required to meet specified targets. The World Bank estimates that the global capital costs of achieving universal access to WASH services by 2030 are US$28.4 billion per year confidence interval [CI]: US$13.8 billion to US$46.7 billion) from 2015 to 2030 for basic WASH and $114 billion per year (CI: US$74 billion to US$166 billion) for safely managed WASH (Hutton and Varughese 2016).[13] Those costs are equivalent to 0.10 percent of global product for basic WASH and 0.39 percent of global product for safely managed WASH, including 140 LMICs. Those needs compare with 0.12 percent of its gross product spent on meeting the MDG water target and making progress toward the sanitation target. Universal basic access by 2030 is feasible at current spending but requires reallocations to sanitation, to rural areas, and to off-track regions. However, substantial further spending is needed to meet the higher standard of safely managed services. The costs as a proportion of gross regional product are shown by MDG region in figure 9.5. Regions most challenged to reach universal access are South Asia and Sub-Saharan Africa.

Many countries also produce investment plans for meeting national targets, thereby focusing on the financing the government will provide. The Organisation for Economic Co-Operation and Development (OECD) has created FEASIBLE, a tool for developing national financing strategies by comparing the costs of meeting national

**Figure 9.5** Costs of Basic and Safely Managed Services as a Percentage of GRP, by Region, with Uncertainty Range

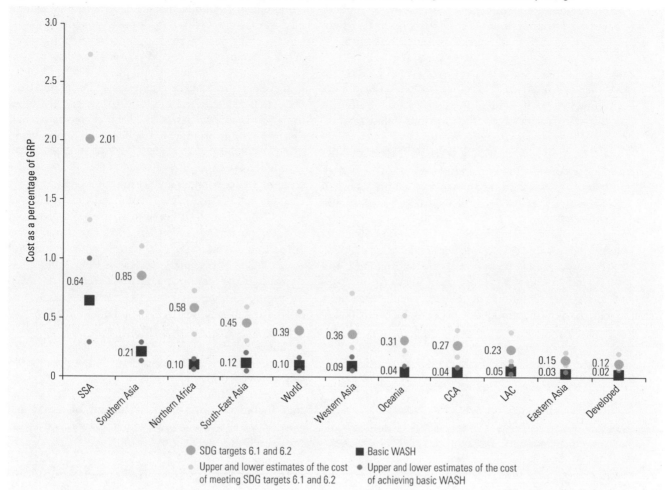

*Source:* Hutton and Varughese 2016.

*Note:* CCA = Caucasus and Central Asia; GRP = gross regional product; LAC = Latin America and the Caribbean; SDG = Sustainable Development Goal; SSA = Sub-Saharan Africa; WASH = water, sanitation, and hygiene. See table 9.2 for details on upper and lower values on variables varied in sensitivity analysis. GRP is based on the aggregated gross domestic product of countries in each region. An economic growth rate of 5 percent is assumed across all regions.

targets with the projected financing available.[14] FEASIBLE has been applied in at least 12 countries (OECD 2011).

A key input to these aggregated studies is the unit costs of WASH provision at the household or community level. Because of climatic, topographical, and socioeconomic differences, the costs of providing service vary highly between studies, contexts, and levels of service. The costs per cubic meter of water and of wastewater services, as well as average monthly household bills, are available for utility services through national regulators, regional associations, and global initiatives (IBNET 2014). Studies commonly compare the cost of different sources of water supply, and they find piped water to be significantly cheaper per unit compared with vendor-supplied water.

However, those studies find monthly expenditure is more similar between the two sources because of higher consumption of piped water than of other water sources (Whittington and others 2009). The IRC WASHCost project calculated benchmark capital and recurrent costs for basic levels of water service in Andhra Pradesh, India; Burkina Faso; Ghana; and Mozambique (Burr and Fonseca 2013). Benchmark capital costs ranged from US$20 per person for boreholes and hand pumps to US$152 for larger water schemes. Benchmark recurrent costs ranged from US$3 to US$15 per person per year, but actual expenditures were substantially lower. Construction cost for equivalent latrines varies widely between settings (Hutton and others 2014). Comparison of alternative sanitation transportation and treatment technologies also provides important policy direction; in general, fecal sludge management is considerably cheaper than sewerage, as in Dakar, Senegal, where it was found to be five times cheaper (Dodane and others 2012). Extrapolating available data from one context to another carries risks. Therefore, simple costing tools and investment in evidence gathering are required so that cost estimates of specific locations can be made.[15]

Ideally, those who determine the costs of water supply and sanitation services would consider the externalities and the long-run cost of supply. One study provides an illustrative example of the full costs of water supply and sanitation (including opportunity costs and environmental costs) with the low costs, varying from a high of US$2.00 per cubic meter to a low of US$0.80 per cubic meter (table 9.5) (Whittington and others 2009).

From a policy perspective, the affordability and willingness to pay for those costs is a critical issue. A global review found that water supply costs as a proportion of household income are significantly higher for poorer populations (Smets 2014) and well above the benchmark of between 3 percent and 5 percent used by some governments and international organizations.

## Benefits

WASH services have a large array of welfare and development benefits. Table 9.6 classifies those benefits under health, convenience, social, educational, reuse, water access, and other.

Those benefits have been evaluated extensively, but few studies evaluate the benefits comprehensively. The most robust scientific studies, such as randomized or matched prospective cohort studies, have been conducted on health effects. But only few of those studies exist, and

economic variables are rarely captured. The majority of economic studies build models filled with data from a mixture of sources. Global studies assessing the economic benefits of improved water supply and sanitation include health economic benefits and convenience time savings (Hutton 2013; Whittington and others 2009). Country studies have also evaluated the value of health and time savings (Pattanayak and others 2010). Regional studies from Southeast Asia assess the water access, reuse, and tourism benefits of improved sanitation as a proportion of avoided damage costs (Hutton and others 2008, 2014).

Willingness-to-pay (WTP) studies have estimated the economic value of water quality improvements, but only very few studies use experimental methods (Null and others 2012). Other studies have assessed WTP to avoid health impacts (Guh and others 2008; Orgill and others 2013) and to receive piped water (Whittington and others 2002). A systematic review of those studies has shown that the economic value derived from the WTP for improved water quality is less than the cost of producing and distributing it (Null and others 2012). Social benefits have been assessed, but few have been expressed in money values except WTP studies, which tend to capture all benefits and make differentiating social from other benefits difficult.

Economic value is associated with river cleanup that includes improved management of municipal wastewater, as well as improved management of industrial discharge, agricultural runoff, and solid waste. The financial viability of WASH services has been expressed in terms of financial returns. The most comprehensive source of data is from projects of multilateral development banks that routinely conduct a financial assessment of WASH services before project approval and that, in some cases, report on the completion of project implementation.

**Table 9.5** Cost Estimates of Improved Water and Sanitation Services

*US$ per cubic meter*

| Cost component | Full cost | Minimal cost |
|---|---|---|
| Opportunity cost of raw water supply | 0.05 | 0.00 ("steal it") |
| Storage and transmission to treatment plant | 0.10 | 0.07 (minimum storage) |
| Treatment to drinking water standards | 0.10 | 0.04 (simple chlorination) |
| Distribution of water to households | 0.60 | 0.24 (PVC pipe) |
| Collection of wastewater from home and conveyance to treatment plant | 0.80 | 0.30 (condominial sewers) |
| Wastewater treatment | 0.30 | 0.15 (simple lagoon) |
| Damages associated with discharge of treated wastewater | 0.05 | 0.00 ("someone else's problem") |
| **Total** | **2.00** | **0.80** |

*Source:* Whittington and others 2009.

*Note:* PVC = polyvinyl chloride. Discount rate used is 6 percent. Using a 3 percent discount rate, the total cost is US$1.80 per cubic meter at full cost and US$0.70 per cubic meter at minimal cost.

**Table 9.6** Benefits of Improved Drinking Water Supply and Sanitation

| Benefit | Water | Sanitation |
|---|---|---|
| Health, burden of disease | • Averted cases of diarrheal disease<br>• Reduced malnutrition, enteropathy, and malnutrition-related conditions (stunting)<br>• Less dehydration from lack of access to water<br>• Less disaster-related health impacts | • Averted cases of diarrheal disease<br>• Averted cases of helminths, polio, and eye diseases<br>• Reduced malnutrition, enteropathy, and malnutrition-related conditions (stunting)<br>• Less dehydration from insufficient water intake because of poor latrine access<br>• Less disaster-related health impacts |
| Health, economic savings | • Costs related to diseases, such as health care, productivity losses, and premature mortality | • Costs related to diseases, such as health care, productivity losses, and premature mortality |
| Convenience time savings | • Saved travel and waiting time for water collection | • Saved travel and waiting time from having nearby private toilet |
| Educational benefits | • Improved educational levels because of higher school enrollment and attendance rates from school water<br>• Higher attendance and educational attainment because of improved health | • Improved educational levels because of higher school enrollment and attendance rates from school sanitation<br>• Higher attendance and educational attainment because of improved health |
| Social benefits | • Leisure and nonuse values of water resources and reduced effort of averted water hauling and gender impacts | • Safety, privacy, dignity, comfort, status, prestige, aesthetics, and gender effects |
| Water access benefits | • Pretreated water at lower costs for averted treatment costs for households | • Less pollution of water supply and hence reduced water treatment costs |
| Reuse | | • Soil conditioner and fertilizer<br>• Energy production<br>• Safe use of wastewater |
| Economic effects | • Incomes from more tourism and business investment<br>• Employment opportunity in water provision<br>• Rise in value of property | • Incomes from more tourism and business investment<br>• Employment opportunity in sanitation supply chain<br>• Rise in value of property |

*Sources:* Adapted from Hutton 2012; Hutton and others 2014.

## Intervention Efficiency: Cost-Benefit Analysis

The discussion of efficiency should distinguish between cost-benefit analysis, which uses a common money metric for all costs and benefits, and cost-effectiveness analysis, which compares interventions for one type of outcome. Reviewed cost-benefit studies are provided in annex 9C.

Efficiency studies can be conducted in two ways (Whittington and others 2009):

- By generating estimates of cost and benefit in specific sites or field studies for the purposes of either evaluating intervention performance or selecting a site for a future project (Kremer and others 2011)
- By using model costs and benefits for specific sites or larger jurisdictions, such as country or global level,

and best-available evidence from multiple sources (Hutton 2013; Whittington and others 2009)

Given the high costs and challenges associated with collecting all the cost and benefit data required for the first approach, it is common practice to combine site-specific values with data extrapolated from other sources (Hutton and others 2014). Table 9.7 shows the most recently available global studies that have modeled selected water supply and sanitation interventions. One important finding from these studies is that lower technology interventions have higher returns than more expensive networked options.

Global studies indicate the projected overall costs and benefits from intervention alternatives, but they are not particularly useful in guiding decisions on

**Table 9.7** Benefit-Cost Ratios from Global Studies

| Study and intervention | Benefit-cost ratio |
| --- | --- |
| *Whittington and others (2009): modeled approach*[a] | |
| Networked water and sewerage services | 0.65 |
| Deep borehole with public hand pump | 4.64 |
| Total sanitation campaign (South Asia) | 3.00 |
| *Household* water treatment (biosand filters) | 2.48 |
| *Hutton (2013): modeled approach*[b] | |
| Improved water supply (JMP definition) | 2.00 |
| Improved sanitation (JMP definition) | 5.50 |

*Sources:* Hutton 2013; Whittington and others 2009.
*Note:* All studies include the value associated with health and convenience time savings.
a. Ranges on each parameter value are then used to conduct Monte Carlo simulation that enables exploration of intervention performance in a range of different settings. Hence, even interventions with a benefit-cost ratio of 2.0 or more are expected to have a benefit-cost ratio of less than 1.0 under some runs of the model.
b. Estimates indicate global averages, and regional averages are available in the paper. A separate working paper provides results for each country (Hutton 2012).

which technology and service level to choose in specific settings. One randomized implementation study in India finds similar health costs between study arms. However, it finds statistically significant savings in time in the intervention group of US$7 per household (US$5 for water and US$2 for sanitation) during the dry season, or roughly 5 percent of monthly cash expenditures (Pattanayak and others 2010). A study from South Africa estimates a benefit-cost ratio of 3.1 for small-scale water schemes (Cameron and others 2011). A study from Indonesia compared three wastewater treatment interventions and finds limited economic rationale for the interventions (Prihandrijanti, Malisie, and Otterpohl 2008). However, a broader cost-benefit study at the river basin level estimated the benefits of cleaning up the Upper Citarum river in Indonesia exceeded costs by 2.3 times (Hutton and others 2013).

Targeting the poor could be justified; children from poorer households are at increased health risk because they live in communities with lower access to improved water and sanitation facilities. A study in Bangladesh, India, and Pakistan estimating the cost per episode for income quintiles shows that costs of an illness represent a higher proportion of income for lower quintiles (Rheingans and others 2012).

The cost efficiency of technologies depends on the local geological setting, population density, and number of households to be served. Large water distribution and sewerage systems may only be cost efficient if they serve large, dense populations. Providing water service on a smaller scale through either communal or in-compound wells or boreholes and onsite household sanitation may be a more appropriate and cost-efficient service level for sparsely populated areas (Ferro, Lentini, and Mercadier 2011).

### Intervention Efficiency: Cost-Effectiveness Analysis

The main outcomes used in cost-effectiveness studies are health and environmental outcomes. When used to compare programs in a sector, cost-effectiveness can be measured by program outcomes, such as the number of latrines constructed, the number of water connections installed, or the percentage of beneficiaries changing behavior. For water supply interventions, health cost-effectiveness studies have been conducted (see annex 9C). Studies focus on improved water supply according to the JMP definition and point-of-use treatment by households or schools. A global study compares water supply interventions at the regional level (Clasen and others 2007).

Figure 9.6 shows the cost per healthy life-year (HLY) gained for four interventions in two regions. It shows that the selected interventions vary by a factor of approximately 2.5 between the most cost-effective (chlorination) and the least cost-effective (ceramic filter). However, all interventions have a cost per HLY that is below the GDP of countries in these regions, thereby indicating a cost-effective use of health resources. Another global study found the incremental costs averted of adding point-of-use water disinfection on top of improved water supply costs resulted in a cost per DALY averted of less than US$25 in Sub-Saharan Africa, of US$63 in India and Bangladesh, and of less than US$210 in South-East Asia and the Western Pacific (Haller, Hutton, and Bartram 2007).

Fewer studies have conducted health cost-effectiveness analyses of sanitation and hygiene interventions. Two global studies by the WHO and World Bank examine the cost-effectiveness of water supply and sanitation combined (Günther and Fink 2011; Haller, Hutton, and Bartram 2007). Using regions defined by epidemiological strata, WHO estimates that the cost in countries with high child and high adult mortality is less than US$530 per DALY averted in the Eastern Mediterranean and Middle East, US$650 in Sub-Saharan Africa, US$1,400 in South and South-East Asia, and US$2,800 in Latin America and the Caribbean. A World Bank study on child mortality reduction estimates the average cost per life year saved in Sub-Saharan African countries is US$1,104 for basic improved water and sanitation

**Figure 9.6** Cost Per HLY Gained from Four Water Supply and Water Quality Interventions in Two World Subregions, US$, 2005

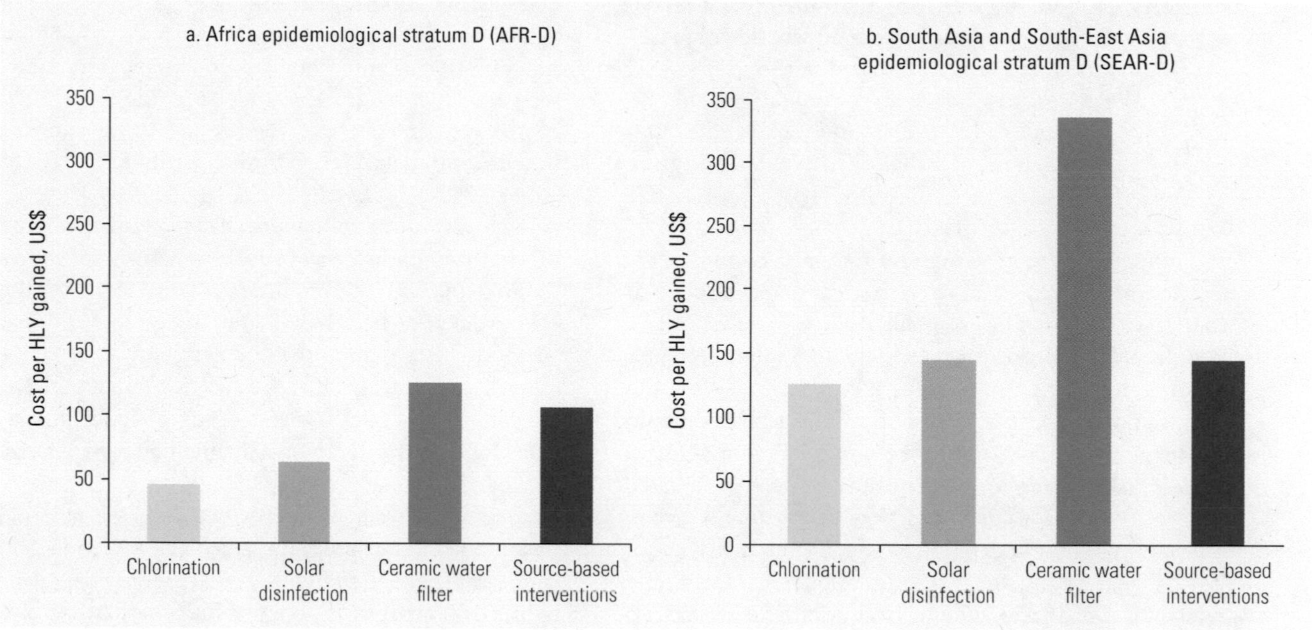

*Source:* Clasen and others 2007.

*Note:* AFR-D = African Region–high child, high adult mortality countries; HLY = healthy life-year; SEAR-D = South-East Asian Region–high child, high adult mortality countries. AFR-D and SEAR-D are part of the World Health Organization's epidemiological subregions.

and is US$995 for privately piped water and flush toilets (Günther and Fink 2011).

In country studies in South-East Asia, the cost per DALY averted of basic sanitation is less than US$1,100 in selected rural areas of Cambodia, China, Indonesia, the Lao People's Democratic Republic, and Vietnam; the exception is in the Philippines, where it is US$2,500 (Hutton and others 2014). Few recent country-specific studies are available on hygiene interventions; one study from Burkina Faso estimates a cost of US$51 per death averted for health education to mothers (Borghi and others 2002).

Sustainability of water supply, sanitation, and hygiene is covered in annex 9D; financing is covered in annex 9E.

## CONCLUSIONS

Although global deaths from diarrhea have declined significantly over the past 20 years, poor water supply, sanitation, and hygiene are still responsible for a significant disease burden. An estimated 842,000 global deaths in 2012 were due to diarrhea caused by poor WASH. Other less well-quantified but important long-term health consequences of poor WASH, such as helminths and enteric dysfunction, remain. Those diseases affect children's nutritional status, thereby inhibiting growth

and mental development. Overall, the health impacts of poor WASH lead to economic consequences of several percent of GDP and continue to significantly affect quality of life and the environment. Furthermore, water stress is a growing phenomenon that will affect at least 2.8 billion people in 48 countries by 2025. Climatic factors are harder to control, but water scarcity can be mitigated by changing water use patterns and reducing pollution of surface waters.

Important progress has been made in achieving the MDG global water and sanitation targets. In September 2015, new global targets for universal access to safe WASH were adopted. At the current rates of progress and using current indicators, achieving those targets will take at least 20 years for water supply and 60 years for sanitation (WHO and UNICEF 2014). Covering the poor and marginalized populations will continue to be a challenge; the remaining unserved populations are likely to be harder to reach as universal access is approached. The service level benchmark of targeting safely managed services will require better policy and regulatory frameworks and more resources. Indeed, as environmental consequences intensify and populations demand a higher quality of service, a higher target for service level will be increasingly required. This demand will raise questions about priorities; countries will face a trade-off between (1) dedicating policy space and spending public subsidies to move populations that are already served higher up the water and sanitation ladder and (2) reaching populations that are not served with basic WASH services. Each country will have its unique set of challenges. The human right to drinking water and sanitation can serve as a reminder that priority should be given to ensuring at least a minimum level of affordable WASH service for all citizens.

Populations are growing and moving, economies are developing and becoming richer, and the climate is changing. Each one has its challenges and opportunities. Population migration to greenfield sites offers a chance of implementing new and appropriate technologies, and selection of cost-effective and affordable technologies in urban planning is essential. Economic growth leads to greater tax revenues for local governments and increased ability to upgrade infrastructure and expand urban renewal. Climate change challenges the delivery of WASH services by affecting rainfall patterns, freshwater availability, and frequency of heat events, and it exacerbates health risks. However, this new threat, when taken seriously, can be an opportunity to overhaul outdated policies and technologies. Furthermore, as nutrient sources for chemical fertilizer become scarcer, price increases will force suppliers to seek alternatives; the price of composted sludge is expected to increase, thereby attracting investments. New research, data, and technologies are increasingly available to present new possibilities for addressing entrenched problems in the WASH sector.

The following research priorities are recommended for immediate attention:

- To adequately address equity considerations in the SDG era, there is a need to understand where poor people live and what their levels of access are. Disaggregated data on the underserved— including slum populations, ethnic groups, women, elderly, and persons with disabilities—can support prioritization. Greater focus is needed on how to increase access in the lagging regions of South Asia and Africa, where a large proportion of the unserved live. At the country level, policy and financial incentives need to be aligned and the economic arguments made for allocating resources to WASH services.
- More evidence is needed to support the emerging understanding of the wider health effects of water, sanitation, and hygiene. Multisectoral approaches will become more important as the complementarities among WASH, health, and nutrition are better understood. Further, rigorously designed and controlled studies are needed to quantify these benefits,

including the measurement of cost-effectiveness to guide policy and program design.
- The social welfare consequences of poor WASH are not well documented but are potentially very large. In particular, a greater understanding is needed of the gender effects of inadequate WASH and of how improved WASH services contribute to gender equality.
- A large part of the remaining challenge of improving access to sanitation and hygiene is behavioral rather than technical. However, little evidence exists on the effectiveness of behavior change using conventional methods at scale or on the transferability of behavior change interventions that are successful in a particular context. A better understanding of habit formation and what leads to sustainable behavior change is needed.
- Innovative delivery platforms that leverage national poverty reduction programs, such as CCT and CDD programs, have the potential to achieve wide coverage at little marginal cost. Such approaches can also provide the methodology and data sources to support targeting areas of poverty in WASH services.
- A better understanding is needed on which WASH interventions work in slum areas and low-income neighborhoods and under what conditions the interventions work.
- A greater understanding is needed of how output-based incentives can be used to improve WASH service delivery and to lead to greater sustainability of services.
- Innovations in subsidies and microfinance are needed to ensure that the poor gain access to improved sanitation. Despite greater availability and lower cost of sanitation goods and services, some people remain too poor to afford adequate water supply and sanitation. Such populations should be identified to receive hardware and financial subsidies.

## ANNEXES

The annexes to this chapter are as follows. They are available at http://www.dcp-3.org/environment.

- Annex 9A. Overview of Studies Presenting Damage Costs of Poor Water, Sanitation, and Hygiene at the National Level
- Annex 9B. Effectiveness of Enabling Environments
- Annex 9C. Cost-Effectiveness and Cost-Benefit Studies on Water, Sanitation, and Hygiene
- Annex 9D. Intervention Sustainability
- Annex 9E. Intervention Financing

## NOTES

World Bank Income Classifications as of July 2014 are as follows, based on estimates of gross national income (GNI) per capita for 2013:

- Low-income countries (LICs) = US$1,045 or less
- Middle-income countries (MICs) are subdivided:
  a) lower-middle-income = US$1,046 to US$4,125
  b) upper-middle-income (UMICs) = US$4,126 to US$12,745
- High-income countries (HICs) = US$12,746 or more.

1. United Nations Human Rights Council, Resolution 18/1, "The Human Right to Safe Drinking Water and Sanitation," adopted September 28, 2011, http://www .worldwatercouncil.org/fileadmin/wwc/Right_to_Water /Human_Rights_Council_Resolution_cotobre_2011.pdf.
2. United Nations Human Rights Council, Resolution 18/1.
3. Whereas no academic literature is available with such examples, national surveys (such as the Demographic and Health Survey or the Multiple Indicator Cluster Survey) show that a higher proportion of households practice unsafe management of children's feces as compared with overall household unimproved sanitation practices.
4. JMP reports for country data and additional breakdowns are available at http://www.wssinfo.org.
5. Characterized by villous atrophy, crypt hyperplasia, increased permeability, inflammatory cell infiltrate, and modest malabsorption.
6. The hidden flow of water if food or other commodities that require water to be produced are traded from one place to another.
7. An odds ratio (OR) is a measure of association between an exposure and an outcome. The OR represents the odds that an outcome will occur given a particular exposure, compared with the odds of the outcome occurring in the absence of that exposure.
8. For more on the Cochrane Library, see http://www .thecochranelibrary.com.
9. For more information on CLTS, see http://www .communityledtotalsanitation.org/page/clts-approach and http://cltsfoundation.org/clts-map.html.
10. The impact evaluation in Senegal was compromised because of contamination of the treatment group with the handwashing with soap intervention group.
11. Examples of results-based approaches include the following: output-based aid (OBA), results-based financing (RBF), pay-for-performance (P4P), program for results (PforR), and conditional-cash transfer (CCT).
12. Accessed March 31, 2014, through the OBA website, https:// www.gpoba.org.
13. *Basic water:* percentage of population using a protected community source or piped water with a total collection time of 30 minutes or less for a round-trip, including queuing (same as JMP improved definition except time criteria has been introduced). *Basic sanitation:* percentage of population using a basic private sanitation facility (same as JMP improved definition). *Basic hygiene:* percentage of population with handwashing facilities with soap and water at home. *Safely managed water:* percentage of population using safely managed drinking water services. Corresponds to population using an improved drinking water source located on the premises, available when needed, and free of fecal and priority chemical contamination. *Safely managed sanitation:* percentage of population using safely managed sanitation services. Includes safe onsite isolation, extraction, conveyance, treatment and disposal, or reuse.
14. For information about the OECD's methodology and FEASIBLE computer model, see http://www.oecd.org/env /outreach/methodologyandfeasiblecomputermodel.htm (accessed November 11, 2015).
15. For example, the IRC International Water and Sanitation Center has developed the WASHCost Calculator (www .ircwash.org/washcost), whereas the World Bank's Economics of Sanitation Initiative has developed an economic assessment toolkit under the Economics of Sanitation Initiative (http://www.wsp.org/esi).

## REFERENCES

Adukia, A. 2014. "Sanitation and Education." PhD thesis, Harvard University, Cambridge, MA.

Ahern, M., R. Kovats, P. Wilkinson, R. Few, and F. Matthies. 2005. "Global Health Impacts of Floods: Epidemiologic Evidence." *Epidemiologic Reviews* 27 (1): 36–46.

Ali, M., A. Nelson, A. Lopez, D. Sack. 2015. "Updated Global Burden of Cholera in Endemic Countries." *PLoS Neglected Tropical Diseases* 9 (6). doi:10.1371/journal .pntd.0003832.

Andres, L., B. Briceno, C. Chase, and J. A. Echenique. 2014. "Sanitation and Externalities: Evidence from Early Childhood Health in Rural India." Policy Research Working Paper 6737, World Bank, Washington, DC.

Atia, A., and A. Buchman. 2009. "Oral Rehydration Solutions in Non-Cholera Diarrhea: A Review." *American Journal of Gastroenterology* 104 (10): 2596–604.

Baker, J. L., ed. 2009. *Opportunities and Challenges for Small Scale Private Service Providers in Electricity and Water Supply: Evidence from Bangladesh, Cambodia, Kenya and the Philippines.* Washington, DC: World Bank and the Public-Private Infrastructure Advisory Facility.

Benova, L., O. Cumming, and O. Campbell. 2014. "Systematic Review and Meta-Analysis: Association between Water and Sanitation Environment and Maternal Mortality." *Tropical Medicine and International Health* 19 (4): 368–87.

Biran, A., M. Jenkins, P. Dabrase, and I. Bhagwat. 2011. "Patterns and Determinants of Communal Latrine Usage in Urban Poverty Pockets in Bhopal, India." *Tropical Medicine and International Health* 16 (7): 854–62.

Biran, A., T. Rabie, W. Schmidt, S. Juvekar, S. Hirve, and others. 2008. "Comparing the Performance of Indicators of Hand-Washing Practices in Rural Indian Households." *Tropical Medicine and International Health* 13 (2): 278–85.

Black, R., L. Allen, Z. Bhutta, L. Caulfield, M. de Onis, and others. 2008. "Maternal and Child Undernutrition: Global and Regional Exposures and Health Consequences." *The Lancet* 371 (9608): 243–60.

Black, R., C. Victora, S. Walker, Z. Bhutta, P. Christian, and others. 2013. "Maternal and Child Undernutrition and Overweight in Low-Income and Middle-Income Countries." *The Lancet* 382 (9890): 427–51.

Blackett, I., P. Hawkins, and C. Heymans. 2014. "The Missing Link in Sanitation Service Delivery: A Review of Fecal Sludge Management in 12 Cities." Water and Sanitation Program Research Brief, World Bank, Washington, DC.

Blencowe, H., S. Cousens, L. Mullany, A. Lee, K. Kerber, and others. 2011. "Clean Birth and Postnatal Care Practices to Reduce Neonatal Deaths from Sepsis and Tetanus: A Systematic Review and Delphi Estimation of Mortality Effect." *BMC Public Health* 11 (Suppl 3): S11.

Borghi, J., L. Guinness, J. Ouedraogo, and V. Curtis. 2002. "Is Hygiene Promotion Cost-Effective? A Case Study in Burkina Faso." *Tropical Medicine and International Health* 7 (11): 960–69.

Briceno, B., A. Coville, and S. Martinez. 2014. "Promoting Handwashing and Sanitation: A Crossover Randomized Experiment in Rural Tanzania." Working Paper, Water and Sanitation Program, World Bank, Washington DC.

Brooker, S., A. Clements, and D. Bundy. 2006. "Global Epidemiology, Ecology and Control of Soil-Transmitted Helminth Infections." *Advances in Parasitology* 62: 221–61.

Brown, J., S. Cairncross, and J. Ensink. 2013. "Water, Sanitation, Hygiene and Enteric Infections in Children." *Archives of Disease in Childhood* 12. doi:10.1136 /archdischild-2011-301528.

Burr, P., and C. Fonseca. 2013. "Applying a Life-Cycle Costs Approach to Water: Costs and Service Levels in Rural and Small Town Areas in Andhra Pradesh (India), Burkina Faso, Ghana and Mozambique." Working Paper 8, IRC International Water and Sanitation Centre, The Hague, the Netherlands.

Cairncross, S. 2004. "The Case for Marketing Sanitation." Field note, Water and Sanitation Program, World Bank, Washington, DC.

Cameron, J., P. Jagals, P. Hunter, S. Pedley, and K. Pond. 2011. "Economic Assessments of Small-Scale Drinking-Water Interventions in Pursuit of MDG Target 7C." *Science of the Total Environment* 410–411: 8–15.

Cameron, L., M. Shah, and S. Olivia. 2013. "Impact Evaluation of a Large-Scale Rural Sanitation Project in Indonesia." Policy Research Working Paper 6360, World Bank, Washington, DC.

Chase, C., and Q.-T. Do. 2012. "Handwashing Behavior Change at Scale: Evidence from a Randomized Evaluation in Vietnam." Policy Research Working Paper 6207, World Bank, Washington, DC.

Checkley, W., G. Buckley, R. Gilman, A. Assis, R. Guerrant, and others. 2008. "Multi-Country Analysis of the Effects of Diarrhoea on Childhood Stunting." *International Journal of Epidemiology* 37 (4): 816–30.

Clasen, T., K. Alexander, D. Sinclair, S. Boisson, R. Peletz, and others. 2005. "Interventions To Improve Water Quality for Preventing Diarrhoea (Review). *The Cochrane Library 2005* (10).

Clasen, T., L. Haller, D. Walker, J. Bartram, and S. Cairncross. 2007. "Cost-Effectiveness of Water Quality Interventions for Preventing Diarrhoeal Disease in Developing Countries." *Journal of Water and Health* 5 (4): 599–608.

Clasen, T., S. Boisson, P. Routray, B. Torondel, M. Bell, and others. 2014. "Effectiveness of a Rural Sanitation Programme on Diarrhoea, Soil-Transmitted Helminth Infection, and Child Malnutrition in Odisha, India: A Cluster-Randomised Trial." *The Lancet Global Health* 2 (11): e645–53.

Corcoran, E., C. Nellemann, E. Baker, R. Bos, D. Osborn, and others. 2011. "Sick Water? The Central Role of Wastewater Management in Sustainable Development." A Rapid Response Assessment, UN HABITAT, GRID-Arendal, United Nations Environment Programme, Arendal, Norway.

Curtis, V., and S. Cairncross. 2003. "Effect of Washing Hands with Soap on Diarrhoea Risk in the Community: A Systematic Review." *The Lancet Infectious Diseases* 3 (5): 275–81.

Curtis, V., B. Kanki, S. Cousens, I. Diallo, A. Kpozehouen, and others. 2001. "Evidence of Behaviour Change following a Hygiene Promotion Programme in Burkina Faso." *Bulletin of the World Health Organization* 79 (6): 518–27.

Dangour, A., L. Watson, O. Cumming, S. Boisson, Y. Che, and others. 2013. "Interventions to Improve Water Quality and Supply, Sanitation and Hygiene Practices, and Their Effects on the Nutritional Status of Children." *Cochrane Database of Systematic Reviews* 8: CD009382. doi:10.1002/14651858 .CD009382.pub2.

Devoto, F., E. Duflo, P. Dupas, W. Pariente, and V. Pons. 2011. "Happiness on Tap: Piped Water Adoption in Urban Morocco." National Bureau of Economic Research (NBER) Working Paper No. 16933, NBER, Cambridge, MA.

Dodane, P.-H., M. Mbéguéré, O. Sow, and L. Strande. 2012. "Capital and Operating Costs of Full-Scale Fecal Sludge Management and Wastewater Treatment Systems in Dakar, Senegal." *Environmental Science and Technology* 46 (7): 3705–11.

Dutto, S. M., M. Lopez Abbate, F. Biancalana, A. Berasategui, and M. Hoffmeyer. 2012. "The Impact of Sewage on Environmental Quality and the Mesozooplankton Community in a Highly Eutrophic Estuary in Argentina." *ICES Journal of Marine Science* 69 (3): 399–409.

Esrey, S. A. 1996. "Water, Waste, and Well-Being: A Multicountry Study." *American Journal of Epidemiology* 143 (6): 608–23.

Esrey, S. A., J. B. Potash, L. Roberts, and C. Shiff. 1991. "Effects of Improved Water Supply and Sanitation on Ascariasis, Diarrhoea, Dracunculiasis, Hookworm Infection, Schistosomiasis, and Trachoma." *Bulletin of the World Health Organization* 69 (5): 609–21.

Ferro, G., E. Lentini, and A. Mercadier. 2011. "Economies of Scale in the Water Sector: A Survey of the Empirical Literature." *Journal of Water, Sanitation and Hygiene for Development* 1 (3): 179–93.

Fisher, J. 2006. "For Her It's the Big Issue: Putting Women at the Centre of Water Supply, Sanitation and Hygiene." Evidence Report, Water Supply and Sanitation Collaborative Council, Geneva.

Fishman, S., L. Caulfield, M. de Onis, M. Blössner, A. Hyder, and others. 2004. "Childhood and Maternal Underweight." In volume 1 of *Comparative Quantification of Health Risks: Global and Regional Burden of Disease due to Selected Major Risk Factors*, edited by M. Ezzati, A. D. Lopez, A. Rodgers, and C. J. L. Murray. Geneva: WHO.

Freeman, M., M. Stocks, O. Cumming, A. Jeandron, J. Higgins, and others. 2014. "Hygiene and Health: Systematic Review of Handwashing Practices Worldwide and Update of Health Effects." *Tropical Medicine and International Health* 19 (8): 906–16.

Galiani, S., P. Gertler, N. Ajzenman, and A. Orsola-Vidal. 2015. "Promoting Handwashing Behavior: The Effects of Large-scale Community and School-level Interventions." *Health Economics* (October 12). doi:10.1002/hec.3273.

Guerrant, R., M. DeBoer, S. Moore, R. Scharf, and A. Lima. 2013. "The Impoverished Gut—A Triple Burden of Diarrhoea, Stunting and Chronic Disease." *Nature Reviews Gastroenterology and Hepatology* 10 (4): 220–29.

Guerrant, R., R. Oriá, S. Moore, M. Oriá, and A. Lima. 2008. "Malnutrition as an Enteric Infectious Disease with Long-Term Effects on Child Development." *Nutrition Reviews* 66 (9): 487–505.

Guh, S., C. Xingbao, C. Poulos, Z. Qi, C. Jianwen, and others. 2008. "Comparison of Cost-of-Illness with Willingness-to-Pay Estimates to Avoid Shigellosis: Evidence from China." *Health Policy and Planning* 23 (2): 125–36.

Günther, I., and G. Fink. 2011. "Water and Sanitation to Reduce Child Mortality: The Impact and Cost of Water and Sanitation Infrastructure." Policy Research Working Paper 5618, World Bank, Washington, DC.

Hales, S., S. Kovats, S. Lloyd, and D. Campbell-Lendrum, eds. 2014. *Quantitative Risk Assessment of the Effects of Climate Change on Selected Causes of Death, 2030s and 2050s.* Geneva: WHO.

Haller, L., G. Hutton, and J. Bartram. 2007. "Estimating the Costs and Health Benefits of Water and Sanitation Improvements at Global Level." *Journal of Water and Health* 5 (4): 467–80.

Hammer, J., and D. Spears. 2013. "Village Sanitation and Children's Human Capital Evidence from a Randomized Experiment by the Maharashtra Government." Policy Research Working Paper 5580, World Bank, Washington, DC.

Hotez, P., D. Bundy, K. Beegle, S. Brooker, L. Drake, and others. 2006. "Helminth Infections: Soil-Transmitted Helminth Infections and Schistosomiasis." In *Disease Control Priorities in Developing Countries*, second edition, edited by D. Jamison, J. Breman, A. Measham, G. Alleyne, M. Claeson, D. Evans, P. Jha, A. Mills, and P. Musgrove. Washington, DC: Oxford University Press and World Bank.

Howard, G., and J. Bartram. 2003. "Domestic Water Quantity, Service Level and Health." Report, WHO/SDE/WSH/03.02, World Health Organization, Geneva.

Humphrey, J. 2009. "Child Undernutrition, Tropical Enteropathy, Toilets, and Handwashing." *The Lancet* 374 (9694): 1032–35.

Hunter, P. R., D. Zmirou-Navier, and P. Hartemann. 2009. "Estimating the Impact on Health of Poor Reliability of Drinking Water Interventions in Developing Countries." *Science of the Total Environment* 407 (8): 2621–24.

Hutton, G. 2012. "Global Costs and Benefits of Drinking-Water Supply and Sanitation Interventions to Reach the MDG Target and Universal Coverage." Report, WHO/HSE/WSH/12.01, World Health Organization, Geneva.

———. 2013. "Global Costs and Benefits of Reaching Universal Coverage of Sanitation and Drinking-Water Supply." *Journal of Water and Health* 11 (1): 1–12.

Hutton, G., S. Kerstens, A. van Nes, and I. Firmansyah. 2013. "Downstream Impacts of Water Pollution in the Upper Citarum River, West Java, Indonesia: Economic Assessment of Interventions to Improve Water Quality." Water and Sanitation Program Technical Paper, World Bank, Washington, DC.

Hutton, G., U. Rodriguez, L. Napitupulu, P. Thang, and P. Kov. 2008. *Economic Impacts of Sanitation in Southeast Asia.* Water and Sanitation Program. Washington, DC: World Bank.

Hutton, G., U.-P. Rodriguez, A. Winara, V. Nguyen, P. Kov, and others. 2014. "Economic Efficiency of Sanitation Interventions in Southeast Asia." *Journal of Water, Sanitation and Hygiene in Development* 4 (1): 23–36.

Hutton, G., and M. Varughese. 2016. *The Costs of Meeting the 2030 Sustainable Development Goal Targets on Drinking Water, Sanitation, and Hygiene.* Water and Sanitation Program. Washington, DC: World Bank.

IBNET (International Benchmarking Network for Water and Sanitation Utilities). 2014. Database. IBNET, World Bank Water and Sanitation Program, Washington, DC. https://www.ib-net.org/.

Ilahi, N., and F. Grimard. 2000. "Public Infrastructure and Private Costs: Water Supply and Time Allocation of Women in Rural Pakistan." *Economic Development and Cultural Change* 49 (1): 45–75.

Jafari, N., A. Shahsanai, M. Memarzadeh, and A. Loghmani. 2011. "Prevention of Communicable Diseases after Disaster: A Review." *Journal of Research in Medical Sciences* 16 (7): 956–62.

Jasper, C., T.-T. Le, and J. Bartram. 2012. "Water and Sanitation in Schools: a Systematic Review of the Health and Educational Outcomes." *International Journal of Environmental Research Public Health* 9 (8): 2772–87.

Jenkins, M., and V. Curtis. 2005. "Achieving the 'Good Life': Why Some People Want Latrines in Rural Benin." *Social Science and Medicine* 61 (11): 2446–59.

Jenkins, M., and B. Scott. 2007. "Behavioral Indicators of Household Decision-Making and Demand for Sanitation and Potential Gains from Social Marketing in Ghana." *Social Science and Medicine* 64 (12): 2427–42.

Koolwal, G., and D. Van de Walle. 2013. "Access to Water, Women's Work, and Child Outcomes." *Economic Development and Cultural Change* 61 (2): 369–405.

Kotloff, K., J. Nataro, W. Blackwelder, D. Nasrin, T. Farag, and others. 2013. "Burden and Aetiology of Diarrhoeal Disease in Infants and Young Children in Developing Countries (The Global Enteric Multicenter Study, GEMS): A Prospective, Case-Control Study." *The Lancet* 382 (9888): 209–22.

Kremer, M., J. Leino, E. Miguel, and A. Zwane. 2011. "Spring Cleaning: A Randomized Evaluation of Source Water Quality Improvement." *Quarterly Journal of Economics* 126 (1): 145–205.

Lanata, C., C. Fischer-Walker, A. Olascoaga, C. Torres, M. Aryee, and others. 2013. "Global Causes of Diarrheal Disease Mortality in Children <5 Years of Age: A Systematic Review." *PLoS One* 8 (9): e72788.

Lim, S., T. Vos, A. Flaxman, G. Danaei, K. Shibuya, and others. 2012. "A Comparative Risk Assessment of Burden of Disease and Injury Attributable to 67 risk factors and Risk Factor Clusters in 21 Regions, 1990–2010: A Systematic Analysis for the Global Burden of Disease Study 2010." *The Lancet* 380 (9859): 2224–60.

Lin, A., B. Arnold, S. Afreen, R. Goto, T. Mohammad Nurul Huda, and others. 2013. "Household Environmental Conditions Are Associated with Enteropathy and Impaired Growth in Rural Bangladesh." *American Journal of Tropical Medicine and Hygiene* 89 (1): 130–37.

Loevensohn, M., L. Mehta, K. Cuming, A. Nicol, O. Cumming, and others. 2015. "The Cost of a Knowledge Silo: A Systematic Re-Review of Water, Sanitation and Hygiene Interventions." *Health Policy and Planning* 30 (5): 660–74.

Lokshin, M., and R. Yemtsov. 2005. "Has Rural Infrastructure Rehabilitation in Georgia Helped the Poor?" *World Bank Economic Review* 19 (2): 311–33.

Lozano, R., M. Naghavi, K. Foreman, S. Lim, and K. Shibuya. 2010. "Global and Regional Mortality from 235 Causes of Death for 20 Age Groups in 1990 and 2010: A Systematic Analysis for the Global Burden of Disease Study 2010." *The Lancet* 380 (9859): 2095–128.

Moriarty, P., C. Batchelor, C. Fonseca, A. Klutse, A. Naafs, and others. 2010. "Ladders for Assessing and Costing Water Service Delivery." WASHCost Working Paper 2, IRC International Water and Sanitation Centre, The Hague, the Netherlands.

Mumssen, Y., L. Johannes, and G. Kumar. 2010. *Output-Based Aid: Lessons Learned and Best Practices.* Washington, DC: World Bank.

Murcott, S. 2012. *Arsenic Contamination in the World: An International Sourcebook 2012.* London: IWA Publishing.

Naujokas, M. F., B. Anderson, H. Ahsan, H. V. Aposhian, J. Graziano, and others. 2013. "The Broad Scope of Health Effects from Chronic Arsenic Exposure: Update on a Worldwide Public Health Problem." *Environmental Health Perspectives* 121 (3): 295–302.

Nicholson, J. A., M. Naeeni, M. Hoptroff, J. R. Matheson, A. J. Roberts, and others. 2013. "An Investigation of the Effects of a Hand Washing Intervention on Health Outcomes and School Absence Using a Randomised Trial in Indian Urban Communities." *Tropical Medicine and International Health* 19 (3): 284–92.

Norman, G., S. Pedley, and B. Takkouche. 2010. "Effects of Sewerage on Diarrhoea and Enteric Infections: A Systematic Review and Meta-Analysis." *The Lancet Infectious Diseases* 10: 536–44.

Null, C., J. G. Hombrado, R. Meeks, M. Edward, and A. P. Zwane. 2012. "Willingness to Pay for Cleaner Water in Less Developed Countries: Systematic Review of Experimental Evidence." Systematic Review No. 6, International Initiative for Impact Evaluation, London.

OECD (Organisation for Economic Co-operation and Development). 2011. "Meeting the Challenge of Financing Water and Sanitation: Tools and Approaches." OECD, Paris.

Olajuyigbe, A. 2010. "Some Factors Impacting on Quantity of Water Used by Households in a Rapidly Urbanizing State Capital in South Western Nigeria." *Journal of Sustainable Development in Africa* 12 (2): 321–37.

Onda, K., J. LoBuglio, and J. Bartram. 2012. "Global Access to Safe Water: Accounting for Water Quality and the Resulting Impact on MDG progress." *International Journal of Environmental Research and Public Health* 9 (3): 880–94.

Orgill, J., A. Shaheed, J. Brown, and M. Jeuland. 2013. "Water Quality Perceptions and Willingness to Pay for Clean Water in Peri-Urban Cambodian Communities." *Journal of Water and Health* 11 (3): 489–506.

Oster, E., and R. Thornton. 2011. "Menstruation, Sanitary Products, and School Attendance: Evidence from a Randomized Evaluation." *American Economic Journal: Applied Economics* 3 (1): 91–100.

Özaltin, E., K. Hill, and S. V. Subramanian. 2010. "Association of Maternal Stature with Offspring Mortality, Underweight, and Stunting in Low- to Middle-Income Countries." *Journal of the American Medical Association* 303 (15): 1507–16.

Patil, S., B. Arnold, A. Salvatore, B. Briceno, S. Ganguly, and others. 2014. "The Effect of India's Total Sanitation Campaign on Defecation Behaviors and Child Health in Rural Madhya Pradesh: A Cluster Randomized Controlled Trial." *PLoS Medicine* 11 (8). doi:10.1371/journal.pmed.1001709.

Pattanayak, S., C. Poulos, J. Yang, and S. Patil. 2010. "How Valuable Are Environmental Health Interventions? Evaluation of Water and Sanitation Programmes in India." *Bulletin of the World Health Organization* 88 (7): 535–42.

Peal, A., B. Evans, and C. van der Voorden. 2010. *Hygiene and Sanitation Software: An Overview of Approaches.* Geneva: Water Supply and Sanitation Collaborative Council.

Petri, W., M. Miller, H. Binder, M. Levine, R. Dillingham, and others. 2008. "Enteric Infections, Diarrhea, and Their Impact on Function and Development." *Journal of Clinical Investigation* 118 (4): 1277–90.

Pickering, A. J., and J. Davis. 2012. "Freshwater Availability and Water Fetching Distance Affect Child Health in Sub-Saharan Africa." *Environmental Science and Technology* 46 (4): 2391–97.

Pickering, A. J., H. Djebbari, C. Lopez, M. Coulibaly, and M. L. Alzua. 2015. "Effect of a Community-Led Sanitation Intervention on Child Diarrhoea and Child Growth in Rural Mali: A Cluster-Randomised Controlled Trial." *The Lancet Global Health* 3 (5): E701–11.

Popkin, B., K. D'Anci, and I. Rosenberg. 2010. "Water, Hydration and Health." *Nutrition Reviews* 68 (8): 439–58.

Potter, A., A. Klutse, M. Snehalatha, C. Batchelor, A. Uandela, and others. 2010. "Assessing Sanitation Service Levels." WASHCost Working Paper 3, IRC International Water and Sanitation Centre, the Hague, the Netherlands.

Prihandrijanti, M., A. Malisie, and R. Otterpohl. 2008. "Cost-Benefit Analysis for Centralized and Decentralized Wastewater Treatment System (Case Study in Surabaya, Indonesia)." In *Efficient Management of Wastewater: Its Treatment and Reuse in Water-Scarce Countries*, edited by I. Al Baz, R. Otterpohl, and C. Wendland, 259–68. Berlin-Heidelberg: Springer.

Prüss-Üstün, A., J. Bartram, T. Clasen, J. Colford, O. Cumming, and others. 2014. "Burden of Diarrheal Disease from Inadequate Water, Sanitation and Hygiene in Low- and Middle-Income Countries: A Retrospective Analysis of Data from 145 Countries." *Tropical Medicine and International Health* 19 (8): 894–905.

Prüss-Üstün, A., and C. Corvalan. 2006. *Preventing Disease through Healthy Environments: Towards an Estimate of the Environmental Burden of Disease.* Geneva: World Health Organization.

———. 2007. "How Much Disease Burden Can Be Prevented by Environmental Interventions?" *Epidemiology* 18 (1): 167–78.

Pullan, R., J. Smith, R. Jasrasaria, and S. Brooker. 2014. "Global Numbers of Infection and Disease Burden of Soil Transmitted Helminth Infections in 2010." *Parasites and Vectors* 7 (37). doi:10.1186/1756-3305-7-37.

Rabalais, N. N., and R. E. Turner, eds. 2013. *Coastal Hypoxia: Consequences for Living Resources and Ecosystems.* Coastal and Estuarine Studies 58. Washington, DC: American Geophysical Union.

Rabie, T., and V. Curtis. 2006. "Handwashing and Risk of Respiratory Infections: A Quantitative Systematic Review." *Tropical Medicine and International Health* 11 (3): 258–67.

Ram, P. 2013. "Practical Guidance for Measuring Handwashing Behavior." Water and Sanitation Program Technical Paper, World Bank, Washington, DC.

Rhee, V., L. Mullany, S. Khatry, J. Katz, S. LeClerq, and others. 2008. "Maternal and Birth Attendant Hand Washing and Neonatal Mortality in Southern Nepal." *Archives of Pediatric and Adolescent Medicine* 162 (7): 603–08.

Rheingans, R., M. Kukla, A. Faruque, D. Sur, A. Zaidi, and others. 2012. "Determinants of Household Costs Associated with Childhood Diarrhea in Three South Asian Settings." *Clinical Infectious Diseases* 55 (Suppl 4): S327–35.

Roaf, V., A. Khalfan, and M. Langford. 2005. "Monitoring Implementation of the Right to Water: A Framework for Developing Indicators." Global Issue Paper No. 14, Heinrich Böll Foundation, Berlin.

Sadoff, C. W., J. W. Hall, D. Grey, J. C. J. H. Aerts, M. Ait-Kadi, and others. 2015. *Securing Water, Sustaining Growth: Report of the GWP/OECD Task Force on Water Security and Sustainable Growth.* Oxford, U.K.: University of Oxford.

Salazar-Lindo, E., S. Allen, D. Brewster, E. Elliott, A. Fasano, and others. 2004. "Intestinal Infections and Environmental Enteropathy: Working Group Report of the Second World Congress of Pediatric Gastroenterology, Hepatology, and Nutrition." *Journal of Pediatric Gastroenterology and Nutrition* 39 (Suppl 2): S662–69.

Schlosser, C. A., K. Strzepek, X. Gao, A. Gueneau, C. Fant, and others. 2014. "The Future of Global Water Stress: An Integrated Assessment." Report No. 254, Massachusetts Institute of Technology Joint Program on the Science and Policy of Global Change, Cambridge, MA.

Schmidt, W.-P., and S. Cairncross. 2009. "Household Water Treatment in Poor Populations: Is There Enough Evidence for Scaling Up Now?" *Environmental Science and Technology* 43 (4): 986–92.

Scott, C., and T. Shah. 2004. "Groundwater Overdraft Reduction through Agricultural Energy Policy: Insights from India and Mexico." *International Journal of Water Resources Development* 20 (2): 149–64.

Sebastian, A., V. Hoffmann, and S. Adelman. 2013. "Menstrual Management in Low-Income Countries: Needs and Trends." *Waterlines* 32 (2): 135–53.

Semmelweis, I. 1983. *The Etiology, Concept and Prophylaxis of Childbed Fever.* Madison, WI: University of Wisconsin Press.

Shah, N. B. 2013. "Microfinance Loans to Increase Sanitary Latrine Sales: Evidence from a Randomized Trial in Rural Cambodia." Policy Brief. International Development Enterprises, Phnom Penh.

Smets, H. 2014. "Quantifying the Affordability Standard." In *The Human Right to Water: Theory, Practice, and Prospects*, edited by M. Langford and A. Russell. Cambridge, U.K.: Cambridge University Press.

Spears, D. 2013. "How Much International Variation in Child Height Can Sanitation Explain?" Policy Research Working Paper 6351, World Bank, Washington, DC.

Spears, D., and S. Lamba. 2013. "Effects of Early-Life Exposure to Sanitation on Childhood Cognitive Skills: Evidence from India's Total Sanitation Campaign." Policy Research Working Paper 6659, World Bank, Washington, DC.

Stanton, B., and J. Clemens. 1987. "Twenty-Four Hour Recall, Knowledge-Attitude-Practice Questionnaires, and Direct Observations of Sanitary Practices: A Comparative Study." *Bulletin of the World Health Organization* 65 (2): 217–22.

Stocks, M., S. Ogden, D. Haddad, D. Addiss, C. McGuire, and others. 2014. "Effect of Water, Sanitation, and Hygiene on the Prevention of Trachoma: A Systematic Review and Meta-Analysis." *PLoS Medicine* 11 (2). doi:10.1371/journal.pmed.1001605.

Strickland, G. 2000. *Hunter's Tropical Medicine and Emerging Infectious Diseases.* 8th ed. Philadelphia, PA: W. B. Saunders Company.

Sumpter, C., and B. Torondel. 2013. "A Systematic Review of the Health and Social Effects of Menstrual Hygiene Management." *PLoS One* 8 (4). doi:10.1371/journal.pone.0062004.

Sy, J., R. Warner, and J. Jamieson. 2014. *Tapping the Markets: Opportunities for Domestic Investments in Water and Sanitation for the Poor.* Washington, DC: World Bank.

Taylor, D. L., T. M. Kahawita, S. Cairncross, and J. H. J. Ensink. 2015. "The Impact of Water, Sanitation and Hygiene Interventions to Control Cholera: A Systematic Review." *PLoS One* 10 (8). doi:10.1371/journal.pone.0135676.

Turner, R., and N. Rabalais. 1991. "Changes in Mississippi River Water Quality This Century and Implications for Coastal Food Webs." *BioScience* 41 (3): 140–47.

UNICEF (United Nations Children's Fund). 1990. *Strategy for Improved Nutrition of Children and Women in Developing Countries: A UNICEF Policy Review.* New York: UNICEF.

———. 2014. *WASH Bottleneck Analysis Tool (WASH-BAT).* New York: UNICEF.

Van den Berg, C., and A. Danilenko. 2010. *The IBNET Water Supply and Sanitation Performance Blue Book: The International Benchmarking Network for Water and Sanitation Utilities Databook.* Water and Sanitation Program. Washington, DC: World Bank.

Victora, C., L. Adair, C. Fall, P. Hallal, R. Martorell, and others. 2008. "Maternal and Child Undernutrition: Consequences for Adult Health and Human Capital." *The Lancet* 371 (9609): 340–57.

Waddington, H., B. Snilstveit, H. White, and L. Fewtrell. 2009. "Water, Sanitation and Hygiene Interventions to Combat Childhood Diarrhoea in Developing Countries." Synthetic Review 001, International Initiative for Impact Evaluation, New Delhi, India.

Whittington, D., Hanemann, W. M., Sadoff, C., and M. Jeuland. 2009. "The Challenge of Improving Water and Sanitation Services in Less Developed Countries." *Foundations and Trends in Microeconomics* 4 (6): 469–607.

Whittington, D., S. Pattanayak, J. Yang and B. Kumar. 2002. "Household Demand for Improved Piped Water Services in Kathmandu, Nepal." *Water Policy* 4 (6): 531–56.

WHO (World Health Organization) and UNICEF (United Nations Children's Fund). 2006. *Meeting the MDG Drinking Water and Sanitation Target: The Urban and Rural Challenge of the Decade.* Geneva: WHO.

———. 2010. *Progress on Drinking Water and Sanitation: 2010 Update.* Geneva: WHO.

———. 2012a. *Rapid Assessment of Drinking-Water Quality (RADWQ): A Handbook for Implementation.* Geneva: WHO

———. 2012b. *Progress on Drinking Water and Sanitation: 2012 Update.* New York: UNICEF and WHO.

———. 2013. *Progress on Drinking Water and Sanitation: 2013 Update.* Geneva: WHO and UNICEF.

———. 2014. *Progress on Drinking Water and Sanitation: 2014 Update.* Geneva: WHO and UNICEF.

———. 2015a. *WASH Post-2015: Proposed Indicators for Drinking Water, Sanitation and Hygiene.* Geneva: WHO and UNICEF.

———. 2015b. *Progress on Drinking Water and Sanitation: 2015 Update and MDG Assessment.* Geneva: WHO and UNICEF.

Wolf, J., A. Prüss-Üstun, O. Cumming, J. Bartram, S. Bonjour, and others. 2014. "Assessing the Impact of Drinking-Water and Sanitation on Diarrhoeal Disease in Low- and Middle-Income Countries: A Systematic Review and Regression Analysis." *Tropical Medicine and International Health* 8 (19).

World Bank. 2009. *The Philippines: Country Environmental Analysis.* Washington, DC: World Bank.

Ziegelbauer, K., B. Speich, D. Mäusezahl, R. Bos, J. Keiser, and others. 2012. "Effect of Sanitation on Soil-Transmitted Helminth Infection: Systematic Review and Meta-Analysis." *PLoS Medicine* 9 (1).

# Chapter 10

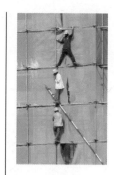

# Interventions to Prevent Injuries and Reduce Environmental and Occupational Hazards: A Review of Economic Evaluations from Low- and Middle-Income Countries

David A. Watkins, Nazila Dabestani, Rachel Nugent, and Carol Levin

## INTRODUCTION

Collectively, unintentional injuries and interpersonal violence accounted for at least 8 percent of deaths and 9 percent of disability-adjusted life years (DALYs) in low- and middle-income countries (LMICs) in 2012 (WHO 2016). Diseases related to air pollution and inadequate water and sanitation measures accounted for 15 percent of attributable deaths and 10 percent of attributable DALYs in LMICs in 2013 (IHME 2015). Millennium Development Goal 7 has inspired steady progress on water- and sanitation-related indicators, although many countries have not yet reached target levels of coverage (Luh and Bartram 2016) or the newer targets for Sustainable Development Goal 6 (UN 2016). Health losses from road traffic injuries (RTIs), interpersonal violence, and outdoor air pollution continue to rise (WHO 2016).

A common feature of the seemingly disparate conditions covered in this volume is that they can be addressed largely through population-based policies and regulations using intersectoral approaches. For example, risks related to most types of injuries can be substantially reduced through educational programs and legal regulations (Ditsuwan and others 2013).

The regulation of air pollution usually occurs within the purview of the public sector environmental agency, as does the provision of clean water and basic sanitation services that are then implemented by public works agencies (Pattanayak and others 2010). Reducing the health risks associated with these environmental hazards involves partnerships between ministries of health and ministries responsible for environment, transportation, and public works. As another example, reduction of occupational hazards is considered the responsibility of employers and employees alike, but it is often monitored and regulated by ministries responsible for labor.

This chapter summarizes the evidence of the costs and benefits of interventions to prevent injuries and reduce occupational and environmental risks in LMICs. Although the interventions reviewed reflect a set of conditions and risk factors more narrow than those covered in this volume, they are the major drivers of disease burden in these cause and risk factor groups in LMICs. The overarching objective of this chapter is to summarize the evidence on value for money to reduce the burden of injuries and environmental and occupational risks in these settings. Evidence on the costs and cost-effectiveness of treating the medical consequences

Corresponding author: David A. Watkins, Department of Medicine, University of Washington, Seattle, Washington, United States; davidaw@uw.edu.

of injury, trauma, and environmental exposures can be found in other volumes of this series.

Although externalities and their policy solutions, such as tradable emissions, that are associated with air and water pollution are critical for human health, this chapter does not review these economic issues as they relate to environmental health. Readers are referred to environmental economics textbooks and manuals for discussions of these issues (Maler and Vincent 2005). This chapter focuses exclusively on studies of costs and cost-effectiveness (including benefit-cost studies) that have been conducted in LMICs.

The economic evidence is modest for injury and ambient environment interventions compared to other conditions, but important lessons can be learned about the types of interventions to receive the highest priority for public investment. Benefit-cost analysis (BCA) is the standard approach in environmental economics. Cost-effectiveness analysis (CEA) is typically applied to health sector interventions, but environmental and other intersectoral interventions—such as development and education—are more suited to BCA because many of the costs and benefits are likely to accrue outside the health sector, and many of these direct benefits can be more easily valued in monetary terms. For example, improved water reduces the risk of morbidity and mortality from diarrheal disease, but it also has many nonhealth benefits, such as its intrinsic value to the consumer and positive effect on tourism. Further, these benefits may even be worth more in monetary terms than the health benefits. This chapter presents CEA and BCA evidence side-by-side with some comments on differences in methods and results.

## METHODS

During July 2015, we systematically searched the literature on costs and cost-effectiveness of interventions to prevent injury and reduce risks in the ambient environment. The search combined terms for the specific injuries and occupational and environmental hazards addressed in this volume, together with economic terms and names of specific LMICs and regions containing LMICs. Our search did not include studies on self-harm, which is treated in volume 4 of this series (Patel and others 2015). Annex 10A contains the search terms and strategy used to identify relevant articles. We were interested in CEAs regardless of perspective. However, we present program costs from the health system or government perspective. The BCAs presented here were conducted from a societal perspective, which is standard in the field.

Our search yielded 4,539 titles through database searches and 31 additional studies through expert consultation. After screening titles and abstracts, we reviewed 161 full-text studies. We included 42 of those studies in the final review on the basis of criteria related to evaluation methods used and quality of the data. Additionally, we considered only those studies published on or after January 1, 2000 (including costs that were collected on or after that date) and pertaining to LMICs (annex 10A). We assessed the quality of included studies using a checklist developed by Drummond and others (2015). Annex 10B provides a flow diagram of the review process.

Among the 42 studies, we identified 16 higher-quality studies. The majority of those studies addressed water, sanitation, and hygiene (WASH); one to two studies were found in each category of injury; and no studies were available on occupational injury. We extracted 41 estimates of intervention costs and 59 estimates of intervention cost-effectiveness, including incremental cost-effectiveness ratios (ICERs), net benefits, and benefit-cost ratios (BCRs). All ICERs, net benefits, and program costs were converted to 2012 U.S. dollars. Costs were first converted to local currency units based on midyear exchange rates in the year that the data were collected. Then they were inflated to 2012 values using the World Bank consumer price index series for the country of the study. Finally, they were converted to U.S. dollars using midyear exchange rates for 2012.

We qualitatively summarized the remaining 26 studies that were of lower quality or used older data sources, but we did not extract quantitative estimates of ICERs or BCRs. In general, an intervention with an ICER less than 1–3 times the per capita gross domestic product of a country was considered cost-effective. An intervention with positive net benefits or a benefit-cost ratio greater than 1 was considered a good investment. Annex 10C provides costs, cost-effectiveness ratios, and descriptive information for each study and a quality assessment score.

## COST-EFFECTIVENESS OF INTERVENTIONS

### Injuries and Occupational Hazards

Economic analyses on injury prevention suggest that interventions to prevent RTIs, drowning, and interpersonal violence are cost-effective and may even be cost saving (table 10.1). A quasi-experimental study by Bishai and others (2008) assessed a traffic enforcement program in Uganda. This program, which focused on reducing speeding, demonstrated a reduction in fatal crashes at a cost of US$944 per death averted (Bishai and others 2008).

**Table 10.1** Results from Economic Evaluations of Injury Prevention Interventions

| Study author (year) | Intervention | Location, perspective[a] | Cost per outcome as presented | Unit of outcome | Currency as presented (year) | Cost per outcome (2012 US$) |
|---|---|---|---|---|---|---|
| Bishai and others (2008) | Traffic enforcement | Uganda, government | 603 | Death averted | U.S. dollar (2005) | 944 |
| Ditsuwan and others (2013) | Checkpoint and media campaign | Thailand, government | 10,400 | DALY averted | Thai baht (2004) | 400 |
| Ditsuwan and others (2013) | Breath testing (selective) | Thailand, government | 13,000 | DALY averted | Thail baht (2004) | 600 |
| Ditsuwan and others (2013) | Breath testing (random) | Thailand, government | 14,300 | DALY averted | Thail baht (2004) | 600 |
| Ditsuwan and others (2013) | Media campaign | Thailand, government | 10,300 | DALY averted | Thai baht (2004) | 400 |
| Ditsuwan and others (2013) | Breath testing (selective) and media campaign | Thailand, government | 12,700 | DALY averted | Thail baht (2004) | 500 |
| Ditsuwan and others (2013) | Breath testing (random) and media campaign | Thailand, government | 13,500 | DALY averted | Thail baht (2004) | 600 |
| Rahman and others (2012) | Anchal drowning prevention program | Bangladesh, societal | 812 | DALY averted | International dollar (2010) | 256 |
| Rahman and others (2012) | SwimSafe drowning prevention program | Bangladesh, societal | 85 | DALY averted | International dollar (2010) | 27 |
| Rahman and others (2012) | Anchal–SwimSafe drowning prevention program (combined) | Bangladesh, societal | 362 | DALY averted | International dollar (2010) | 114 |
| Jan and others (2011) | Microfinance and gender training (trial period) | South Africa, government | 7,688 | DALY averted | U.S. dollar (2004) | 9,826 |
| Jan and others (2011) | Microfinance and gender training (scale-up period) | South Africa, government | 2,307 | DALY averted | U.S. dollar (2004) | 2,948 |

*Note:* DALY = disability-adjusted life year.

a. "Perspective" refers to the perspective from which costs were estimated.

A study in Thailand modeled the cost-effectiveness of several hypothetical interventions for RTIs, including checkpoints, media campaigns, and breath testing, alone or in combination. Compared to the null set, all interventions were very cost-effective; all interventions were cost saving when treatment costs averted were included in the ICER calculations (Ditsuwan and others 2013).

A quasi-experimental study (Rahman and others 2012) addressed drowning prevention in rural Bangladesh. The intervention had two components. The first program, Anchal, focused on direct supervision of children ages 1–5 years at child care centers near bodies of water. The second program, SwimSafe, focused on teaching children ages 4–12 years about basic swimming, safety, and rescue of others from drowning. Both Anchal and SwimSafe were very cost-effective; when their results were combined and extrapolated to a program that would apply to the entire population of rural Bangladesh, they cost approximately US$114 per DALY averted (Rahman and others 2012).

Interpersonal violence is the intentional use of physical force or power against other persons by an individual or small group of individuals (chapter 5 in this volume, Mercy and others 2017). A modeling study by Elliot and Harris (2001) estimated the costs and benefits of landmine clearance in postconflict Mozambique. They found negative net benefits and recommended against landmine clearance. Despite ongoing calls for and guidance on conducting economic evaluations for intimate partner violence (IPV) (Duvvury and others 2013), only a single study included in this review focused on IPV. This study, by Jan and others (2011), evaluated a trial of microfinance to reduce IPV in South Africa. In the South African economic context, ICERs for this program were favorable in both the trial and a subsequent scale-up period (Jan and others 2011).

Additional global and regional studies and modeling approaches using a set of assumptions and secondary data sources provide insights into the potential economic costs and benefits of injury prevention. Bishai and Hyder (2006) found that increased enforcement, speed bumps, bicycle helmets, motorcycle helmets, and childproof containers to prevent poisoning were cost-effective in most world regions. Chisholm and others (2012) conducted an RTI prevention study using the World Health Organization–Choosing Interventions That Are Cost-Effective (WHO-CHOICE) approach. Focusing on WHO regions, the authors found that (1) bicycle helmets; (2) a combination of speed limits, drunk-driving laws, and motorcycle helmet use; and (3) a combination of speed limits, drunk-driving laws, seatbelt laws, bicycle helmet use, and motorcycle helmet use were cost-effective in high-mortality Sub-Saharan African countries, such as Kenya and Tanzania. They also found that a combination of speed limits, impaired driving laws, seatbelt laws, and motorcycle helmet use—with or without bicycle helmet use—were cost-effective in high-mortality Asian countries, such as India and Nepal. Finally, using a preevaluation–postevaluation strategy, Stevenson and others (2008) found that a seatbelt use program was cost-effective in Guangzhou City, China.

Additionally, two regional analyses using the WHO-CHOICE model provide evidence on the cost-effectiveness of measures to prevent occupational injury. In the first study, training programs were more cost-effective than

engineering and ergonomics programs in all WHO regions (Lahiri, Markkanen, and Levenstein 2005). In the second study, engineering controls were more cost-effective than masks and respirators to prevent silicosis (a frequent cause of occupational lung injury) in the Western Pacific, including China (Lahiri and others 2005). Finally, a study by Guimaraes, Ribeiro, and Renner (2012) looked at ergonomic changes in footwear manufacturing facilities in Brazil; their intervention had a BCR of 7.2.

### Environmental Hazards

The limited evidence on economic evaluation for improved air quality comes from Mexico and focuses on reducing pollution from small-scale industry and automobiles (table 10.2). Blackman and others (2000) investigated different ways of reducing pollution from brick kilns, which are a significant contributor to industrial pollution by the small-scale informal sector. Their analysis used an air dispersion model for pollution and assumed a linear relationship between particulate concentration and health outcomes. Net benefits, measured in total dollars per population, were greatest for the strategies focused on retrofitting kilns or using natural gas. Relocating kilns to less densely populated areas or instituting no-burn days had lower net benefits (Blackman and others 2000). In another study, Stevens, Wilson, and Hammitt (2005) assessed a variety of methods for retrofitting vehicles to reduce air pollution. They used a box model with

**Table 10.2** Results from Economic Evaluations of Ambient Environment Interventions: Benefit-Cost Analyses

| Study author (year) | Intervention | Location | Net benefit as presented | Currency as presented (year) | Net benefit (2012 US$) |
|---|---|---|---|---|---|
| Blackman and others (2000) | NMSU kiln | Mexico | 46,810,286 | U.S. dollar (1999) | 73,761,533 |
| Blackman and others (2000) | Natural gas | Mexico | 47,063,087 | U.S. dollar (1999) | 74,159,885 |
| Blackman and others (2000) | Relocation | Mexico | 26,759,571 | U.S. dollar (1999) | 42,166,522 |
| Blackman and others (2000) | No-burn days | Mexico | 905,308 | U.S. dollar (1999) | 1,426,543 |
| Stevens, Wilson, and Hammitt (2005) | Catalyzed DPF | Mexico | 400–1,700 | U.S. dollar (2000) | 500–2,300 |
| Stevens, Wilson, and Hammitt (2005) | Active regeneration DPF | Mexico | 100–8,100 | U.S. dollar (2000) | 100–10,800 |
| Stevens, Wilson, and Hammitt (2005) | Diesel oxidation catalyst | Mexico | 100–2,600 | U.S. dollar (2000) | 100–3,500 |

*Note:* DPF = diesel particulate filter; NMSU = New Mexico State University.

health outcomes informed by concentration-response coefficients from cohort studies in the United States. Despite the cost of the retrofit, all interventions had impressive net benefits that ranged from US$100 to nearly US$11,000 per vehicle retrofitted.

The largest number of economic evaluations of environmental health interventions address water and sanitation and highlight a range of interventions at the population, community, and household levels (tables 10.3 and 10.4). One quasi-experimental study that assessed a hygiene education initiative in Burkina Faso (Borghi and others 2002) found this program to be modestly cost-effective at approximately US$1,100 per death averted. A randomized, controlled trial looked at home-based education and provision of filters, specifically targeting households affected by human immunodeficiency virus/acquired immune deficiency syndrome (HIV/AIDS) in Uganda. The ICER for this program was more than US$2,000 per DALY averted, which is not considered cost-effective in the Ugandan context by Shrestha and others (2006).

The nine remaining water and sanitation evaluations are derived from public works programs affecting environmental health. Günther and Fink (2011) developed a model using Demographic and Health Survey data from 38 countries that demonstrated the relative cost-effectiveness of both basic improved water and sanitation and privately piped water and toilets. Three benefit-cost analyses of improved water and sanitation

in different settings demonstrated favorable BCRs (ranging from 1.9 to 5.1) for a variety of interventions, including filters, piped water, and boreholes, as well as private latrines and community-based sanitation practices (Cameron and others 2011; Hutton and others 2014; Whittington and others 2009). The study by Cameron and others (2011) used preintervention and postintervention data from their study site to estimate health outcomes, whereas the other two studies used static (equation-based) models of health outcomes. Another study (World Bank 2013) used a water quality simulation model to assess wastewater treatment strategies in Indonesia. This study demonstrated favorable BCRs for all approaches except one that focused only on large industries. Finally, two multicountry studies that used static (equation-based) models of health outcomes demonstrated wide variation in BCRs by country. However, all the water and sanitation strategies—alone or in combination—were generally a good return on investment (Hutton 2012; Hutton, Haller, and Bartram 2007).

Further findings based on the WHO-CHOICE and other models compare cost-effectiveness of various community-wide and household prevention approaches for water treatment and reduction of indoor air pollution. One study found that household water treatments were generally more cost-effective than piped water supply and sewage connections in

**Table 10.3** Results from Economic Evaluations of Ambient Environment Interventions: Cost-Effectiveness Analyses

| Study author (year) | Intervention | Location, perspective[a] | Cost per outcome as presented | Unit of outcome | Currency as presented (year) | Cost per outcome (2012 US$) |
|---|---|---|---|---|---|---|
| Borghi and others (2002) | Hygiene promotion | Burkina Faso, government | 657 | Death averted | U.S. dollar (1999) | 1,113 |
| Shrestha and others (2006) | Improved water among households affected by HIV/AIDS | Uganda, government | 1,252 | DALY averted | U.S. dollar (2004) | 2,066 |
| Günther and Fink (2011) | Basic improved water and sanitation in Sub-Saharan African countries | Multiple, government | 1,104 | LY saved | U.S. dollar (2007) | n.a. |
| Günther and Fink (2011) | Privately piped water and flush toilets | Multiple, government | 995 | LY saved | U.S. dollar (2007) | n.a. |
| Günther and Fink (2011) | Improved water and sanitation | Multiple, government | 3,281 | LY saved | U.S. dollar (2007) | n.a. |
| Günther and Fink (2011) | Privately piped water and flush toilets in other LMICs | Multiple, government | 3,188 | LY saved | U.S. dollar (2007) | n.a. |

*Note:* HIV/AIDS = human immunodeficiency virus/acquired immune deficiency syndrome; DALY = disability-adjusted life year; LMICs = low- and middle-income countries; LY = life year; n.a. = not applicable. Costs were estimated for multiple countries and then aggregated; no cost deflator is available for this grouping.

a. "Perspective" refers to the perspective from which costs were estimated.

**Table 10.4** Results from Economic Evaluations of Ambient Environment Interventions: Benefit-Cost Analyses

| Study author (year) | Intervention | Location | Benefit-cost ratio[a] | Currency used (year) |
|---|---|---|---|---|
| Cameron and others (2011) | Improved water | South Africa | 3.1 | South African rand (2008) |
| Hutton and others (2014) | Community sewage system (urban) | East Asia and Pacific | 1.9 | U.S. dollar (2008) |
| Hutton and others (2014) | Private wet pit latrine (rural) | East Asia and Pacific | 5.1 | U.S. dollar (2008) |
| Whittington and others (2009) | Borehole and public hand pump | Multiple | 3.3 | U.S. dollar (2007) |
| Whittington and others (2009) | Community-led total sanitation program | Multiple | 3.0 | U.S. dollar (2007) |
| Whittington and others (2009) | Biosand filter | Multiple | 3.0 | U.S. dollar (2007) |
| Whittington and others (2009) | Large dam | Multiple | 3.7 | U.S. dollar (2007) |
| World Bank (2013) | Treatment of domestic wastewater | Indonesia | 2.3 | Indonesian rupiah (2010) |
| World Bank (2013) | Treatment of industrial wastewater, differentiating all industries or large industries only | Indonesia | 0.6 | Indonesian rupiah (2010) |
| World Bank (2013) | Treatment of domestic and industrial wastewater | Indonesia | 2.0 | Indonesian rupiah (2010) |
| World Bank (2013) | Treatment of domestic and industrial wastewater and recycling of industrial wastewater | Indonesia | 2.3 | Indonesian rupiah (2010) |
| Hutton, Haller, and Bartram (2007) | Improved water | Multiple | 4.4–31.6 | n.a. |
| Hutton, Haller, and Bartram (2007) | Improved water and sanitation | Multiple | 5.5–45.5 | n.a. |
| Hutton, Haller, and Bartram (2007) | Improved water and sanitation and universal basic access | Multiple | 5.2–45.0 | n.a. |
| Hutton, Haller, and Bartram (2007) | Universal basic access and point-of-use treatment | Multiple | 5.7–40.7 | n.a. |
| Hutton, Haller, and Bartram (2007) | Regulated piped water supply and sewer connection | Multiple | 2.1–11.8 | n.a. |
| Hutton (2012) | Universal access to improved sanitation | Multiple | 2.8–8.0 | n.a. |
| Hutton (2012) | Universal access to improved drinking water sources | Multiple | 0.6–3.7 | n.a. |
| Hutton (2012) | Universal access to improved sanitation and improved drinking water sources | Multiple | 2.0–5.3 | n.a. |

*Note:* n.a. = not applicable. Costs were estimated for multiple countries and then aggregated; no cost deflator is available for this grouping. Net benefits and benefit-cost ratios are presented from a societal perspective.

a. Benefit-cost ratios are presented as given in the article because they are independent of currency inflation and exchange rates.

different world regions (Haller, Hutton, and Bartram 2007). Within the household, two studies found that using home-based water filter techniques was ultimately more cost-effective than boiling water (Clasen and others 2007; Clasen and others 2008). A study by Larsen (2003) found that providing safe sanitation facilities was more cost-effective than providing safe water supplies, which was more cost-effective than hygiene improvement strategies. Finally, Jeuland and Pattanayak (2012) developed a model for use in conducting multiple sensitivity analyses related to cookstove interventions. A major finding is that uptake levels of interventions and other assumptions greatly alter the estimated net benefits to households; in some cases, households are worse off with improved cookstoves (Jeuland and Pattanayak 2012).

## PROGRAM COSTS

### Injuries and Occupational Hazards

The estimated costs of the injury prevention program derived from the cost-effectiveness and benefit-cost studies are presented in table 10.5. The RTI prevention interventions in Thailand and Uganda cost less than US\$1 per capita. However, the combined drowning prevention program in Bangladesh and the IPV prevention program cost more than US\$20 per capita per participant, owing to the higher resource needs and training required to conduct these programs. Mine clearance was very expensive, at more than US\$14,000 per hectare, which is part of the reason the program had net negative benefits.

### Environmental Hazards

Table 10.6 summarizes the costs of programs to reduce environmental risks. Air pollution control, despite being cost-effective, was relatively expensive in Mexico. Water and sanitation programs also required large investments over a long time horizon, with the exception of personal point-of-use technologies. Special attention was paid in these studies to the recurrent costs of WASH infrastructure, which in many cases were a substantial contributor to overall costs and might be borne by households. However, these large costs appeared to be outweighed by the economic benefits. A collection of studies on water and sanitation demand not included in this

**Table 10.5** Program Costs of Injury Prevention Interventions

| Study author (year) | Intervention | Location, perspective[a] | Cost as presented | Unit of cost | Currency as presented (year) | Cost (2012 US$) |
|---|---|---|---|---|---|---|
| Bishai and others (2008) | Traffic enforcement | Uganda, government | 0.45 | Per vehicle per year | U.S. dollar (2005) | 0.70 |
| Ditsuwan and others (2013) | Sobriety checkpoints by metropolitan police | Thailand, government | 0.27 | Per capita per year | Thai baht (2004) | 0.01 |
| Ditsuwan and others (2013) | Sobriety checkpoints by traffic police | Thailand, government | 5.29 | Per capita per year | Thai baht (2004) | 0.23 |
| Ditsuwan and others (2013) | Media campaign on drink-driving | Thailand, government | 2.86 | Per capita per year | Thai baht (2004) | 0.12 |
| Rahman and others (2012) | Anchal drowning prevention program | Bangladesh, societal | 60.50 | Per capita first year | International dollar (2010) | 19.07 |
| Rahman and others (2012) | Anchal drowning prevention program | Bangladesh, societal | 50.74 | Per capita second year onward | International dollar (2010) | 16.00 |
| Rahman and others (2012) | SwimSafe drowning prevention program | Bangladesh, societal | 13.46 | Per capita per year | International dollar (2010) | 4.24 |
| Elliot and Harris (2001) | Mine clearance | Mozambique, societal | 6,176.50 | Per hectare | U.S. dollar (1996) | 14,249.00 |
| Jan and others (2011) | Microfinance and gender training (trial period) | South Africa, government | 42.93 | Per capita per 2 years | U.S. dollar (2004) | 54.87 |
| Jan and others (2011) | Microfinance and gender training (scale-up) | South Africa, government | 12.88 | Per capita per 2 years | U.S. dollar (2004) | 16.46 |

a. "Perspective" refers to the perspective from which costs were estimated.

**Table 10.6** Program Costs of Ambient Environment Interventions

| Study author (year) | Intervention | Location, perspective[a] | Cost as presented | Unit of cost | Currency as presented (year) | Cost (2012 US$) |
|---|---|---|---|---|---|---|
| *Air pollution* | | | | | | |
| Blackman and others (2000) | NMSU kiln | Mexico, societal | 175,214.00 | Per year | U.S. dollar (1999) | 276,094.00 |
| Blackman and others (2000) | Natural gas | Mexico, societal | 249,553.00 | Per year | U.S. dollar (1999) | 393,234.00 |
| Blackman and others (2000) | Relocation | Mexico, societal | 350,429.00 | Per year | U.S. dollar (1999) | 552,190.00 |
| Blackman and others (2000) | No-burn days | Mexico, societal | 24,692.00 | Per year | U.S. dollar (1999) | 38,909.00 |
| Stevens, Wilson, and Hammitt (2005) | Catalyzed DPF | Mexico, societal | 270.00 | Per vehicle per year | U.S. dollar (2000) | 360.00 |
| Stevens, Wilson, and Hammitt (2005) | Active regeneration DPF | Mexico, societal | 600.00 | Per vehicle per year | U.S. dollar (2000) | 800.00 |
| Stevens, Wilson, and Hammitt (2005) | Diesel oxidation catalyst | Mexico, societal | 90.00 | Per vehicle per year | U.S. dollar (2000) | 120.00 |
| *Water, Sanitation, and Hygiene* | | | | | | |
| Borghi and others (2002) | Hygiene promotion | Burkina Faso, government | 8.11 | Per capita | U.S. dollar (1999) | 13.73 |
| Cameron and others (2011) | Improved water | South Africa, societal | 153.31 | Per capita per year | South African rand (2008) | 2.58 |
| Shrestha and others (2006) | Improved water among households affected by HIV/AIDS | Uganda, government | 2.19 | Per capita per year | U.S. dollar (2004) | 3.61 |
| Whittington and others (2009) | Borehole and public hand pump | Multiple, societal | 2.00 | Per house per month | U.S. dollar (2007) | n. a. |
| Whittington and others (2009) | Community-led total sanitation program | Multiple, societal | 0.39 | Per house per month | U.S. dollar (2007) | n. a. |
| Whittington and others (2009) | Biosand filter | Multiple, societal | 1.25 | Per house per month | U.S. dollar (2007) | n. a. |
| Whittington and others (2009) | Large dam | Multiple, societal | 3,743,000.00 | Per 75 years | U.S. dollar (2007) | n. a. |
| World Bank (2013) | Treatment of domestic wastewater | Indonesia, societal | 888,000,000,000.00 | Per 20 years | Indonesian rupiah (2010) | 109,000,000.00 |
| World Bank (2013) | Treatment of industrial wastewater, differentiating all industries or large industries only | Indonesia, societal | 172,000,000,000.00 | Per 20 years | Indonesian rupiah (2010) | 21,000,000.00 |

*table continues next page*

**Table 10.6** Program Costs of Ambient Environment Interventions (continued)

| Study author (year) | Intervention | Location, perspective[a] | Cost as presented | Unit of cost | Currency as presented (year) | Cost (2012 US$) |
|---|---|---|---|---|---|---|
| World Bank (2013) | Treatment of domestic and industrial wastewater | Indonesia, societal | 1,059,000,000,000.00 | Per 20 years | Indonesian rupiah (2010) | 130,000,000.00 |
| World Bank (2013) | Treatment of domestic and industrial wastewater and recycling of industrial wastewater | Indonesia, societal | 1,164,000,000,000.00 | Per 20 years | Indonesian rupiah (2010) | 143,000,000.00 |
| Günther and Fink (2011) | Basic sanitation (latrines) | Multiple, government | 600.00–965.00 | Per house per lifetime | U.S. dollar (2007) | n.a. |
| Günther and Fink (2011) | Basic improved water | Multiple, government | 309.00–545.00 | Per house per lifetime | U.S. dollar (2007) | n.a. |
| Günther and Fink (2011) | Flush toilets | Multiple, government | 2,099.00–2,400.00 | Per house per lifetime | U.S. dollar (2007) | n.a. |
| Günther and Fink (2011) | Privately piped water | Multiple, government | 1,623.00–2,509.00 | Per house per lifetime | U.S. dollar (2007) | n.a. |

*Note:* HIV/AIDS = human immunodeficiency virus/acquired immune deficiency syndrome; DPF = diesel particulate filter; NMSU = New Mexico State University; n.a. = not applicable. Costs were estimated for multiple countries and then aggregated; no cost deflator is available for this grouping.

a. "Perspective" refers to the perspective from which costs were estimated.

review suggests that despite the high cost of water and sanitation infrastructure, households in LMICs are generally willing to pay a substantial amount for these goods and services (Dutta and Tiwari 2005; Pattanayak and others 2010).

Some recent studies can inform the costs of these programs, although data may be incomplete or out of date. For example, a study by Banerjee and others (2007) found that social marketing of safe water systems resulted in economies of scale and greater financial sustainability. A study by Crocker and Bartram (2014) looked at the cost of routine water quality testing in seven countries. They documented great heterogeneity and economic inefficiencies in existing monitoring practices and proposed ways of optimizing monitoring. A study by Dodane and others (2012) demonstrated that in urban Senegal, sewer-based systems were more expensive, less feasible, and no more effective than more commonly used on-site waste management systems.

## OTHER ECONOMIC ASPECTS OF INJURIES AND ENVIRONMENTAL HEALTH

Prevention of injury is likely to have more economic benefits than those described in the cost-effectiveness studies here. Injury often leads to disability, which can be permanent. From a human capital perspective, injury leads to foregone wages and hinders economic growth and development (Nguyen and others 2016). Gender-based violence, in particular, can hinder women's economic opportunities and impede gender equity, leading to consequences for overall economic growth (Duvvury and others 2013). Occupational injury may have deleterious effects on both employees and employers, but in practice, costs often fall exclusively on employees. In countries where trauma care is financed predominantly by out-of-pocket funds, injuries can have catastrophic or impoverishing effects on households (Nguyen and others 2016). Preventing injury in these settings can reduce the risk of medical impoverishment (Olson and others 2016).

The rationale for government intervention to prevent environmental exposures stems from the concept of internalizing externalities or reducing the social costs associated with private decisions. Such social costs include negative effects on the environment. The BCA approach used in most environmental health evaluations reviewed should, in principle, include an estimate of the environmental (nonhealth) benefits of scaling up WASH and addressing air pollution. In practice, however, many of these benefits are undervalued. For example, households appear to place a high intrinsic value (willingness-to-pay) on WASH services, but when these services are not present, households face high coping costs related to unreliable water supply (Dutta and Tiwari 2005). In such cases, public sector regulation can improve economic efficiency. Empirical evidence suggests that in most settings, people are willing to pay substantial amounts to mitigate negative externalities in the injury and environmental health domains (Ortuzar, Cifuentes, and Williams 2000).

## LIMITATIONS IN EVIDENCE

Our review has summarized the recent economic evaluations that focus on preventing injuries and reducing environmental hazards in LMICs. The absolute number of studies on such hazards in LMICs published since 2000 is small in comparison to other areas of health. However, there are a few additional studies from LMICs published before 2000; these were reviewed in chapters 42 and 43 of *Disease Control Priorities in Developing Countries* (second edition) (Bruce and others 2006; Kjellstrom and others 2006).

Despite broad recognition of the problem and many effective interventions, there is surprisingly little economic literature on the prevention of RTIs in LMICs. Evidence from high-income countries shows that investments in promoting or establishing helmet laws, vehicle inspections, seatbelt use, and, to a lesser extent, speed limits appear to be good value for money (Waters, Hyder, and Phillips 2004). Many of these approaches would likely be effective in LMICs. However, the costs, affordability, and cost-effectiveness may vary, depending on country context and the amount of government and regulatory infrastructure in place to implement and scale up these interventions.

Similarly, there are few economic analyses on prevention of falls, burns, poisoning, or injuries from forces of nature in LMICs. Given the increasing burden of injuries (in particular, falls) and of interpersonal violence in LMICs, this area will be important for future research. Studies in high-income countries have demonstrated that regulatory and legal interventions are cost-effective, but the social and legal differences compared to LMICs make these studies difficult to generalize (Waters and others 2004). Further, the most neglected area for economic analysis by far is occupational injury. We found no high-quality studies in LMICs in this area, but we anticipate that the productivity benefits of addressing occupational hazards in

these settings will be impressive and warrant further investigation.

With respect to environmental risks, the evidence is compelling for scaling up WASH interventions, particularly basic sanitation measures and point-of-use water quality interventions. Piped water and other large-scale infrastructure projects can be good value for money from a societal standpoint (that is, including the intrinsic value individuals place on having piped water independent of its health effect). However, these projects require more substantial up-front investments and may be infeasible as a first step for low-income countries. Whether WASH infrastructure should be a high priority for other sectoral reasons (that is, besides the health benefits) for governments of low-income countries is unclear.

Unfortunately, little economic evidence exists on control of outdoor air pollution in LMICs outside of Mexico, and there are essentially no economic studies published after 2000 on control of indoor air pollution. In contrast, outdoor air pollution—which, in the near future, is expected to supplant the burden of indoor air pollution in LMICs—has been the focus of many epidemiological studies and economic evaluations in high-income countries. These analyses can serve as a first step to informing policy in LMICs. (See, for example, the economic evaluations conducted by the U.S. Environmental Protection Agency [2011].) Analyses of outdoor air pollution policies in LMICs will be of utmost importance given trends in urbanization and the potential for mitigating climate change. We note that a discussion of the economics of climate change is particularly challenging and is outside the scope of this review. See chapter 8 in this volume (Ebi, Hess, and Watkiss 2017) for a discussion of potential global costs and benefits of mitigating climate change.

Even more difficult than evaluating health sector interventions, economic evaluations of cross-sectoral interventions with multiple types of costs and benefits face serious methodological challenges, given the difficulty of valuing and combining the direct and indirect benefits of reducing personal injury and promoting environmental health. The literature is concentrated in several areas, especially RTI interventions and structural WASH interventions. Both areas suggest quite positive results, but do not fully account for social benefits. For RTIs, an accounting for downstream health effects of injury is lacking. For environmental exposures, the key issue is the difficulty of capturing and measuring benefits across sectors. In these cases, we are likely to be underestimating the benefits of such interventions and therefore underinvesting in environmental health protection.

## CONCLUSIONS

We have identified several areas in injury prevention and environmental and occupational health where a good economic case might be made for action. Yet important methodological challenges remain, as well as unanswered questions and conditions for which no literature exists. If one considers the human capital and other social costs associated with these diseases and risk factors, more research in this area is urgently needed to inform the design and implementation of intersectoral policies.

## ANNEXES

The annexes to this chapter are as follows. They are available at http://www.dcp-3.org/environment.

- Annex 10A. Search Terms Used to Identify Relevant Literature
- Annex 10B. Flow Chart of Identification, Screening, and Eligibility of Included Studies
- Annex 10C. List of Included Studies, Main Findings, and Quality Assessment

## NOTE

World Bank Income Classifications as of July 2014 are as follows, based on estimates of gross national income (GNI) per capita for 2013:

- Low-income countries (LICs) = US$1,045 or less
- Middle-income countries (MICs) are subdivided:
  a) lower-middle-income = US$1,046 to US$4,125
  b) upper-middle-income (UMICs) = US$4,126 to US$12,745
- High-income countries (HICs) = US$12,746 or more.

All intervention costs in this chapter have been converted into 2012 US$, using the World Bank consumer price index or regional inflation rates, unless otherwise noted.

## REFERENCES

Banerjee, A., D. McFarland, R. Sinh, and R. Quick. 2007. "Cost and Financial Sustainability of a Household-Based Water Treatment and Storage Intervention in Zambia." *Journal of Water and Health* 5 (3): 385–95.

Bishai, D., B. Asiimwe, S. Abbas, A. Hyder, and W. Bazeyo. 2008. "Cost-Effectiveness of Traffic Enforcement: Case Study from Uganda." *Injury Prevention* 14: 223–27.

Bishai, D., and A. Hyder. 2006. "Modeling the Cost Effectiveness of Injury Interventions in Lower and Middle Income Countries: Opportunities and Challenges." *Cost Effectiveness and Resource Allocation* 4 (2): 1–11.

Blackman, A., S. Newbold, J. Shih, and J. Cook. 2000. "The Benefits and Costs of Informal Sector Pollution Control: Mexican Brick Kilns." Discussion Paper 00-46, Resources for the Future, Washington, DC.

Borghi, J., L. Guinness, J. Ouedraogo, and V. Curtis. 2002. "Is Hygiene Promotion Cost-Effective? A Case Study in Burkina Faso." *Tropical Medicine and International Health* 7 (11): 960–69.

Bruce, N., E. Rehfuess, S. Mehta, G. Hutton, and K. Smith. 2006. "Indoor Air Pollution." In *Disease Control Priorities in Developing Countries* (second edition), edited by D. T. Jamison, J. G. Bremen, A. R. Measham, G. Alleyne, M. Claeson, D. B. Evans, P. Jha, A. Mills, and P. Musgrove. Washington, DC: World Bank.

Cameron, J., P. Jagals, P. Hunter, S. Pedley, and K. Pond. 2011. "Economic Assessments of Small-Scale Drinking-Water Interventions in Pursuit of MDG Target 7C." *Science of the Total Environment* 410–11: 8–15.

Chisholm, D., H. Naci, A. Hyder, N. Tran, and M. Peden. 2012. "Cost Effectiveness of Strategies to Combat Road Traffic Injuries in Sub-Saharan Africa and South East Asia: Mathematical Modelling Study." *BMJ* 344: c612.

Clasen, T., C. McLaughlin, N. Nayaar, S. Boisson, R. Gupta, and others. 2008. "Microbiological Effectiveness and Cost of Disinfecting Water by Boiling in Semi-Urban India." *American Society of Tropical Medicine and Hygiene* 79 (3): 407–13.

Clasen, T., D. Thao, S. Boisson, and O. Shipin. 2007. "Microbiological Effectiveness and Cost of Boiling to Disinfect Drinking Water in Rural Vietnam." *Environmental Science and Technology* 42 (12): 4255–61.

Crocker, J., and J. Bartram. 2014. "Comparison and Cost Analysis of Drinking Water Quality Monitoring Requirements versus Practice in Seven Developing Countries." *International Journal of Environmental Research and Public Health* 11: 7333–46.

Ditsuwan, V., J. Veerman, M. Bertram, and T. Vos. 2013. "Cost-Effectiveness of Interventions for Reducing Road Traffic Injuries Related to Driving under the Influence of Alcohol." *Value in Health* 16: 23–30.

Dodane, P., M. Mbeguere, O. Sow, and L. Strande. 2012. "Capital and Operating Costs of Full-Scale Fecal Sludge Management and Wastewater Treatment Systems in Dakar, Senegal." *Environmental Science and Technology* 46: 3705–11.

Drummond, M. F., M. J. Schulpher, K. Claxton, G. L. Stoddart, and G. W. Torrance. 2015. *Methods for the Economic Evaluation of Health Care Programmes*, fourth edition. Oxford, U.K.: Oxford University Press.

Dutta, V., and A. Tiwari. 2005. "Cost of Services and Willingness to Pay for Reliable Urban Water Supply: A Study from Delhi, India." *Journal of Water Science and Technology* 5 (6): 135–44.

Duvvury, N., A. Callan, P. Carney, and S. Raghavendra. 2013. "Intimate Partner Violence: Economic Costs and Implications for Growth and Development." Working Paper 82532, World Bank, Washington, DC.

Ebi, K. L., J. J. Hess, and P. Watkiss. 2017. "Health Risks and Costs of Climate Variability and Change." In *Disease Control Priorities* (third edition): Volume 7, *Injury Prevention and Environmental Health*, edited by C. N. Mock, R. Nugent, O. Kobusingye, and K. R. Smith. Washington, DC: World Bank.

Elliot, G., and G. Harris. 2001. "A Cost-Benefit Analysis of Landmine Clearance in Mozambique." *Development Southern Africa* 18 (5): 625–33.

Guimaraes, L., J. Ribeiro, and J. Renner. 2012. "Cost-Benefit Analysis of a Socio-Technical Intervention in a Brazilian Footwear Company." *Applied Ergonomics* 43: 948–57.

Günther, I., and G. Fink. 2011. "Water and Sanitation to Reduce Child Mortality: The Impact and Cost of Water and Sanitation Infrastructure." Policy Research Working Paper 5618, World Bank, Washington, DC.

Haller, L., G. Hutton, and J. Bartram. 2007. "Estimating the Costs and Health Benefits of Water and Sanitation Improvements at Global Level." *Journal of Water and Health* 5 (4): 467–81.

Hutton, G. 2012. *Global Costs and Benefits of Drinking-Water Supply and Sanitation Interventions to Reach the MDG Target and Universal Coverage.* Geneva: World Health Organization.

Hutton, G., L. Haller, and J. Bartram. 2007. "Global Cost-Benefit Analysis of Water Supply and Sanitation Interventions." *Journal of Water and Health* 5 (4): 481–502.

Hutton, G., U. Rodriguez, A. Winara, N. Anh, K. Phyrum, and others. 2014. "Economic Efficiency of Sanitation Interventions in Southeast Asia." *Journal of Water, Sanitation and Hygiene for Development* 4 (1): 23–36.

IHME (Institute for Health Metrics and Evaluation). 2015. "Global Burden of Disease Study 2013 (GBD 2013) Data Downloads." IHME, Seattle. http://ghdx.healthdata.org/global-burden -disease-study-2013-gbd-2013-data-downloads.

Jan, S., G. Ferrari, C. Watts, J. Hargreaves, J. Kim, and others. 2011. "Economic Evaluation of a Combined Microfinance and Gender Training Intervention for the Prevention of Intimate Partner Violence in Rural South Africa." *Health Policy and Planning* 26: 366–72.

Jeuland, M., and S. K. Pattanayak. 2012. "Benefits and Costs of Improved Cookstoves: Assessing the Implications of Variability in Health, Forest and Climate Impacts." *Plos One* 7 (2): e30338.

Kjellstrom, T., M. Lodh, T. McMichael, G. Ranmuthugala, R. Shrestha, and others. 2006. "Air and Water Pollution: Burden and Strategies for Control." In *Disease Control Priorities in Developing Countries* (second edition), edited by D. T. Jamison, J. G. Bremen, A. R. Measham, G. Alleyne, M. Claeson, D. B. Evans, P. Jha, A. Mills, and P. Musgrove. Washington, DC: World Bank.

Lahiri, S., C. Levenstein, D. Nelson, and B. Rosenberg. 2005. "The Cost Effectiveness of Occupational Health Interventions: Prevention of Silicosis." *American Journal of Industrial Medicine* 48: 503–14.

Lahiri, S., P. Markkanen, and C. Levenstein. 2005. "The Cost Effectiveness of Occupational Health Interventions: Preventing Occupational Back Pain." *American Journal of Industrial Medicine* 48: 515–29.

Larsen, B. 2003. "Hygiene and Health in Developing Countries: Defining Priorities through Cost-Benefit Assessments." *International Journal of Environmental Health Research* 13: S37–46.

Luh, J., and J. Bartram. 2016. "Drinking Water and Sanitation: Progress in 73 Countries in Relation to Socioeconomic Indicators." *Bulletin of the World Health Organization* 94: 111–21.

Maler, K. G., and J. R. Vincent, eds. 2005. *Handbook of Environmental Economics: Economywide and International Environmental Issues,* third edition. Amsterdam: North Holland.

Mercy, J. A., S. D. Hillis, A. Butchart, M. A. Bellis, C. L. Ward, and others. 2017. "Interpersonal Violence: Global Impact and Paths to Prevention." In *Disease Control Priorities* (third edition): Volume 7, *Injury Prevention and Environmental Health*, edited by C. N. Mock, R. Nugent, O. Kobusingye, and K. R. Smith. Washington, DC: World Bank.

Nguyen, H., R. Ivers, S. Jan, A. Martiniuk, L. Segal, and others. 2016. "Cost and Impoverishment 1 Year after Hospitalisation due to Injuries: A Cohort Study in Thai Binh, Vietnam." *Injury Prevention* 22 (1): 33–39.

Olson, Z., J. A. Staples, C. N. Mock, N. P. Nguyen, A. M. Bachani, and others. 2016. "Helmet Regulation in Vietnam: Impact on Health, Equity, and Medical Impoverishment." *Injury Prevention* 22 (4): 233–38.

Ortuzar, J. D., L. A. Cifuentes, and H. C. W. L. Williams. 2000. "Application of Willingness-to-Pay Methods to Value Transport Externalities in Less Developed Countries." *Environment and Planning A* 32 (11): 2007–18.

Patel, V., D. Chisholm, T. Dua, R. Laxminarayan, and M. E. Medina-Mora, eds. 2015. *Disease Control Priorities* (third edition): Volume 4, *Mental, Neurological, and Substance Use Disorders.* Washington, DC: World Bank.

Pattanayak, S., C. Poulos, J. Yang, and S. Patil. 2010. "How Valuable Are Environmental Health Interventions? Evaluation of Water and Sanitation Programmes in India." *Bulletin of the World Health Organization* 88: 535–42.

Rahman, F., S. Bose, M. Linnqn, A. Rahman, S. Mashreky, and others. 2012. "Cost-Effectiveness of an Injury and Drowning Prevention Program in Bangladesh." *Pediatrics* 130 (6): 1–10.

Shrestha, R., E. Marseille, J. Kahn, J. Lule, C. Pitter, and others. 2006. "Cost-Effectiveness of Home-Based Chlorination and Safe Water Storage in Reducing Diarrhea among HIV-Affected Households in Rural Uganda." *American Journal of Tropical Medicine and Hygiene* 74 (5): 884–90.

Stevens, G., A. Wilson, and J. Hammitt. 2005. "A Benefit-Cost Analysis of Retrofitting Diesel Vehicles with Particulate Filters in the Mexico City Metropolitan Area." *Risk Analysis* 25 (4): 1–17.

Stevenson, M., D. Hendrie, R. Ivers, Z. Su, and R. Norton. 2008. "Reducing the Burden of Road Traffic Injury: Translating High-Income Country Interventions to Middle-Income and Low-Income Countries." *Injury Prevention* 14: 2848–49.

UN (United Nations). 2016. *Sustainable Development Goals: 17 Goals to Transform Our World. Goal 6: Ensure Access to Water and Sanitation for All.* New York: UN. http://www.un .org/sustainabledevelopment/water-and-sanitation.

U.S. EPA (United States Environmental Protection Agency). 2011. "The Benefits and Costs of the Clean Air Act from 1990 to 2010: Final Report–Rev. A." Office of Air and Radiation, U.S. EPA, Washington, DC.

Waters, H. R., A. A. Hyder, and T. L. Phillips. 2004. "Economic Evaluation of Interventions to Reduce Road Traffic Injuries: A Review of the Literature with Applications to Low and Middle-Income Countries." *Asia-Pacific Journal of Public Health* 16 (1): 23–31.

Waters, H. R., A. A. Hyder, Y. Rajkotia, S. Basu, and J. A. Rehwinkel. 2004. *The Economic Dimensions of Interpersonal Violence.* Geneva: World Health Organization.

Whittington, D., M. Shanemann, C. Sadoff, and M. Jeuland. 2009. "The Challenge of Improving Water and Sanitation Services in Less Developed Countries." *Foundations and Trends in Microeconomics* 4 (6–7): 469–609.

WHO (World Health Organization). 2016. *Global Health Estimates 2012.* Geneva: WHO. http://www.who.int /healthinfo/global_burden_disease/en/.

World Bank. 2013. "Downstream Impacts of Water Pollution in the Upper Citarum River, West Java, Indonesia: Economic Assessment of Interventions to Improve Water Quality." Technical Paper 85194, World Bank, Washington, DC.

# 11

# Helmet Regulation in Vietnam: Impact on Health, Equity, and Medical Impoverishment

Zachary Olson, John A. Staples, Charles N. Mock,
Nam Phuong Nguyen, Abdulgafoor M. Bachani,
Rachel Nugent, and Stéphane Verguet

## INTRODUCTION

Road traffic injury (RTI) accounts for a substantial and increasing burden of mortality, morbidity, and health care costs in developing nations. Globally, road traffic is responsible for 1.3 million fatal and 78 million nonfatal injuries each year (WHO 2013a; World Bank and IHME 2014). In the Western Pacific, RTI is the leading cause of mortality for people ages 15–49 years (WHO 2013b). Direct economic costs are estimated to exceed US$500 billion worldwide and are anticipated to grow in tandem with motorization of the developing world (WHO 2004; World Bank and IHME 2014). The potentially substantial out-of-pocket (OOP) medical costs associated with traffic injury may result in catastrophic expenditures (expenditures that crowd out a significant portion of household expenditures) and subsequent impoverishment (Wagstaff 2010).

In response to the growing burden of traffic injury, the government of Vietnam passed comprehensive legislation mandating the use of motorcycle helmets in 2007. This legislation extended the mandatory use of helmets to all riders on all roads, substantially increased penalties for failure to wear a helmet, and provided for increased enforcement (Passmore, Nguyen, and others 2010). As a result, helmet use increased from 30 percent to 93 percent of riders within months (Hung, Stevenson, and Ivers 2006; Nguyen, Passmore, and others 2013). Studies in other settings have examined the influence of helmet use policies on aggregate health, but the distribution of benefits and equity improvements resulting from such regulatory changes remains understudied and uncertain (Ngo and others 2012; Passmore, Tu, and others 2010).

Traffic injury can lead to substantial and potentially impoverishing health expenditures (Wagstaff 2010). Legislation mandating helmet use is one non–health sector policy that may protect individuals against this financial risk. In nations with universal health coverage, helmet regulation may also reduce government spending for traffic injuries and thus free up health spending for other conditions. Defining the magnitude of the health and financial benefits attributable to Vietnam's comprehensive helmet policy might bolster the case for a similar policy in neighboring countries (for example, Cambodia) and in other low-and-middle-income countries.

Extended cost-effectiveness analysis (ECEA) incorporates the dimensions of equity and financial risk protection into economic evaluations (Verguet, Laxminarayan, and Jamison 2014; Verguet and others 2013, 2015). In this

Corresponding author: Zachary Olson, School of Public Health, University of California, Berkeley, CA, United States; zolson@berkeley.edu. Zachary Olson and John Staples contributed equally to the work.

chapter, a simulation model is used to perform an ECEA examining the influence that Vietnam's 2007 helmet legislation has had in four areas:

- Road traffic deaths and nonfatal injuries
- Individuals' direct costs of acute care treatment for motorcycle injuries
- Individuals' income losses from missed work
- Individuals' financial risk.

## METHODS

### Design

For the period of interest, the annual number of nonfatal traffic injuries reported by Vietnam's National Traffic Safety Committee is not disaggregated by type of road user and generally lacks consistency and credibility. For example, the number of nonfatal traffic injuries reported by police in 2007 (10,300) is drastically different from the number noted in health data reports for the same year (445,000) (WHO 2009). To address this discrepancy, the model developed for this chapter uses secondary data to simulate the benefits accruing from the 2007 comprehensive helmet policy. After ensuring consistency of the model with reported reductions in total road traffic deaths (National Traffic Safety Committee 2014; Passmore, Nguyen, and others 2010), an ECEA was performed to estimate the distribution of health benefits and costs across income groups. Conceptually, the study period includes a one-year pre-policy baseline period (July 2006 to June 2007), a six-month transition period during which the majority of the helmet policy legislation was introduced and came into effect (June to December 2007), and a one-year post-policy evaluation period (January to December 2008).

### Setting

At the midpoint of the study period, Vietnam was a lower-middle-income country with a population of about 84 million and per capita gross domestic product (GDP) of about US$1,200 (World Bank 2012). About 95 percent of registered vehicles were motorized two-wheel vehicles (WHO 2013c). Prior to the 2007 legislation, the incidence of road traffic deaths was estimated to be 14 per 100,000 people per year (WHO 2009). About 55 percent of health care costs were paid out of pocket (Tien and others 2011; WHO 2010).

Prior to 2007, Vietnam had limited motorcycle helmet legislation with incomplete implementation and enforcement. Comprehensive legislation that made helmet use compulsory for all motorcycle riders and passengers on all roads was introduced in June 2007, came into force for government workers in September 2007, and came into force for the general public in December 2007 (Passmore, Nguyen, and others 2010). Legislation introduced in September 2007 increased the fines for failure to wear a helmet from US$2–US$5 to US$11–US$22 per offense, the latter range representing about 30 percent of average monthly income per capita (Government of Vietnam 2007; Passmore, Nguyen, and others 2010). At that time, the majority of Vietnamese households were willing to pay the average market price of US$17 for a standard helmet (Pham and others 2008).

### Variables

In the simulation, all input parameters were abstracted from academic studies and from reports issued by governmental and nongovernmental agencies (table 11.1; see also annex 11A, table 11A.1). The output estimates of primary interest were traffic deaths averted, nonfatal traffic injuries averted, individuals' OOP acute care medical costs averted, and individuals' income losses averted during the one-year post-policy period. Costs were viewed from the individuals' perspective, including both OOP acute care costs and income losses. Estimation of subacute and chronic outpatient medical costs was not possible, as reliable input parameters were not available. All costs are in 2012 U.S. dollars and were converted using consumer price indexes and exchange rates as reported by the World Bank (2012).

### Major Assumptions

According to the National Traffic Safety Committee (2014), the number of registered motorcycles in Vietnam increased from 21 million in 2007 to 25 million in 2008. However, for simplicity, the model assumes that the number of registered motorcycles remained static at the pre-policy level during the study period. This assumption makes the estimates more conservative but substantially improves their interpretability and generalizability. Furthermore, the effectiveness of motorcycle helmets in Vietnam was assumed to be equivalent to the estimated effectiveness of helmets in high-income countries (HICs). However, major concerns have been raised regarding the proliferation of substandard helmets in Vietnam (Hung, Stevenson, and Ivers 2008; WHO 2015; Yu and others 2011). Given the lack of local data regarding the effectiveness of substandard helmets, this crucial issue was addressed in a separate sensitivity analysis. For the main analysis, the distribution of fatal and nonfatal traffic injuries across income quintiles was assumed to reflect the distribution of motorcycle ownership across quintiles,

**Table 11.1** Model Input Parameters

| Parameter | Estimate (range) | References |
|---|---|---|
| Population of Vietnam | 84,000,000 | World Bank 2012 |
| Pre-policy RTI deaths | 13,000 | WHO 2009 |
| Pre-policy nonfatal RTIs | 445,000 | WHO 2009 |
| % of RTI deaths attributable to motorcycles | 58 (51–73) | Hoang and others 2008; Ngo and others 2012; Pham and others 2008; |
| % of nonfatal RTIs attributable to motorcycles | 59 (51–75) | Hoang and others 2008; Hung, Stevenson, and Ivers 2006; Ngo and others 2012; Nguyen, Passmore, and others 2013; Pham and others 2008 |
| % of nonfatal motorcycle RTIs with head injury | 21 (10–32) | Nguyen, Ivers, and others 2013 |
| Pre-policy helmet use (%) | 30 (20–40) | Hung, Stevenson, and Ivers 2006; Nguyen, Passmore, and others 2013 |
| Postpolicy helmet use (%) | 93 (83–98) | Nguyen, Passmore, and others 2013 |
| Average direct acute care cost of nonfatal RTI with a helmet (US$) | 436 (366–506) | Nguyen, Ivers, and others 2013 |
| Average direct acute care cost of nonfatal RTI without a helmet (US$) | 559 (416–702) | Nguyen, Ivers, and others 2013 |
| Expected increase in treatment cost for each US$10 increase in income (%) | 1 | Nguyen, Ivers, and others 2013 |
| Income loss (number of weeks) | 32 | Hoang and others 2008 |
| Mean per capita income, by quintile (US$) | 305, 530, 777, 1,185, 2,730 | GSO 2010 |
| Distribution of motorcycle ownership by quintile (%) | 20, 35, 54, 73, 94 | GSO, NIHE, and ORC Macro 2006 |
| Relative risk of death, helmet vs. no helmet | 0.58 (0.50–0.79) | Liu and others 2008 |
| Relative risk of injury, helmet vs. no helmet | 0.31 (0.25–0.66) | Liu and others 2008 |
| Per capita cost of policy implementation (US$) | 0.29 | Chisholm and others 2012 (correspondence from Dan Chisholm) |

*Note:* RTI = road traffic injury. Table 11A.1 in the annex provides the detailed rationale and additional sources for selection of point estimates and ranges.

as obtained from the Vietnamese Demographic and Health Survey. This assumption also was explored in sensitivity analyses (GSO, NIHE, and ORC Macro 2006).

### Consequences for Health

To simulate the impact on health consequences, the number of deaths and nonfatal head injuries attributable to motorcycles in the one-year baseline period was estimated, as was the pre-policy proportion of motorcycle riders using helmets. Helmet effectiveness (expressed as the relative risk of head injury among riders wearing helmets compared to riders not wearing helmets) was estimated using published odds ratios. By accounting for the increase in the proportion of helmeted riders

following the comprehensive helmet policy, the number of deaths and head injuries averted within each quintile during the one-year post-policy evaluation period was simulated (annex tables 11A.3–11A.4 and equations 11A.1–11A.4).

### Consequences for Cost and Affordability

The OOP acute care costs averted by the policy were simulated by subtracting the expected OOP costs of hospitalization in the post-policy period from the expected OOP cost in the baseline period. The expected cost was derived from published estimates on average cost for injury with and without a helmet, taking into account variations in the severity and type of injury based on helmet use (Nguyen, Ivers, and others 2013). These changes in costs were then multiplied by the estimated change in incidence of motorcycle injuries (see annex 11A, equation 11A.5 in table 11A.5).

Empirical research has shown variations in the average direct acute care cost of treatment by income group in Vietnam (Nguyen, Ivers, and others 2013). The average direct acute care cost of treatment in each income quintile was derived by combining the estimated quintile-specific monthly income per capita with the reported 1 percent increase in the cost of treating a traumatic brain injury for every US$10 increase in monthly income per capita (GSO 2010; Nguyen, Ivers, and others 2013). Income losses were calculated by multiplying monthly per capita income by the Vietnamese average absence from work of eight months following traumatic brain injury (Hoang and others 2008).

Two measures of financial risk protection were calculated: cases of poverty averted and catastrophic health expenditures averted. Both measures reflect the reduction in financial hardship that may occur when an injury is averted or when the cost of treatment is reduced. Cases of poverty averted were defined as the number of individuals who, as a result of the helmet policy, would no longer fall below the national poverty line because of a traffic injury. In the baseline model, 21 percent of the population is living in poverty (World Bank 2012). Cases of catastrophic health expenditures averted were defined as the number of people who, as a result of the policy, would no longer be paying more than 25 percent of their annual income per capita on direct acute care costs. The threshold for a catastrophic health expenditure varies depending on the literature, but it generally lies between 2.5 percent and 15 percent of household income or between 10 percent and 45 percent of disposable income (Wagstaff and van Doorslaer 2003). For a population of $P$ individuals with a certain income distribution,[1] the number of people injured before the intervention in each quintile was multiplied by the probability that they would face poverty or a catastrophic health expenditure. The same estimate was recalculated using the post-intervention injury rate and costs. Subtraction yielded the number of cases of poverty or catastrophic health expenditure that were averted in the population (see annex 11A, equation 11A.6 in table 11A.5).

The government's cost of implementing the comprehensive helmet legislation in Vietnam was approximated by multiplying the estimated costs per capita of implementing the legislation in South-East Asia (including legislation and program management, media, enforcement, and helmet purchase) by the population of Vietnam (Wagstaff and van Doorslaer 2003).[2]

## Sensitivity Analysis

A univariate sensitivity analysis was performed on key model inputs to test their influence on the findings. Upper and lower bounds for the inputs were obtained from published studies wherever possible and were otherwise derived from available data or plausibly estimated (annex 11A, table 11A.1). One critical sensitivity analysis explored the impact of substandard helmets in Vietnam, accounting for less safe designs (half-head or cap style), failure to meet quality standards, and inadequate fastening of chin straps. Each safety deficit was assumed to halve the reduction in relative risk of death or injury provided by the helmet, and this was combined with the approximate population prevalence of each deficit to estimate a lower bound of population-level helmet effectiveness (see annex 11A, table 11A.1 and figure 11A.9).

Additional sensitivity analyses were performed to evaluate the influence of model input distributional assumptions on the distribution of health and financial benefits across income quintiles (annex 11A, table 11A.2). The distribution of motorcycle deaths and nonfatal injuries across quintiles, the distribution of pre-policy helmet use, and the distribution of post-policy helmet use across quintiles were varied in these analyses, first alone and then by multivariate sensitivity analysis.

## RESULTS

The results of the analysis are presented in table 11.2.

Assuming that helmets in Vietnam are as effective as helmets in HIC, the simulation estimates that the 2007 helmet policy prevented approximately 2,200 deaths and 29,000 head injuries, saved individuals US$18 million in direct acute care costs, and averted US$29 million in individual income losses in the year following its introduction (table 11.2). Countrywide implementation of the policy cost the government an estimated US$24 million, although this cost was offset by revenue arising from the collection of fines and enforcement (Chisholm and others 2012). From a government perspective (which accounts for implementation costs only), the helmet policy cost about US$11,000 per death averted or US$800 per nonfatal injury averted. From a societal perspective (which sums individuals' OOP direct acute care cost savings, individuals' averted income losses, and government's implementation costs), the policy saved approximately US$11,000 per death averted or US$800 per nonfatal injury averted.

The main distributional analysis assumed that the distribution of traffic injury reflected the distribution of motorcycle ownership across income quintiles and

**Table 11.2** Estimated Reduction in Death, Injury, and Cost Attributable to the Mandatory Helmet Legislation in Vietnam

| Indicator | Pre-policy estimate (attributable to motorcycles) | Estimated absolute reduction (range)[a] | Estimated relative reduction (%) (range)[a] |
|---|---|---|---|
| Deaths | 7,400 | 2,200 (1,000–2,700) | 29 (14–37) |
| Nonfatal head injuries | 54,100 | 29,000 (12,700–44,500) | 54 (23–82) |
| Direct acute care costs for nonfatal head injuries (US$, millions) | 35 | 18 (8–28) | 52 (24–81) |
| Income losses following death or nonfatal head injury (US$, millions) | 63 | 29 (11–40) | 46 (18–64) |
| Direct acute care costs plus income losses (US$, millions) | 98 | 48 (24–72) | 49 (24–73) |

a. Values in parentheses represent lower and upper bounds obtained on univariate sensitivity analyses.

**Figure 11.1** Deaths and Nonfatal Head Injuries Averted as a Result of the Helmet Policy in Vietnam, by Income Quintile (1 = Poorest, 5 = Richest)

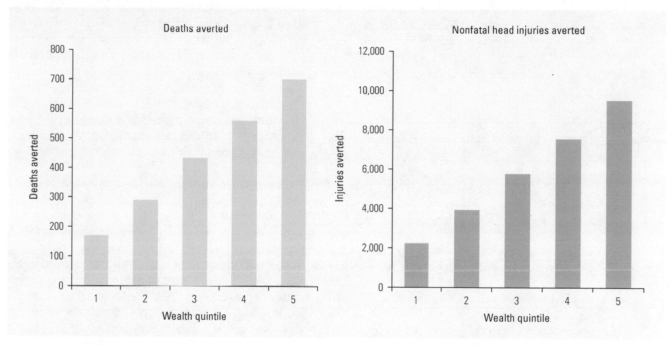

found that the wealthiest quintiles own the greatest number of motorcycles and thus accrue a larger share of the health and financial benefits (in absolute terms) from the 2007 helmet policy (figure 11.1). With regard to financial risk protection, traffic injury is so expensive to treat that any injury averted also would avert catastrophic health expenditures (figures 11.2 and 11.3). In other words, both before and after the policy, traffic injury leads to health expenditures that exceed 25 percent of per capita income, amounting to more than 22,000 cases of catastrophic health expenditure averted.

The helmet legislation likely has averted poverty for persons in the second and third income quintiles, amounting to nearly 11,000 cases of poverty averted. Persons in the first quintile are poor already, and the cost is not so high that those in the fourth and fifth quintiles will be thrust into poverty.

Table 11.2 presents the lower and upper values obtained in a univariate sensitivity analysis. The sensitivity analysis that accounted for substandard and inadequately fastened helmets yielded the lowest estimates of deaths and injuries averted, a finding with

**Figure 11.2** Out-of-Pocket Costs Averted as a Result of the Helmet Policy in Vietnam, by Income Quintile (1 = Poorest, 5 = Richest) *2012 US$, millions*

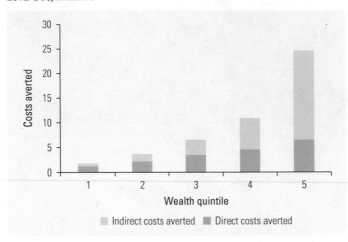

**Figure 11.3** Financial Risk Protection Afforded as a Result of the Helmet Policy in Vietnam, by Income Quintile (1 = Poorest, 5 = Richest)

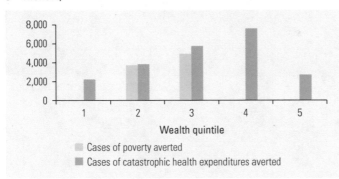

*Note:* No data are available for cases of poverty averted for quintiles 1, 4, and 5.

clear implications for policy and enforcement. Deaths, injuries, and OOP costs averted were extremely sensitive to variation in the proportion of motorcycle injuries anticipated to cause head injury. Direct costs of acute care averted also were highly sensitive to variation in the average costs of acute care for crash victims with and without helmets. The univariate sensitivity analyses, along with those for poverty and catastrophic health expenditures averted, are presented graphically in the annex (figures 11A.1–11A.5 and 11A.9).

Distributional sensitivity analyses demonstrated that the distribution of health benefits is highly sensitive to variation in the pre-policy distribution of motorcycle injury across quintiles. Both health and financial benefits accrue disproportionately to the poor

under conditions of perfectly equitable pre-policy motorcycle injury and death. This finding is amplified when occurring in conjunction with highly inequitable pre-policy helmet use (with highest use among the wealthy) and perfectly equitable post-policy helmet use (annex 11A, figures 11A.6–11A.8).

## DISCUSSION

Assuming that helmets in Vietnam are as effective as those in HIC, the 2007 comprehensive helmet policy prevented approximately 2,200 deaths and 29,000 head injuries, saved individuals US$18 million in direct acute care costs, and averted US$29 million in individual income losses in the year following its introduction. The combination of anticipated health and financial benefits makes a comprehensive helmet policy strongly preferable to the pre-policy status quo. These findings suggest that similar comprehensive legislation and enforcement should be considered in countries where motorcycles are pervasive, yet helmet use is less common.

In the simulations, the relative reduction in motorcycle crash deaths fell from 29 percent to 14 percent after accounting for the proliferation of less-effective helmets in Vietnam. Policy makers wanting to enact an effective comprehensive helmet law might consider making provisions for adequate regulatory enforcement of manufacturers, retailers, and motorcycle riders to ensure that helmets are of adequate quality and appropriately fastened.

The results of the ECEA suggest that the wealthy likely accrued a large share of the absolute health and financial benefits resulting from the helmet use legislation. This finding was dependent on the assumption that the risk of RTI tracked with motorcycle ownership. In contrast, under all of the conditions tested, the legislation was likely to have prevented a greater number of cases of poverty resulting from motorcycle accidents among the near poor and middle-income quintiles. This supports the conclusion that injury prevention also is poverty prevention among individuals of lesser wealth. In settings with universal health insurance, cost savings from a comprehensive helmet policy (potentially substantial, as the wealthy are known to use a disproportionate share of public health care) might also be freed up for use on other health priorities (Wagstaff 2010).

The validity of the model's estimates are supported by the results of prior research. The findings anticipate a 29 percent reduction in deaths from motorcycle accidents and a 17 percent reduction in deaths from all traffic accidents. These results are similar to the 36 percent reduction in deaths from motorcycle accidents generally anticipated with helmet legislation and the 18 percent reduction in deaths from all traffic accidents reported in Vietnam in the year following introduction of the helmet legislation (Passmore, Nguyen, and others 2010; Passmore, Tu, and others 2010). The results also are in harmony with the results of regional evaluations of helmet use legislation (Chiu and others 2000; Ichikawa, Chadbunchachai, and Marui 2003; Tsai and Hemenway 1999).

## Limitations

Several limitations are related to the model and its inputs. First, the modeling study estimated the anticipated effectiveness and cost-effectiveness of the 2007 comprehensive helmet policy in Vietnam but did not directly measure the benefits or costs. The published academic literature has not yet articulated the observed benefits and costs of this policy, despite the crucial importance of these values for evaluating policy success. Second, many of the inputs used (including pre-policy deaths and injuries attributable to motorcycles, acute care costs, and policy implementation costs) were not directly available and had to be derived or estimated from published reports. The use of academic and non-governmental reports rather than government surveillance data improves the quality of data but diminishes the local applicability of the results. Third, the main analysis ignored the influence of substandard helmets in Vietnam because of the absence of reliable estimates of the relative effectiveness of the substandard helmets, particularly in a setting with relatively low traffic speeds (Ackaah and others 2013).[3]

The analysis was also limited by several assumptions made in constructing the model. The assumption that the number of motorcycles on the road was the same before and after the policy rendered the estimated benefits more conservative, interpretable, and generalizable (Le and Blum 2013). Changes in the prevalence of speeding and alcohol use, increased enforcement of traffic laws not related to helmets, changes in road maintenance and congestion, and other secular trends were ignored. The cost estimates did not account for a potential increase in nonhead injuries among riders whose lives were saved by helmet use. The simulated number of deaths averted represents less than 10 percent of the simulated number of injuries averted, so the potential increase in nonhead injuries was anticipated to be minimal. Lastly, insufficient information made estimating the higher costs for individuals and the higher revenue for government resulting from improved enforcement and higher fines resulting from the helmet policy impossible.

The potential for impoverishment resulting from helmet infraction fines was assumed to be uncommon and relatively inconsequential.

## Cost-Effectiveness

The results suggest that Vietnam's 2007 helmet legislation was cost-effective. Large health and financial benefits accrued to the wealthy, yet the policy also provided significant health benefits and substantial financial risk protection to Vietnam's poorest citizens. As countries develop and more individuals acquire motorcycles, we are likely to see a reversal in the distribution of benefits from helmet legislation. Increased ridership among the poor will increase the risk of injury, yet improved helmets are likely to be worn only by the wealthy. The issues of road traffic safety are only going to grow as motorcycles become more accessible throughout the region. Fortunately, most countries have implemented helmet legislation. Others, such as Cambodia, have recently expanded their policies to include passengers and children. The implications of road safety policy go well beyond health, as our analysis has shown. Policy makers wishing to account for such effects may want to use ECEA to understand the likely influence of policy on equity.

## AUTHOR CONTRIBUTIONS AND ACKNOWLEDGMENTS

This chapter is based on the following article: Olson, Z., J. A. Staples, C. N. Mock, N. P. Nguyen, A. M. Bachani, and others. 2016. "Helmet Regulation in Vietnam: impact on Health, Equity, and Medical Impoverishment." *Injury Prevention* 1–6. Epub January 4, 2016. doi:10.1136 /injuryprev-2015-041650.

Zachary Olson, John A. Staples, Charles N. Mock, Rachel Nugent, and Stéphane Verguet were responsible for the design of the study. Olson and Staples had full access to all of the data and take responsibility for the integrity of the data and the accuracy of the data analysis. They also prepared the initial draft of the manuscript. All authors contributed to data interpretation, revised the manuscript, and provided approval for submission.

The study was funded with support from the Bill and Melinda Gates Foundation to the Disease Control Priorities Network. Olson was funded in part by National Institute of Child Health and Human Development grant T32-HD007275. No funding organization was involved in the design and conduct of the study; collection, management, analysis, and interpretation of the data; preparation, review, and approval of the manuscript; or decision to submit the manuscript for analysis.

The authors thank Dan Chisholm, Jonathan Passmore, Dean Jamison, Carol Levin, Beth E. Ebel, Mara K. Hansen, Jenny Nguyen, Clint Pecenka, and Alex Quistberg for their insightful comments.

## ANNEX

The annex to this chapter is as follows. It is available at http://dcp-3.org/environment.

- Annex 11A. Supplementary Tables and Figures on the Effects of Vietnam's Mandatory Helmet Legislation on Health, Equity, and Medical Impoverishment

## NOTES

World Bank Income Classifications as of July 2014 are as follows, based on estimates of gross national income (GNI) per capita for 2013:

- Low-income countries (LICs) = US$1,045 or less
- Middle-income countries (MICs) are subdivided:
  a) lower-middle-income = US$1,046 to US$4,125
  b) upper-middle-income (UMICs) = US$4,126 to US$12,745
- High-income countries (HICs) = US$12,746 or more.

1. A proxy for individual income was extracted from the income distribution of Vietnam derived from its GDP per capita (US$1,200 in 2012 US$) and its Gini index (0.36) (Salem and Mount 1974; World Bank 2012).
2. This number was derived by Dan Chisholm, Jonathon Passmore, and Nguyen Phuong Nam using the same model cited (Chisholm and others 2012).
3. See also *Viet Nam News* 2014.

## REFERENCES

Ackaah, W., F. Afukaar, W. Agyemang, T. Thuy Anh, A. R. Hejar, and others. 2013. "The Use of Non-Standard Motorcycle Helmets in Low- and Middle-Income Countries: A Multicentre Study." *Injury Prevention* 19 (3): 158–63.

Chisholm, D., H. Naci, A. A. Hyder, N. T. Tran, and M. Peden. 2012. "Cost-Effectiveness of Strategies to Combat Road Traffic Injuries in Sub-Saharan Africa and South East Asia: Mathematical Modelling Study." *BMJ* 344: e612.

Chiu, W. T., C. Y. Kuo, C. C. Hung, and M. Chen. 2000. "The Effect of the Taiwan Motorcycle Helmet Use Law on Head Injuries." *American Journal of Public Health* 90 (5): 793–96.

Government of Vietnam. 2007. "Resolution on a Number of Urgent Countermeasures to Curb Traffic Safety and Alleviate Traffic Congestion." Resolution 32/2007/NQ-CP (June 29, 2007), Government of Viet Nam, Hanoi.

GSO (General Statistics Office). 2010. *Vietnam Household Living Standards Survey.* Hanoi: Statistical Publishing House.

GSO, NIHE (National Institute of Hygiene and Epidemiology), and ORC Macro. 2006. *Vietnam Population and AIDS Indicator Survey 2005.* Calverton, MD: GSO, NIHE, and ORC Macro.

Hoang, H., T. Pham, T. Vo, P. Nguyen, C. Doran, and others. 2008. "The Costs of Traumatic Brain Injury Due to Motorcycle Accidents in Hanoi, Vietnam." *Cost Effectiveness and Resource Allocation* 6 (1): 17.

Hung, D. V., M. R. Stevenson, and R. Q. Ivers. 2006. "Prevalence of Helmet Use among Motorcycle Riders in Vietnam." *Injury Prevention* 12 (6): 409–13.

———. 2008. "Motorcycle Helmets in Vietnam: Ownership, Quality, Purchase Price, and Affordability." *Traffic Injury Prevention* 9 (2): 135–43.

Ichikawa, M., W. Chadbunchachai, and E. Marui. 2003. "Effect of the Helmet Act for Motorcyclists in Thailand." *Accident Analysis and Prevention* 35 (2): 183–89.

Le, L. C., and R. W. Blum. 2013. "Road Traffic Injury among Young People in Vietnam: Evidence from Two Rounds of National Adolescent Health Surveys, 2004–2009." *Global Health Action* 6: 1–9.

Liu, B., R. Ivers, R. Norton, S. Boufous, S. Blows, and others. 2008. "Helmets for Preventing Injury in Motorcycle Riders." *Cochrane Database of Systematic Reviews* 1: CD004333.

National Traffic Safety Committee. 2014. "Vietnam Road Traffic Injury Official Estimates." National Traffic Safety Committee, Hanoi.

Ngo, A. D., C. Rao, N. P. Hoa, D. G. Hoy, K. T. Q. Trang, and others. 2012. "Road Traffic Related Mortality in Vietnam: Evidence for Policy from a National Sample Mortality Surveillance System." *BMC Public Health* 12 (July): 561.

Nguyen, H., R. Q. Ivers, S. Jan, A. L. Martiniuk, Q. Li, and others. 2013. "The Economic Burden of Road Traffic Injuries: Evidence from a Provincial General Hospital in Vietnam." *Injury Prevention* 19 (2): 79–84.

Nguyen, H. T., J. Passmore, P. V. Cuong, and N. P. Nguyen. 2013. "Measuring Compliance with Viet Nam's Mandatory Motorcycle Helmet Legislation." *International Journal of Injury Control and Safety Promotion* 20 (2): 192–96.

Passmore, J., L. H. Nguyen, N. P. Nguyen, and J. M. Olive. 2010. "The Formulation and Implementation of a National Helmet Law: A Case Study from Viet Nam." *Bulletin of the World Health Organization* 88 (10): 783–87.

Passmore, J., N. T. Tu, M. A. Luong, N. D. Chinh, and N. P. Nam. 2010. "Impact of Mandatory Motorcycle Helmet Wearing Legislation on Head Injuries in Viet Nam: Results of a Preliminary Analysis." *Traffic Injury Prevention* 11 (2): 202–5.

Pham, K. H., W. X. L. Thi, D. J. Petrie, J. Adams, and C. M. Doran. 2008. "Households' Willingness to Pay for a Motorcycle Helmet in Hanoi, Vietnam." *Applied Health Economics and Health Policy* 6 (2–3): 137–44.

Salem, A. B. Z., and T. D. Mount. 1974. "A Convenient Descriptive Model of Income Distribution: The Gamma Density." *Econometrica* 42 (6): 1115–27.

Tien, T. V., H. T. Phuong, I. Mathauer, and N. T. K. Phuong. 2011. *A Health Financing Review of Viet Nam with a Focus on Social Health Insurance.* Geneva: World Health Organization.

Tsai, M., and D. Hemenway. 1999. "Effect of the Mandatory Helmet Law in Taiwan." *Injury Prevention* 5 (4): 290–91.

Verguet, S., R. Laxminarayan, and D. T. Jamison. 2014. "Universal Public Finance of Tuberculosis Treatment in India: An Extended Cost-Effectiveness Analysis." *Health Economics* 24 (3): 318–32.

Verguet, S., S. Murphy, B. Anderson, K. A. Johansson, R. Glass, and others. 2013. "Public Finance of Rotavirus Vaccination in India and Ethiopia: An Extended Cost-Effectiveness Analysis." *Vaccine* 31 (42): 4902–10.

Verguet, S., Z. D. Olson, J. B. Babigumira, D. Desalegn, K. A. Johansson, and others. 2015. "Health Gains and Financial Risk Protection Afforded by Public Financing of Selected Interventions in Ethiopia: An Extended Cost-Effectiveness Analysis." *The Lancet Global Health* 3 (5): e288–96.

*Viet Nam News*. 2014. "Police Struggle to Identify Substandard Helmets." *Viet Nam News*, July 2. http://vietnamnews.vn /society/256910/police-struggle-to-identify-substandard -helmets.html.

Wagstaff, A. 2010. "Measuring Financial Protection in Health." In *Performance Measurement for Health System Improvement: Experiences, Challenges, and Prospects*, edited by P. C. Smith, E. Mossialos, I. Papanicolas, and S. Leatherman, 114–37. Cambridge, U.K.: Cambridge University Press.

Wagstaff, A., and E. van Doorslaer. 2003. "Catastrophe and Impoverishment in Paying for Health Care: With Applications to Vietnam 1993–1998." *Health Economics* 12 (11): 921–34.

WHO (World Health Organization). 2004. *World Report on Road Traffic Injury Prevention*. Geneva: WHO. http://www .who.int/violence_injury_prevention/publications/road _traffic/world_report/en/.

———. 2009. "Road Safety Status: Country Profile, Vietnam." WHO, Geneva. http://www.who.int/violence_injury _prevention/road_safety_status/country_profiles/viet_nam.pdf.

———. 2010. *World Health Statistics 2010*. Geneva: WHO. http://www.who.int/whosis/whostat/EN_WHS10_Full .pdf.

———. 2013a. *Global Status Report on Road Safety 2013*. Geneva: WHO. http://www.who.int/violence_injury _prevention/road_safety_status/2013/en/index.html.

———. 2013b. "Road Safety Fact Sheet, Western Pacific Region." WHO, Geneva. http://www.wpro.who.int/mediacentre /factsheets/fs_20130627/en/.

———. 2013c. "Road Safety Status: Country Profile, Vietnam." WHO, Geneva. http://www.who.int/violence_injury _prevention/road_safety_status/2013/country_profiles /viet_nam.pdf.

———. 2015. *Study on Motorcycle Helmet Quality in Viet Nam*. WHO and Hanoi School of Public Health. http:// www.wpro.who.int/vietnam/topics/injuries/helmet_quality _vietnam.pdf.

World Bank. 2012. *World Development Indicators*. Washington, DC: World Bank. http://data.worldbank.org/data-catalog /world-development-indicators.

World Bank and IHME (Institute for Health Metrics and Evaluation). 2014. *Transport for Health: The Global Burden of Disease from Motorized Road Transport*. Seattle, WA: IHME.

Yu, W. Y., C. Y. Chen, W. T. Chiu, and M. R. Lin. 2011. "Effectiveness of Different Types of Motorcycle Helmets and Effects of Their Improper Use on Head Injuries." *International Journal of Epidemiology* 40 (3): 794–803.

# Chapter 12

# Household Energy Interventions and Health and Finances in Haryana, India: An Extended Cost-Effectiveness Analysis

Ajay Pillarisetti, Dean T. Jamison, and Kirk R. Smith

## INTRODUCTION

Approximately 40 percent of the world's population relies on solid fuels, including wood, dung, grass, crop residues, and coal, for cooking (Bonjour and others 2013). Household air pollution (HAP) arising from this use of solid fuels results in 3 million to 4 million deaths yearly from acute lower respiratory infection (ALRI) in children and chronic obstructive pulmonary disease (COPD), ischemic heart disease (IHD), stroke, and lung cancer in adults. This burden constitutes approximately 5 percent of global mortality, ranking highest among all environmental risk factors contributing to global ill health (Forouzanfar and others 2015; Smith and others 2014).

In India, the reliance on solid fuels and the estimated related burden of disease are pronounced. An estimated 770 million individuals—approximately 70 percent of the total population (Government of India 2011)—living in 160 million households continue to use solid fuels as a primary energy source for cooking (Venkataraman and others 2010). Among all risk factors contributing to ill health in India, exposure to HAP from cooking ranks second for mortality, with approximately 925,000 premature deaths yearly; it ranks third for lost disability-adjusted life years (DALYs), amounting to approximately 25 million lost

DALYs per year (Forouzanfar and others 2015).[1] An estimated 4 percent of the deaths occur in children under age five years because of pneumonia, which overall accounts for 12 percent of total child deaths in India.

Attempts to reduce this burden fall into two primary categories: (1) those that seek to make biomass combustion cleaner and more efficient, and (2) those that seek to replace biomass use with liquid fuels or electricity (Foell and others 2011; Smith and Sagar 2015). Private and public sector actors have taken action in India to reduce this large burden of disease. Private sector endeavors include research, development, marketing, and distribution of biomass stoves by large multinational corporations, such as Philips and BP, and smaller Indian and international firms, such as Envirofit, Greenway, First Energy, BioLite, and Prakti. In all cases, the evaluations of the viability of these interventions for long-term use, which would be required to reduce exposures and thus the health burden, have been mixed (Brooks and others 2016; Pillarisetti and others 2014; Sambandam and others 2015).

The government of India has undertaken a number of policy initiatives to address HAP through improved biomass combustion, beginning in the 1980s with a failed National Programme on Improved Chulhas

Corresponding author: Ajay Pillarisetti, Division of Environmental Health Sciences, School of Public Health, University of California, Berkeley, CA, United States; ajaypillarisetti@gmail.com.

(Kishore and Ramana 2002) and continuing in 2010 with a National Biomass Cookstoves Initiative. More recently, two innovative programs—the Give It Up (GIU) and Smokeless Village (SV) campaigns—are seeking to bring clean cooking via liquefied petroleum gas (LPG) to the rural poor (Smith and Sagar 2015). Both GIU, which encourages better-off Indian households to voluntarily give up their LPG subsidies and redirects those subsidies one-for-one to below-poverty-line (BPL) families, and SV, which connects every household in a village to LPG, occur in close collaboration with India's three national oil companies. In mid-2016, Indian Prime Minister Narendra Modi introduced Pradhan Mantri Ujjwala Yojana (Ujjwala), a program to extend the GIU and SV campaigns by making free LPG connections available to all BPL households. This policy will affect approximately 50 million households.[2] These programs have the potential to substantially reduce the mortality and morbidity associated with the use of solid fuels for cooking, if one assumes near-complete transitions to clean fuels (Smith and Sagar 2015).

This chapter describes an extended cost-effectiveness analysis (ECEA) of policies designed to promote uptake of hypothetical HAP control interventions aligned with three national government programs:

- A low-cost, mud chimney stove, as was promoted in the National Programme on Improved Chulhas that operated from about 1983 to 2002 (We evaluate this program under the same current conditions as the other programs.)
- An advanced combustion cookstove, like that being promoted in the current National Biomass Cookstoves Initiative
- A transition to LPG being promoted in the national Give It Up campaign.

Our scenarios simplify complex behavioral issues by assuming full use of all intervention stoves in order to estimate best-case health and welfare benefits of clean cooking transitions. We evaluate the sensitivity of our use assumption in annex 12A. Our goal is to indicate the types of policy-relevant analyses that are possible using ECEA and the magnitude of potential benefits of LPG adoption.

Traditional economic cost-effectiveness analyses, such as that by Mehta and Shahpar (2004), focus on the U.S. dollars spent per death or per DALY averted. ECEA also considers the financial implications of policies across wealth strata of a population (introduced in Verguet, Laxminarayan, and Jamison 2015), in this case, by income quintile. ECEAs assess the consequences of financial or other policies that influence the aggregate uptake of an intervention and its health and financial consequences across income groups. Verguet, Laxminarayan and Jamison (2015), for example, looked at public finance and enhanced borrowing capacity as policies to affect tuberculosis treatment in India. Verguet and others (2015) assessed the consequences of a policy to increase tobacco taxes in China. Including distributional analysis by income quintile enables novel policy evaluations, as well as an evaluation of the GIU campaign.

This ECEA focuses on policies to reduce exposure to HAP in Haryana, India. This state has a population of 20 million, about 55 percent of whom use solid fuels for cooking, although significant heterogeneity exists between both rural and urban areas and between available datasets for analyses. In addition, we benefit from the availability of published continuous exposure-response relationships for HAP-related diseases and a fuel gathering–based time metric, allowing us to quantify the potential earnings gained by use of a stove that improves fuel efficiency.[3]

## Review of Economic Analyses of Household Energy Interventions

Existing peer-reviewed literature on the costs, benefits, and cost-effectiveness of HAP interventions is sparse (Jeuland, Pattanayak, and Bluffstone 2015). A limited number of global (Hutton and others 2006; Hutton, Rehfuess, and Tediosi 2007; Jeuland and Pattanayak 2012; Mehta and Shahpar 2004) and geography-specific (Arcenas and others 2010; Aunan and others 2013; Malla and others 2011; Pant 2011) economic evaluations exists. A short review follows.

Mehta and Shahpar (2004) found wide variation in the cost-effectiveness of improved stoves and LPG and propane interventions across the World Health Organization subregions, but their analysis did not consider the cost of illness and treatment or potential non-health benefits of transitioning to cleaner cooking. Hutton and others (2006) and Hutton, Rehfuess, and Tediosi (2007) performed a global cost-benefit analysis of eight scenarios that reduced exposure through a transition to either clean fuels or clean biomass stoves and considered benefits including improved health, decreased emissions of climate-altering pollutants, fewer lost work days, and time savings. They found that both the clean fuel transition and the improved stove transition had favorable cost-benefit ratios of 4.3 and approximately 60, respectively. Unlike Hutton and others (2006) and Mehtha and Shahpar (2004), both of which used regional scale inputs, Jeuland and Pattanayak (2012) modeled costs and benefits from household and societal perspectives for clean fuel and clean stove technologies. They found that transitions away from traditional cooking yield variable results; some interventions have high probabilities of net costs to households and societies. Their modeling indicates that LPG, kerosene, and improved charcoal stoves have the highest probability of net positive benefits at household and societal scales. They note that the findings are sensitive to a number of factors, including emission rates and fuel costs.

Cost-benefit analysis has been applied in a number of geography-specific studies, including in Nepal (Malla and others 2011; Pant 2011), China (Aunan and others 2013), the Western Pacific region (Arcenas and others 2010), and Kenya and Sudan (Malla and others 2011). Malla and others (2011) found that across three separate interventions in Nepal (smoke hood), Kenya (LPG or smoke hoods), and Sudan (LPG), benefits exceeded costs over the 10-year intervention period, although there was significant heterogeneity among study sites. They note, however, that the effect of monetized health benefits was relatively small across all sites, compared to time and fuel savings. In China, Aunan and others (2013) evaluated transitions in no-chimney or chimney stove homes to either second-generation improved cookstoves or community-scale pellet stoves. In all cases, benefit-cost ratios were positive (central estimate range of 3.3–14.7), and the largest ratios occurred by switching away from chimneyless stoves. Only health benefits were monetized. Similarly, Pant (2011) and Arcenas and others (2010) used cost-of-illness and value of a statistical life, respectively, to assess the effect of household energy transitions by using survey data. Pant (2011) modeled the effect of a transition from dung fuel to biogas, noting the health cost per household—driven by medication expenses— to be 61.3 percent higher in dung-burning households than the cost of fuel in biogas households.

## Clean Fuel Intervention Costs

Interventions considering either fuels—such as LPG or natural gas—or electricity must contend with both upfront and recurrent costs. In India, before 2015, every cylinder of LPG sold to household customers was subsidized at the point of sale, regardless of the income of the household. In 2015, the government announced that cylinders would be sold at full price to all consumers, but that households would have subsidies transferred directly to their bank accounts—the PAHAL scheme (Tripathi, Sagar, and Smith 2015). Among others goals, this policy sought to prevent small and medium enterprises from being able to buy subsidized fuel intended for households from the black market. Current subsidies are approximately one-fourth of the cost of a cylinder, although they vary with the market price of LPG.

As part of the GIU campaign, in addition to the redistribution of the subsidy to the poor, the corporate social responsibility funds of the three national oil companies were used to cover the upfront costs of the regulator and cylinder deposits—a subsidy of approximately 2,000 rupees (Rs) (approximately US$30) made available to BPL households, an official category that varies somewhat by state. Some states also provide a stove to families receiving the GIU benefit. According to the Ministry of Petroleum (2016), 10 million middle-income households had given up their LPG subsidy as of May 1, 2016 (Smith and Sagar 2015). Ujjwalla extends this by providing the same subsidy to all BPL households through use of a new allotment of about US$1.2 billion of Indian government funds (*Times of India* 2016).

## Estimation of Health Benefits of Clean Cooking

Understanding improved health attributable to a HAP-reducing intervention, such as a transition to LPG, relies on complex exposure science and behavioral processes. The relationship between exposure to HAP and health is nonlinear and is described through a set of integrated-exposure response (IER) (Burnett and others 2014) curves that link exposure to particulate matter with an effective diameter of less than 2.5 micrometers ($PM_{2.5}$, a key component of combustion-generated air pollution) with a number of health endpoints. IERs currently exist for ALRI, IHD, stroke, lung cancer, and COPD. The IERs integrate exposure data from a range of $PM_{2.5}$ sources, including HAP, active tobacco smoking, secondhand tobacco smoke, and ambient air pollution.

The continuous nature of the exposure-response relationships allows modeling of the potential health benefits of a reduction in exposure to $PM_{2.5}$ attributable to a specific intervention by disease type (Pillarisetti, Mehta, and Smith 2016). However, quantifying exposure reductions is challenging and relies on either expensive and intrusive monitoring of individuals or sophisticated modeling of pollution levels and time-activity patterns. Exposure reductions are complicated by issues of compliance or *stove stacking*, the phenomenon of continuing to use the traditional cooking technology even though a new technology or fuel has come into the household (Brooks and others 2016; Johnson and Chiang 2015; Pillarisetti and others 2014; Ruiz-Mercado and others 2011; Sambandam and others 2015; Smith and others 2015). However, this situation is not unusual in health interventions, where provision of a healthier technology needs to be followed by policies to encourage long-term use and elimination of the unhealthy behavior (for example, with condoms, bednets, and latrines). In a sense, then, the analyses here represent an efficacy approach—the best that could be achieved for each intervention.

To address these issues and others, we have developed (1) an online tool that uses the IERs and relevant background data to estimate the potential effect of an intervention known as the Household Air Pollution Intervention Tool (HAPIT) (Pillarisetti, Mehta, and Smith 2016) and (2) standard protocols to use HAPIT to estimate averted ill health (Smith and others 2014).

## METHODS

### Estimation of Reductions in Morbidity and Mortality Resulting from HAP Interventions

This chapter uses a modified version of HAPIT (based on the version described in Pillarisetti, Mehta, and Smith [2016] but modified to facilitate evaluation of multiple scenarios at a subnational scale) to estimate the averted deaths and DALYs attributable to an intervention over a five-year period. Briefly, HAPIT uses national background health data and the methods and databases developed as part of the Comparative Risk Assessment (Lim and others 2012), a component of the Global Burden of Disease Study 2010 (GBD 2010) (Lozano and others 2012), to determine pre- and post-intervention population attributable fractions. The burden of disease averted can then be determined by multiplying the background disease-specific burden by the difference in population attributable fractions. Notably, therefore, HAPIT incorporates exposure-response functions for five separate diseases associated with air pollution in recent international assessments based on synthesizing results from multiple individual epidemiological studies in a number of countries. It estimates the effect of interventions based on the background conditions of each of the diseases in the country considered (in this case, India). Pillarisetti, Mehta, and Smith (2016) provide a detailed explanation of HAPIT and its underlying calculations.

Background disease data for Haryana were not readily accessible. Instead, underlying disease burden data for India from the GBD 2010 were scaled by the proportion of the population living in Haryana. To estimate background disease characteristics by income quintile (table 12.1) in Haryana, we distributed premature deaths for children and adults and DALYs according to the fraction of all solid fuel–using households in Haryana residing in a specific income quintile, as determined through analysis of the Indian Human Development Survey (IHDS) 2005–06 (Barik and Desai 2014; Desai, Vanneman, and National Council of Applied Economic Research 2005). The uncertainty in the background disease estimates

provided by the Institute for Health Metrics and Evaluation in the Global Burden of Disease Study 2010 is used to bound estimates of averted DALYs and deaths attributable to an intervention.

We also evaluated two additional modes of distributing background disease (annex 12A). In the first, disease data were split on the basis of the overall percentage of Haryana's population in each quintile, calculated by multiplying the number of households per quintile by the number of people per household. In the second, we assumed (1) that all quintiles had equal populations and age distributions and (2) that solid fuel use (SFU) linearly decreased as wealth increased, beginning at 90 percent in quintile (Q) 1 and ending at 60 percent SFU in Q5.

### Evaluation of the Consequences of Policy

We evaluate the effect of policies leading to 100 percent penetration and adoption of three interventions—a simple mud chimney stove; a fan-assisted, forced-draft semi-gasifier, also known as a blower stove; and an expansion of LPG—on exposure to $PM_{2.5}$ and subsequent ill health in Haryana, India (table 12.2). Although each scenario is grounded in either past or ongoing policy initiatives (discussed in the introduction), we focus on a simulation of potential benefits of these policies under aspirational conditions. We did, however, assess the sensitivity of our findings to the assumption of full adoption (annex 12A) by modeling a scenario with high adoption of chimney stoves (90 percent) and moderate adoption of blower stoves (65 percent) and LPG stoves (50 percent).

Simple mud chimney stoves cost approximately US$10 (Dutta and others 2007), while blower stoves cost approximately US$60. We assume that chimney stoves have low maintenance costs and work for one year and then provide no benefit, which is consistent with surveys in India. Similarly, blower stoves have low yearly maintenance costs, but they need to be replaced once every three years. The transition to LPG incurs a number of costs, including the cost of the LPG stove (approximately US$20), and the connection fee, security deposit, and administrative costs for the first cylinder (approximately US$30). Cylinder refills cost approximately US$8.70 per cylinder unsubsidized and US$6.60 per cylinder subsidized. Families use approximately nine cylinders per year, on average, across India. Total costs to the government are described in table 12.5 later in this chapter.

Using exposure models developed with data from India, we assume the pre-intervention exposure to $PM_{2.5}$ for adults is 337 micrograms per cubic meter ($\mu g/m^3$)

**Table 12.1** Background Disease Burden in India and in Haryana, India, by Income Quintile

| | ALRI[a] | | COPD[b] | | IHD[b] | | Lung Cancer[b] | | Stroke[b] | | Solid fuel use (%) | Population (millions) |
|---|---|---|---|---|---|---|---|---|---|---|---|---|
| | Deaths | DALYs (thousands) | Deaths | DALYs (thousands) | Deaths | DALYs (thousands) | Deaths | DALYs (thousands) | Deaths | DALYs (thousands) | | |
| India | 200,000 | 17,000 | 910,000 | 26,000 | 1,100,000 | 26,000 | 83,000 | 2,100 | 610,000 | 12,000 | 63 | 1,000 |
| Haryana | 4,600 | 400 | 21,000 | 600 | 26,000 | 600 | 1,900 | 50 | 14,000 | 280 | 55[2] | 20 |
| Q1 (Poorest) | 1,000 | 90 | 4,600 | 130 | 5,700 | 130 | 420 | 10 | 3,100 | 60 | 89 | |
| Q2 | 1,000 | 90 | 4,800 | 140 | 6,000 | 140 | 440 | 10 | 3,200 | 65 | 90 | |
| Q3 | 1,000 | 90 | 4,600 | 130 | 5,700 | 130 | 420 | 10 | 3,100 | 60 | 88 | 4 |
| Q4 | 780 | 70 | 3,600 | 100 | 4,400 | 100 | 320 | 10 | 2,400 | 50 | 66 | |
| Q5 (Wealthiest) | 730 | 60 | 3,400 | 95 | 4,200 | 100 | 310 | 10 | 2,200 | 45 | 62 | |

*Sources:* Global Burden of Disease Study 2010, India country profile (IHME 2015) (disease burden data); IHDS 2005–06 (Desai, Vanneman, and National Council of Applied Economic Research 2005) (population data); Census of India 2011 (Government of India 2011) (solid fuel use).

*Note:* ALRI = acute lower respiratory infection; COPD = chronic obstructive pulmonary disease; DALYs = disability-adjusted life years; IHD = ischemic heart disease; Q = quintile.

a. ALRI in children under age five years. Apportioned by the percentage of all solid fuel–using households in each quintile

b. Chronic outcomes in adults.

**Table 12.2** Potential Interventions in Haryana, India

| Intervention | Description | Target population | Existing coverage,[a] % (quintile) | Proposed coverage[b] (%) | Exposure reduction (%) | Reduction in biomass fuel use (%) |
|---|---|---|---|---|---|---|
| Chimney stove | A simple mud-brick chimney stove with two potholes | $3.4 \times 10^6$ households in Haryana | 11 (Q1), 10 (Q2), 12 (Q3), 24 (Q4), 28 (Q5) | 100 | 50 | 15 |
| Blower stove | A single pothole semi-gasifier stove | $2.6 \times 10^6$ households using unclean fuels[c] | | 100 | 63 | 42 |
| LPG | Fuel stored as liquid under slight pressure, burned as a gas | | | 100 | 90 | 100 |

*Sources:* IHDS 2005–06 (Desai, Vanneman, and National Council of Applied Economic Research 2015) (chimney stove, blower stove, and LPG); Census of India 2011 (Government of India 2011) (chimney stove); Bailis and others 2007 (chimney stove); Sambandam and others 2015 (blower stove).

*Note:* LPG = liquefied petroleum gas.

a. Coverage equals the percentage of households in Haryana currently using an equivalent or better technology. For LPG, this includes households using LPG, electricity, or biogas but does not indicate exclusive use of these clean cooking technologies.

b. This comprises the total population (that does not currently have an equivalent or better cooking technology) to cover by a specific intervention.

c. Unclean fuels include the following Census of India 2011 categories: firewood, crop residue, and cowdung cake; coal, lignite, and charcoal; and kerosene. Eighty-five percent of these households are rural.

and 150 μg/m³ for children (Balakrishnan and others 2013; Northcross and others 2010; Pillarisetti, Mehta, and Smith 2016; Smith and others 2014). We scale the central estimate of exposure by the respective exposure reduction (table 12.2) attributable to a given intervention. For this analysis, we estimate intervention costs and benefits across five years, child health gains accrue instantly at the start of each year, and adult health gains are weighted using the U.S. Environmental Protection Agency cessation lag (U.S. EPA 2004) model. For simplicity, averted deaths and DALYs are reported in total. For all evaluated interventions, we consider deployments only in households using biomass fuels in traditional cookstoves.

## Household Expenditures

We assume households take responsibility for replacing stoves after their useful lifetime has passed. For this analysis, households replace a blower stove once during the five years of the evaluation, a useful lifetime for this class of interventions consistent with evidence from the literature (Pillarisetti and others 2014; Sambandam and others 2015). We assume that a gas stove needs no replacement during the five years of this assessment and that households do not replace their chimney stove after the first year, consistent with findings from the National Programme on Improved Chulhas (Venkataraman and others 2010).

We also assume that the averted ill health attributable to this publicly financed intervention results in lower household medical expenditures. Expenditures averted are based on the probability of seeking care for acute and chronic conditions and the combined inpatient and outpatient costs of such visits, including drugs, hospital visits, and transportation to and from clinics. To calculate the expenditure averted by complete adoption of an intervention, we scale the cost of hospital or doctor visits and related expenditures by the relative reduction in DALYs attributable to an intervention separately for acute (ALRI) and chronic (COPD, IHD, stroke, and lung cancer) conditions. For example, for a hypothetical intervention that reduces DALYs associated with chronic diseases by 10 percent, we assume a 10 percent reduction in health care–related expenditure on chronic diseases.

Treatment-seeking behaviors and associated costs are derived from IHDS (Desai, Vanneman, and National Council of Applied Economic Research 2005) and IHDS summary documents (Barik and Desai 2014). Approximately 94 percent of households across India seek treatment for short-term illnesses, defined as fever, cough, and diarrhea. This figure is consistent with Haryana data extracted from IHDS databases and is applied equally for all quintiles. Similarly, we apply national treatment-seeking percentages by quintile to the chronic illnesses of concern. Treatment-seeking behaviors and associated costs[4] by quintile are described in table 12.3.

Additionally, we translate the increase in fuel efficiency attributable to an intervention into weekly time savings by multiplying the increase in fuel

**Table 12.3** Treatment-Seeking Behaviors and Associated Costs

| Disease | Behavior and cost | Q1 | Q2 | Q3 | Q4 | Q5 |
|---|---|---|---|---|---|---|
| Acute diseases (ALRI) | Treatment (%) | 94 | 94 | 94 | 94 | 94 |
| | Median cost (US$) | 17 | 14 | 10 | 18 | 12 |
| Chronic diseases (IHD, COPD, lung cancer, stroke) | Treatment (%) | 88 | 86 | 90 | 94 | 95 |
| | Median cost (US$) | 19 | 20 | 22 | 24 | 38 |

*Sources:* Data extracted from IHDS data (Desai, Vanneman, and National Council of Applied Economic Research 2005) and summary documents (Barik and Desai 2014).
*Note:* ALRI = acute lower respiratory infection; COPD = chronic obstructive pulmonary disease; IHD = ischemic heart disease; Q = quintile.

**Table 12.4** Intervention Financial Parameters per Unit

| | Government | | | Household | | | |
|---|---|---|---|---|---|---|---|
| Intervention | Stove (US$) | One-time costs, US$ (quintile)[a] | Yearly costs, US$ (quintile)[b] | Stove (US$) | One-time costs, US$ (quintile) | Yearly costs, US$ (quintile)[b] | Time savings, hours per year (quintile) |
| Chimney | 10 | 5 | n.a. | n.a. | n.a. | 1 | 25 (Q1), 19 (Q2), 20 (Q3), 15 (Q4), 14 (Q5) |
| Blower | 60 | 10 | n.a. | n.a. | 60 | 5 | 72 (Q1), 53 (Q2), 56 (Q3), 41 (Q4), 40 (Q5) |
| LPG status quo | 0 | 0 | 33 | 20 | 30 (Q1), 30 (Q2), 30 (Q3), 30 (Q4), 30 (Q5) | 46 (Q1), 46 (Q2), 46 (Q3), 46 (Q4), 46 (Q5) | 170 (Q1), 126 (Q2), 134 (Q3), 97 (Q4), 96 (Q5) |
| LPG–GIU[c] | 0 | 30 (Q1), 30 (Q2), 0 (Q3), 0 (Q4), 0 (Q5) | 33 (Q1), 33 (Q2), 0 (Q3), 0 (Q4), 0 (Q5) | 20 | 0 (Q1), 0 (Q2), 30 (Q3), 30 (Q4), 30 (Q5)[d] | 46 (Q1), 46 (Q2), 80 (Q3), 80 (Q4), 80 (Q5) | |

*Note:* GIU = Give It Up; LPG = liquefied petroleum gas; n.a. = not applicable; Q = quintile.
a. For LPG scenarios, one-time costs are the LPG connection costs. Current prices are available at IndianOil Corporation, https://indane.co.in/connection_tarrifs.php; US$1.00 = 68.13 rupees (Rs). For biomass stoves, one-time costs represent the cost of implementation.
b. For LPG scenarios, yearly costs are the cost of the fuel subsidy to the government and the cost of the fuel to the households. The analysis assumes that houses use nine cylinders per year at an unsubsidized cost of US$8.80 (Rs 600.00) per cylinder; that Haryana has 3.35 million homes; and that the per cylinder subsidy is approximately US$3.70 (Rs 250.00). For biomass stoves, yearly costs are stove maintenance costs borne by the household.
c. India's national oil companies cover connection costs for 60 percent of households; connection costs to the household apply only for the upper three quintiles.
d. The subsidy provided to existing LPG users is redirected to the lower-income quintiles.

efficiency relative to the base case scenario by the time spent collecting fuel. We place a monetary value on this gained time using the Mahatma Gandhi National Rural Employment Guarantee Act's guaranteed wage of Rs 251 (US$$3.70) per day, for up to 100 days, in Haryana.[5,6] Accordingly, a household's yearly total averted expenditure as the result of an intervention is the sum of the wage earned during time previously spent collecting fuel and the avoided health expenditure, minus any cost to the household of the intervention (for example, stove maintenance or replacement or fuel costs):

$$Averted\ expenditure = \left( \frac{Time\ savings(hrs)}{8\ hrs/day} \times Wage \right)$$

$$+\ Averted\ medical\ expenditure$$

$$-\ Intervention\ cost$$

### Government Costs

The government incurs costs from providing the intervention. The provision cost of chimney and blower stoves includes the upfront cost of the intervention and a one-time cost of deployment. For the LPG intervention, we consider a policy pathway mimicking the ongoing Give It Up campaign. In this scenario, subsidies are provided to all solid fuel–using households in only the lower two income quintiles (Q1 and Q2 in tables and figures); the subsidy given to existing LPG users in the upper three income quintiles is redirected to the lower two quintiles. Because subsidies are being retargeted, the net cost to the government is zero; the upper-income quintiles absorb the additional costs. However, we assume the connection costs borne by the corporate social responsibility funds from oil companies for the lower two income quintiles could be used elsewhere by these companies, which are owned largely by the government, and thus represent a cost to the government. All households pay for their own

LPG stove and for their LPG fuel. This analysis assumes that houses use nine cylinders per year at an unsubsidized cost of US$8.80 (Rs 600.00) per cylinder and that the per cylinder subsidy is approximately US$3.70 (Rs 250.00). Table 12.4 summarizes the per unit private and public intervention costs.

All analyses were carried out using R 3.1 statistical software (R Foundation 2015); plots were generated using the ggplot2 system (Wickham 2009).

## RESULTS

Under the assumptions of the analysis, the intervention pathways described result in reductions in ill health attributable to using solid fuel for cooking. The scale of those reductions varies both among interventions and among quintiles; all interventions show higher reductions in ill health in the poorest three quintiles (figure 12.1 and table 12.5). The costs to the government of the five-year programs vary widely among interventions: the chimney stove intervention costs approximately US$39 million, and the blower stove intervention costs approximately US$180 million. At these prices, a life saved by the chimney stove costs the government approximately US$20,000 and the cost of an averted DALY is US$520, whereas a life saved by the blower stove costs US$10,000 and an averted DALY costs US$275. Complete replacement of traditional stoves in solid fuel–using households in Haryana results

**Figure 12.1** Averted Deaths and DALYs for Three Classes of Interventions in Haryana, India, by Income Quintile

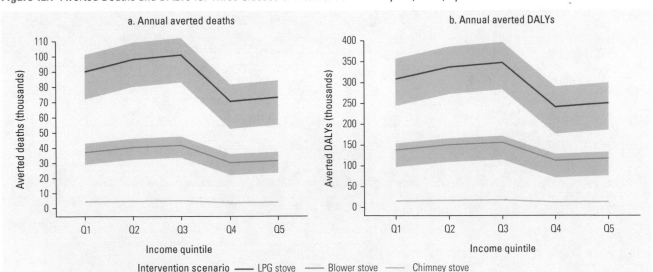

*Note:* DALYs = disability-adjusted life years; LPG = liquefied petroleum gas; Q = quintile. Shaded areas account for uncertainty in background disease conditions and indicate the minimum and maximum avoidable burden. The relatively constant shape of the lines for each scenario is a byproduct of high solid fuel use across all income quintiles (range 60 percent to 90 percent) and the increasing number of people per household with increasing income, despite an approximately equal number of homes in each quintile.

**Table 12.5** Five-Year Government Intervention Costs, Costs to Households, Household Expenditures Averted, and Deaths and DALYs Averted for Chimney Stove, Blower Stove, and LPG Intervention Pathways

| | Q1<br>N = 669,000<br>SFU = 595,000 | Q2<br>N = 670,000<br>SFU = 604,000 | Q3<br>N = 671,000<br>SFU = 592,000 | Q4<br>N = 671,000<br>SFU = 445,000 | Q5<br>N = 670,000<br>SFU = 418,000 |
|---|---|---|---|---|---|
| *Chimney stove* | | | | | |
| Government costs | 8,900,000 | 9,100,000 | 8,900,000 | 6,700,000 | 6,300,000 |
| Household maintenance costs | 3,000,000 | 3,000,000 | 3,000,000 | 2,200,000 | 2,000,000 |
| Household expenditures averted | 6,700,000 | 4,900,000 | 5,100,000 | 2,800,000 | 2,600,000 |
| Deaths averted | 420 | 450 | 470 | 340 | 350 |
| DALYs averted | 16,000 | 17,000 | 18,000 | 13,000 | 14,000 |
| *Blower stove* | | | | | |
| Government costs | 42,000,000 | 42,000,000 | 41,000,000 | 31,000,000 | 29,000,000 |
| Household maintenance and stove replacement costs | 50,000,000 | 51,000,000 | 50,000,000 | 38,000,000 | 36,000,000 |
| Household expenditures averted | 52,000,000 | 27,000,000 | 31,000,000 | 8,300,000 | 8,500,000 |
| Deaths averted | 3,700 | 4,100 | 4,200 | 3,000 | 3,200 |
| DALYs averted | 140,000 | 150,000 | 160,000 | 110,000 | 120,000 |
| *LPG–GIU pathway* | | | | | |
| Government costs | 18,000,000 | 18,000,000 | 0 | 0 | 0 |
| Fuel cost to households | 150,000,000 | 150,000,000 | 270,000,000 | 200,000,000 | 190,000,000 |
| Household expenditures averted | 95,000,000 | 36,000,000 | −72,000,000 | −91,000,000 | −84,000,000 |
| Deaths averted | 9,100 | 9,900 | 10,000 | 7,000 | 7,300 |
| DALYs averted | 310,000 | 340,000 | 350,000 | 240,000 | 250,000 |

*Note:* DALYs = disability-adjusted life years; GIU = Give It Up; LPG = liquefied petroleum gas; Q = quintile; SFU = solid fuel use. Fuel cost to households includes the up-front, one-time stove costs and recurrent maintenance and fuel costs. Household expenditures averted are the sum of the hourly wages accrued and the medical costs averted minus the cost to the households. For the LPG-GIU pathway, subsidy retargeting has different implications for solid fuel users versus current LPG users. Solid fuel users assume the additional full cost of unsubsidized LPG, while current LPG users assume only the difference between the full, unsubsidized LPG cost and the subsidized cost.

in 2,000 averted deaths and 77,000 averted DALYs for the chimney stove and 18,100 averted deaths and 676,000 averted DALYs for the blower stove.

The LPG pathway, in which the government pays for connection charges from the allocation of corporate social responsibility funds, costs approximately US$36 million, or approximately US$11 per home when averaged across all homes or US$30 per home when averaged across only the lower two income quintiles. This policy pathway assumes that all higher-income households (n ~ 2,000,000) give up their subsidy and that the reclaimed subsidy can be targeted to solid fuel–using households (n ~ 1,340,000) in the lower-income quintiles, effectively not altering the cost to the government. Under this scheme, an averted death costs the government US$825 and an averted DALY costs US$25. Over the five-year evaluation period, 1,484,000 DALYs and 44,000 deaths are averted.

The LPG stove averts the most deaths and DALYs across all income quintiles, per US$100,000 spent (figure 12.2). The figure panels for the LPG intervention evenly split the costs between all income quintiles, though the only additional expenditure by the government is for the bottom two quintiles.

Figure 12.3 depicts the trends in expenditures averted by households by quintile. Notably, households in the poor quintiles avoid more private expenditure than do households in the upper quintiles. This finding is most pronounced for the blower and LPG stoves. The described LPG intervention, in which the richest households receive no subsidy for fuel, simulates the GIU campaign and results in a net cost to these households, which must pay the full, unsubsidized price for their fuel and their one-time connection costs. The national oil companies cover connection costs for poor households, which also receive subsidized fuel.

**Figure 12.2** Averted Deaths and DALYs per US$1 Million Spent for Three Classes of Interventions in Haryana, India, over Five-Year Intervention Lifetime, by Income Quintile

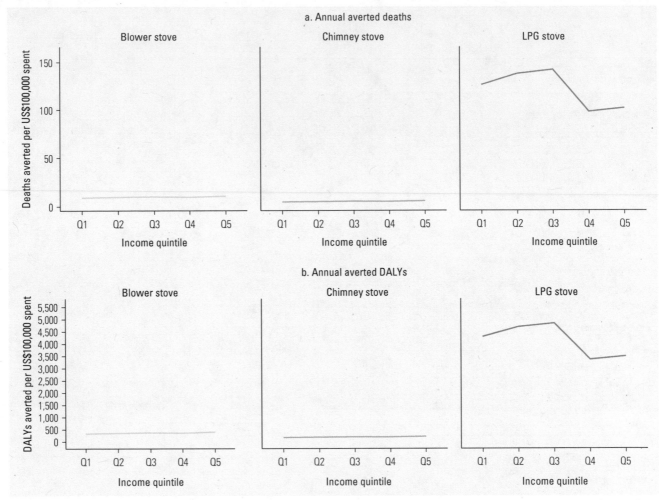

*Note:* DALYs = disability-adjusted life years; LPG = liquefied petroleum gas; Q = quintile. Panels represent intervention classes. For the LPG scenario, gas subsidies given up by income quintiles 4 and 5 result in no expense to the government for the intervention in these quintiles; the subsidy is retargeted evenly to income quintiles 1, 2, and 3.

## DISCUSSION

We present results from ECEAs of policies designed to achieve high uptake of three hypothetical classes of HAP interventions in Haryana, India. The classes of interventions presented match historical modes of household energy programs, first attempted with chimney stoves, then with blower-assisted biomass stoves, and, most recently, with a transition to truly clean cooking using LPG. By evaluating multiple types of interventions, we are able to compare cheap, poorly performing chimney stoves with intermediate (blower) and modern (LPG) options.

Our approach is novel in several ways:

- It seems to be the first ECEA to date evaluating household energy policies.

- It takes into account the earning potential of individuals who save time by transitioning to more efficient stoves, which require less fuel and less time spent collecting fuel.
- It uses a continuous exposure-response function to estimate health benefits of interventions with different exposure reduction potentials.
- It evaluates a current LPG policy pathway that mimics the ongoing retargeting of LPG fuel subsidies.

By considering earnings and medical expenses averted as a result of these interventions, we hope to present a more rigorous and multidimensional set of options for policy makers to evaluate and consider as they seek to reduce the significant health burden associated with exposure to smoke arising from use of solid fuel combustion for cooking. Unlike many other ECEAs, we present both averted deaths and averted DALYs, a combined metric of both morbidity and mortality.

Our findings indicate that from the perspective of avoiding ill health, the evaluated LPG scenario outperforms attempts to make biomass combustion clean, although it imposes an additional fuel cost on households. Our findings show, however, that the added cost of subsidized fuel—at least for the poorest income quintiles—is more than covered by the monetary values of saved time and avoided healthcare. This striking finding, however, is heavily influenced by the assumption that use of time previously spent collecting fuel is repurposed for productive economic return, which may not be true in these settings. The income quintile–based consequences of these policy pathways are complicated by the underlying distributions of SFU and disease burden. Using those distributional consequences alone to make policy decisions would favor less effective interventions and ignore the significant health burden remaining from adoption of such technology. In contrast, the financial protection provided by the LPG policy pathways benefits the poor, who receive subsidized fuel, free LPG connections, and reduced health care costs and who stand to gain the most in wages. This inverse relationship between those quintiles that receive an advantage from health benefits versus financial benefits is not uncommon to ECEA (Pecenka and others 2015); it reveals the methodology's ability to highlight multiple policy-relevant facets masked by traditional cost-effectiveness analysis. It also indicates an area of ongoing concern. Public financing of interventions such as those that are targeted to quintiles and that are modeled to benefit the most may have unintended consequences.

Strikingly, retargeting the subsidy—as is happening in India under the Give It Up campaign—significantly increases the cost-effectiveness of interventions targeting the poorest income quintiles. This finding suggests that such an approach—especially when considered in light of the considerable financial risk protection afforded by targeting the lower-income quintiles—may be a way to quickly and efficiently move resources to those most vulnerable to both the health and the financial effects of SFU for cooking.

Despite these clear distributional benefits, less profound difference exists among quintiles than originally anticipated, which explains the relatively constant values across quintiles seen in figures 12.1, 12.2, and 12.3. We believe this is due in part to relatively high SFU numbers across all quintiles and an increasing number of people per household as wealth increases, resulting in a skewed distribution of background disease rates.

**Figure 12.3** Averted Private Expenditure for Each Class of Intervention over the Proposed Five-Year Intervention Lifetime

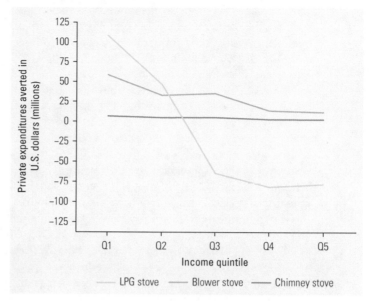

*Note:* LPG = liquefied petroleum gas; Q = quintile. Negative values indicate net costs to households. However, the upper quintiles are voluntarily giving up their subsidy in the GIU campaign. Annex 12A, figure 7 shows the per household costs and savings by income quintile and intervention scenario.

We conducted a sensitivity analysis to evaluate the effect of a hypothetical scenario with an equal number of people per quintile and linearly decreasing SFU as wealth increases. Under these conditions, the effects of all three scenarios were most profound for the poorer income quintiles.

Our analysis has a number of limitations. First, we present only a small number of potential household energy intervention scenarios under ideal use scenarios, none of which considers an additional benefit in the form of reducing the herd or the neighborhood effect; that is, by swapping out entire communities, wider gains in exposure reduction could occur. We assume that households transition fully to the cleaner technology in all three cases and do not revert to older technologies even partially. We address this shortcoming in part by evaluating the effects of adoption rates less than 100 percent and the effects of variation in exposure that may represent suboptimal intervention performance or use of both old and new interventions. We find that the overall trends in our findings are robust to these types of changes (annex 12A). We chose this framing to indicate the potential effects of statewide adoption and use of LPG, realizing that such a transition will take time and must contend with issues of stove stacking. We acknowledge that such a framing does not contend with issues of the perceived costs of fuel versus potential health savings and wage gains, which may be viewed independently by household decision makers.

Second, our study uses older IHDS data from 2005–06. Newer data—either from IHDS itself or from other national surveys—may provide more up-to-date numbers on the penetration of LPG in Haryana and on treatment-seeking behaviors and related costs. We also recognize that our mapping of BPL households to IHDS income quintiles 1 and 2 may not match the current reality. However, to our knowledge, unlike other surveys, IDHS has the benefit of providing a single source from which to gather almost all parameters needed for this analysis, thereby preventing potentially problematic comparison among surveys with different sampling frames. Similarly, we use national data on treatment-seeking behavior for Haryana; data from IHDS at the state level were unrealistically homogenous across income quintiles.

Our quantification of the monetary value of time savings does not account for behavioral aspects related to job-seeking behavior or any potential rebound effects of adoption of cleaner cooking technologies. We acknowledge that small daily or weekly time savings may not be large enough and (1) that a search for a job via the Mahatma Gandhi National Rural Employment Guarantee Act is warranted, (2) that employment opportunities exist for the modeled time savings, or (3) that household members who experience time savings might engage in employment versus other household or leisure-related activities. We assume that people will successfully seek employment in the national program and that the time saved by shifting away from biomass can be utilized productively—findings that may not hold and warrant further investigation. Our approach does offer an empirical money metric of time savings based on an ongoing program in Haryana and India at large. Thus, it is based on a documented rural wage rate.

We assume universal adoption of the cleaner cooking technology in Haryana for the main scenarios described in this chapter. This assumption is highly optimistic because older, more polluting stoves are often not abandoned immediately when a cleaner one of any kind is adopted; studies have shown that even the best modern biomass stoves often do not perform well over time in reducing pollution exposures. However, LPG is essentially always clean. We bound our chimney stove scenario by assuming that it breaks down after one year and is not rebuilt, which has often occurred with the inexpensive models widely deployed in India. An alternative approach would be to build in regular replacement of these stoves, or perhaps to move to the much more expensive and robust chimney stoves that have been successfully used in other countries and subregions. For example, in China and Mexico and in Central America, chimney stoves that function for a decade or more are not uncommon, but costs are at least 15 times greater.

Because of the need to purchase fuel, the financial conditions of the biomass and LPG scenarios are fundamentally different, but we attempt to explore them here in the same analysis. In doing so, we evaluated the current LPG subsidy system as a given and took only the extra costs of LPG connections in the GIU campaign as the cost of the LPG expansion, thereby assuming that the shift of subsidy from the middle class to the poor did not itself incur any change in government expenditures; that is, there were no transactional costs to the government. The framing in a different country without any current LPG subsidy, however, might be quite different. Although the funds for connections currently come from the required social responsibility funds of the national oil companies, we assign these as government expenditures because they could have been used for other purposes. Finally, in the absence of information, we assumed no operational costs to the government to design, promote, manage, and evaluate the large-scale disseminations that would be needed in all three scenarios.

Solid fuel–using households in upper income quintiles (Q3, Q4, and Q5) absorb a significant fuel costs in our modeled LPG intervention, as they move from no LPG to full-price LPG. The large number of solid fuel–using households in the wealthier income quintiles suggests that future subsidies and LPG-promoting programs may wish to address these households using a sliding subsidy, as suggested by Tripathi, Sagar, and Smith (2015). Ongoing LPG programs in India do not currently have a provision to target these households.

Future analyses of this type should investigate alternate methods of apportioning underlying data from national data to state-level data and into disease quintiles. Furthermore, although partitioning by SFU is reasonable in our example, it may mask behavioral patterns related to solid fuel use that we did not anticipate and differences between quintiles that impact disease distributions.

Beyond methodological and data limitations, we assume the status quo remains constant with respect to international LPG prices and related subsidies. This assumption ensures analytic tractability, but it may not hold, given the volatility in oil prices globally. India is undergoing a rapid, policy-driven transformation that is dramatically increasing access to LPG for communities previously reliant on solid fuels. Although these ongoing changes may alter the calculus behind the results, they highlight the need for being able to perform multifaceted analyses that consider more than simply basic cost-effectiveness to estimate the potential effects of large programs—precisely the type of evaluation facilitated by ECEA.

## CONCLUSIONS

Exposure to HAP from solid cookfuel, mainly as biomass, causes an estimated 925,000 deaths yearly in India today. The number of people most affected—700 million to 800 million—has not declined in 30 years, despite considerable economic development and the growth of clean fuel use for the middle class. Other approaches are clearly needed to address this health hazard.

Three types of national policies have been initiated to address the health, social, and environmental effects of inefficient household biomass use. In the 1980s and 1990s, households relied on inexpensive stoves made locally with simple materials but without much improvement in smoke emissions, although often including a chimney. Around 2010, a new program was initiated that promised to develop and promote biomass stoves that produced far less pollution emissions, but usually this program did not incorporate chimneys. Starting in 2014, the national GIU campaign began to greatly expand access to a clean modern fuel, LPG, for BPL families by using innovative financing and promotional modalities. Newer initiatives—including the Smokeless Village program and the recently announced Ujjwala program—continue this trend of making clean cooking available widely across India. This chapter has evaluated each of the approaches separately for their cost-effectiveness in hypothetical deployments in the same northern Indian state, Haryana. We believe these types of modeling exercises are instructive and help target further, field-based studies evaluating the effect of programs.

Lowering household exposures to air pollution can decrease both health and financial burdens not only by reducing medical costs, but also by averting household expenditures or avoiding lost wage earnings. The scale of the reduction—and the amount of disease burden left untouched by each of them—varies widely among the three intervention options, however, although cost-effectiveness varies less widely. More modest reductions from chimney stoves, for example, are to some extent matched by more modest costs.

The innovative policy of Ujjwala, extending out of the GIU campaign, starts by retargeting existing LPG subsidies away from the middle class to the poor. This approach can result in highly cost-effective health improvements in the poorest quintiles of the population. It is accompanied by some shift of costs to the middle class, but, notably, by their agreement and without a net increase in government expenditures. By being the cleanest of the options examined, LPG also has the potential to achieve the greatest health benefits. Compared to the other two fuels, LPG also benefits from a familiar long-lived cooking technology that has a well-established repair and refill system in place in the region, although it requires reliable extension to additional populations.

To be effective, however, any intervention program must focus not only on providing access to the intervention but also on enhancing use over the long term, including continuing to pay for subsidized fuel and repair and replacement of the stoves. Only when use of the traditional polluting biomass stoves is greatly reduced over time and replaced by LPG or another equally clean alternative will full health benefits be secured.

## ANNEX

The annex to this chapter is as follows. It is available at http://www.dcp-3.org/environment.

- Annex 12A. Supporting Information

## ACKNOWLEDGMENTS

The authors thank Rachel Nugent, Zachary Olson, Charles N. Mock, and two anonymous reviewers for their thoughtful comments and suggestions.

## NOTES

World Bank Income Classifications as of July 2014 are as follows, based on estimates of gross national income (GNI) per capita for 2013:

- Low-income countries (LICs) = US$1,045 or less
- Middle-income countries (MICs) are subdivided:
  a) lower-middle-income = US$1,046 to US$4,125
  b) upper-middle-income (UMICs) = US$4,126 to US$12,745
- High-income countries (HICs) = US$12,746 or more.

1. We use the DALY that was first widely deployed in the GBD 2010. It is not adjusted by age weighting or discounting. It cannot be directly compared to previous versions that did so.
2. Policy measures to increase access to LPG among the rural poor in India are advancing rapidly. The programs mentioned in this chapter are up to date as of July 2016.
3. Our analysis does not include any assessment of outdoor air pollution and the reduction in emissions from the household sector, which account for an estimated 25–50 percent of ambient small particle exposures in India (Chafe and others 2014; Lelieveld and others 2015).
4. We use IHDS questions about cough and fever in the past month as a proxy for ALRI. The total number of households reporting this proxy for ALRI per quintile is multiplied by 12 to obtain the number of cases per quintile per year and then divided by the total number

of households in the quintile to determine the number of cases per household per year. The per case cost estimate is multiplied by the number of cases per household by quintile to determine the yearly cost.

5. See http://www.haryanarural.gov.in/guidelines/MGNREGS /1025MGNREGS_wage_notification_2015_16.pdf.
6. See http://www.haryanarural.gov.in/detail-nrega.htm#bnote.

## REFERENCES

Arcenas, A., J. Bojö, B. R. Larsen, and F. Ruiz Ñunez. 2010. "The Economic Costs of Indoor Air Pollution: New Results for Indonesia, the Philippines, and Timor-Leste." *Journal of Natural Resources Policy Research* 2 (1): 75–93.

Aunan, K., L. W. H. Alnes, J. Berger, Z. Dong, L. Ma, and others. 2013. "Upgrading to Cleaner Household Stoves and Reducing Chronic Obstructive Pulmonary Disease among Women in Rural China: A Cost-Benefit Analysis." *Energy for Sustainable Development* 17 (5): 489–96.

Bailis, R., V. Berrueta, C. Chengappa, K. Dutta, R. Edwards, and others. 2007. "Performance Testing for Monitoring Improved Biomass Stove Interventions: Experiences of the Household Energy and Health Project." *Energy for Sustainable Development* 11 (2): 57–70.

Balakrishnan, K., S. Ghosh, B. Ganguli, S. Sambandam, N. Bruce, and others. 2013. "State and National Household Concentrations of PM2.5 from Solid Cookfuel Use: Results from Measurements and Modeling in India for Estimation of the Global Burden of Disease." *Environmental Health* 12: 77.

Barik, D., and S. Desai. 2014. "Determinants of Private Healthcare Utilisation and Expenditure Patterns in India." In *India Infrastructure Report 2013|14: The Road to Universal Health Coverage*, edited by S. B. A. S. Ghosh, 52–64. New Delhi: Orient Blackswan Private Limited.

Bonjour, S., H. Adair-Rohani, J. Wolf, N. G. Bruce, S. Mehta, and others. 2013. "Solid Fuel Use for Household Cooking: Country and Regional Estimates for 1980–2010." *Environmental Health Perspectives* 121 (7): 784–90.

Brooks, N., V. Bhojvaid, M. A. Jeuland, J. J. Lewis, O. Patange, and others. 2016. "How Much Do Alternative Cookstoves Reduce Biomass Fuel Use? Evidence from North India." *Resource and Energy Economics* 43: 153–71.

Burnett, R. T., C. A. Pope 3rd, M. Ezzati, C. Olives, S. S. Lim, and others. 2014. "An Integrated Risk Function for Estimating the Global Burden of Disease Attributable to Ambient Fine Particulate Matter Exposure." *Environmental Health Perspectives* 122 (4): 397–403.

Chafe, Z. A., M. Brauer, Z. Klimont, R. Van Dingenen, S. Mehta, and others. 2014. "Household Cooking with Solid Fuels Contributes to Ambient PM2.5 Air Pollution and the Burden of Disease." *Environmental Health Perspectives* 122 (12): 1314–20.

Desai, S, R. Vanneman, and National Council of Applied Economic Research, New Delhi. 2005. India Human Development Survey (IHDS). ICPSR22626-v11. Ann Arbor, MI: Inter-University Consortium for Political and Social Research, 2016-02-16. http://doi.org/10.3886/ICPSR 22626.v11.

Dutta, K., K. N. Shields, R. Edwards, and K. R. Smith. 2007. "Impact of Improved Biomass Cookstoves on Indoor Air Quality near Pune, India." *Energy for Sustainable Development* 11: 19–32.

Foell, W., S. Pachauri, D. Spreng, and H. Zerriffi. 2011. "Household Cooking Fuels and Technologies in Developing Economies." *Energy Policy* 39 (12): 7487–96.

Forouzanfar, M., L. Alexander, H. R. Anderson, V. F. Bachman, S. Biryukov, and others. 2015. "Global, Regional, and National Comparative Risk Assessment of 79 Behavioural, Environmental and Occupational, and Metabolic Risks or Clusters of Risks in 188 Countries, 1990–2013: A Systematic Analysis for the Global Burden of Disease Study 2013." *The Lancet* 386 (10010): 2287–323.

Government of India. 2011. Census of India 2011: Houses, Household Amenities, and Assets. Registrar General and Census Commissioner, New Delhi.

Hutton, G., E. Rehfuess, and F. Tediosi. 2007. "Evaluation of the Costs and Benefits of Interventions to Reduce Indoor Air Pollution." *Energy for Sustainable Development* 11 (4): 34–43.

Hutton, G., E. Rehfuess, F. Tediosi, and S. Weiss. 2006. *Evaluation of the Costs and Benefits of Household Energy and Health Interventions at Global and Regional Levels.* Geneva: World Health Organization.

Institute for Health Metrics and Evaluation (IHME). 2015. GBD Compare. Seattle, WA: IHME, University of Washington. http://vizhub.healthdata.org/gbd-compare.

Jeuland, M. A., and S. K. Pattanayak. 2012. "Benefits and Costs of Improved Cookstoves: Assessing the Implications of Variability in Health, Forest and Climate Impacts." *PLoS One* 7 (2): e30338–15.

Jeuland, M. A., S. K. Pattanayak, and R. Bluffstone. 2015. "The Economics of Household Air Pollution." *Annual Review of Resource Economics* 7 (1): 81–108.

Johnson, M. A., and R. A. Chiang. 2015. "Quantitative Guidance for Stove Usage and Performance to Achieve Health and Environmental Targets." *Environmental Health Perspectives* 123 (8): 820–26.

Kishore, V., and P. V. Ramana. 2002. "Improved Cookstoves in Rural India: How Improved Are They? A Critique of the Perceived Benefits from the National Programme on Improved Chulhas (NPIC)." *Energy* 27 (1): 47–63.

Lelieveld, J., J. S. Evans, M. Fnais, D. Giannadaki, and A. Pozzer. 2015. "The Contribution of Outdoor Air Pollution Sources to Premature Mortality on a Global Scale." *Nature* 525 (7569): 367–71.

Lim, S. S., T. Vos, A. D. Flaxman, G. Danaei, K. Shibuya, and others. 2012. "A Comparative Risk Assessment of Burden of Disease and Injury Attributable to 67 Risk Factors and Risk Factor Clusters in 21 Regions, 1990–2010: A Systematic Analysis for the Global Burden of Disease Study 2010." *The Lancet* 380 (9859): 2224–60.

Lozano, R., M. Naghavi, K. Foreman, S. Lim, K. Shibuya, and others. 2012. "Global and Regional Mortality from 235 Causes of Death for 20 Age Groups in 1990 and 2010:

A Systematic Analysis for the Global Burden of Disease Study 2010." *The Lancet* 380 (9859): 2095–28.

Malla, M. B., N. Bruce, E. Bates, and E. Rehfuess. 2011. "Applying Global Cost-Benefit Analysis Methods to Indoor Air Pollution Mitigation Interventions in Nepal, Kenya and Sudan: Insights and Challenges." *Energy Policy* 39 (12): 7518–29.

Mehta, S., and C. Shahpar. 2004. "The Health Benefits of Interventions to Reduce Indoor Air Pollution from Solid Fuel Use: A Cost-Effectiveness Analysis." *Energy for Sustainable Development* 8 (3), 53–59.

Ministry of Petroleum, Government of India. 2016. "My LPG. in." http://mylpg.in/index.aspx.

Northcross, A., Z. Chowdhury, J. McCracken, E. Canuz, and K. R. Smith. 2010. "Estimating Personal PM2.5 Exposures Using CO Measurements in Guatemalan Households Cooking with Wood Fuel." *Journal of Environmental Monitoring* 12: 873–78.

Pant, K. P. 2011. "Cheaper Fuel and Higher Health Costs among the Poor in Rural Nepal." *AMBIO* 41 (3): 271–83.

Pecenka, C. J., K. A. Johansson, S. T. Memirie, D. T. Jamison, and S. Verguet. 2015. "Health Gains and Financial Risk Protection: An Extended Cost-Effectiveness Analysis of Treatment and Prevention of Diarrhoea in Ethiopia." *BMJ Open* 5: e006402.

Pillarisetti, A., S. Mehta, and K. R. Smith. 2016. "HAPIT, the Household Air Pollution Intervention Tool, to Evaluate the Health Benefits and Cost-Effectiveness of Clean Cooking Interventions." In *Broken Pumps and Promises: Incentivizing Impact in Environmental Health*, edited by E. Thomas, 147–70. Cham, Switzerland: Springer International Publishing AG.

Pillarisetti, A., M. Vaswani, D. Jack, K. Balakrishnan, M. N. Bates, and others. 2014. "Patterns of Stove Usage after Introduction of an Advanced Cookstove: The Long-Term Application of Household Sensors." *Environmental Science and Technology* 48 (24): 14525–33.

R Foundation for Statistical Computing. 2015. *R: A Language and Environment for Statistical Computer.* Vienna: R Foundation for Statistical Computing. http://www.R-project.org.

Ruiz-Mercado, I., O. Masera, H. Zamora, and K. R. Smith. 2011. "Adoption and Sustained Use of Improved Cookstoves." *Energy Policy* 39: 7557–66.

Sambandam, S., K. Balakrishnan, S. Ghosh, A. Sadasivam, S. Madhav, and others. 2015. "Can Currently Available Advanced Combustion Biomass Cook-Stoves Provide Health Relevant Exposure Reductions? Results from Initial Assessment of Select Commercial Models in India." *Ecohealth* 12 (1): 25–41.

Smith, K. R., N. Bruce, K. Balakrishnan, H. Adair-Rohani, J. Balmes, and others. 2014. "Millions Dead: How Do We Know and What Does It Mean? Methods Used in the Comparative Risk Assessment of Household Air Pollution." *Annual Review of Public Health* 35: 185–206.

Smith, K. R., A. Pillarisetti, L. D. Hill, D. Charron, S. Delapena, and others. 2015. "Proposed Methodology: Quantification of a Saleable Health Product (aDALYs) from Household Cooking Interventions." Household Energy, Climate, and Health Research Group, University of California, Berkeley, and Berkeley Air Monitoring Group, Berkeley, for the World Bank.

Smith, K. R., and A. D. Sagar. 2015. "Making the Clean Available: Escaping India's Chulha Trap." *Energy Policy* 75: 410–14.

*Times of India.* 2016. "PM to Launch Rs 8,000 Crore Scheme for Free LPG Connections to Poor." April 22.

Tripathi, A., A. D. Sagar, and K. R. Smith. 2015. "Promoting Clean and Affordable Cooking." *Economic Political Weekly* 48: 81–84.

U.S. EPA (United States Environmental Protection Agency). 2004. "Advisory on Plans for Health Effects Analysis in the Analytical Plan for EPA's Second Prospective Analysis: Benefits and Costs of the Clean Air Act, 1990–2020." EPA-SAB-COUNCIL-ADV-04-002, Advisory Council on Clean Air Compliance Analysis, U.S. EPA, Washington, DC.

Venkataraman, C., A. D. Sagar, G. Habib, N. Lam, and K. R. Smith. 2010. "The Indian National Initiative for Advanced Biomass Cookstoves: The Benefits of Clean Combustion." *Energy for Sustainable Development* 14: 63–72.

Verguet, S., C. L. Gauvreau, S. Mishra, M. MacLennan, S. M. Murphy, and others. 2015. "The Consequences of Tobacco Tax on Household Health and Finances in Rich and Poor Smokers in China: An Extended Cost-Effectiveness Analysis." *The Lancet Global Health* 3 (4): e206–16.

Verguet, S., R. Laxminarayan, and D. T. Jamison. 2015. "Universal Public Finance of Tuberculosis Treatment in India: An Extended Cost-Effectiveness Analysis." *Health Economics* 24 (3): 318–32.

Wickham, H. 2009. *ggplot2: Elegant Graphics for Data Analysis.* New York: Springer.

# Chapter 13

# Costs and Benefits of Installing Flue-Gas Desulfurization Units at Coal-Fired Power Plants in India

Maureen L. Cropper, Sarath Guttikunda, Puja Jawahar, Kabir Malik, and Ian Partridge

## INTRODUCTION

Coal-fired power plants, in addition to emitting greenhouse gases, are a major source of local pollution and health damages throughout the world. China, the United States, and other countries that rely on coal for electricity production regulate emissions from coal-fired power plants, primarily for health reasons. In the United States, the 1990 Clean Air Act Amendments caused many power plants to switch to low-sulfur coal or to install flue-gas desulfurization units (FGD units, or scrubbers). Subsequent tightening of sulfur dioxide ($SO_2$) regulations has caused more plants to scrub their emissions. In 2010, power plants with FGD units accounted for 60 percent of the electricity generated from coal in the United States (Schmalensee and Stavins 2013). By 2013, 95 percent of China's coal-fired generating capacity had been fitted with FGD units (Ministry of Environmental Protection 2014).

India, which relies on coal to generate 76 percent of its electricity (CEA 2015), did not regulate $SO_2$ emissions from coal-fired power plants until December 2015. That lack of regulation may have been due, in part, to the low sulfur content of Indian coal (Chikkatur and Sagar 2007). Indian coal is approximately 0.5 percent sulfur by weight, similar to Powder River Basin (PRB) coal in the United States (Lu and others 2013). However, the population exposed to $SO_2$ emissions from power plants in India is much greater than that in the United States, as is

the amount of coal burned to generate a kilowatt hour (kWh) of electricity. Recent studies suggest serious health effects associated with $SO_2$ emissions from Indian power plants. Guttikunda and Jawahar (2014) estimate that Indian power plants caused more than 80,000 deaths in 2011; they attribute 30–40 percent of these deaths to $SO_2$. Cropper and others (2012) suggest that as many as 60 percent of the deaths associated with coal-fired power plants in India may be attributable to $SO_2$ emissions rather than to directly emitted particulate matter or oxides of nitrogen (NOx).

This chapter analyzes the health benefits and the costs of installing FGD units at each of the 72 coal-fired power plants in India, plants that in 2009 constituted 90 percent of coal-fired generating capacity. We estimate the health benefits of one FGD unit by estimating $SO_2$ emissions from a plant without an FGD unit and then translating those emissions into changes in ambient air quality. This is accomplished using an Eulerian photochemical dispersion model (CAMx) that allows $SO_2$ to form fine sulfate particles (smaller than 2.5 micrometers in diameter [$PM_{2.5}$]) in the atmosphere. The impacts of $PM_{2.5}$ on premature mortality are estimated for ischemic heart disease, stroke, lung cancer, chronic obstructive pulmonary disease (COPD), and acute lower respiratory infection (ALRI) using the integrated exposure response (IER) coefficients in Burnett and others (2014).

Corresponding author: Maureen Cropper, Department of Economics, University of Maryland, College Park, MD, United States; cropper@econ.umd.edu.

We assume that a scrubber will reduce SO₂ emissions by 90 percent. The annual reductions in premature mortality and associated life years lost resulting from use of scrubbers are combined with an estimate of annualized capital and operating costs to compute the cost per statistical life saved and cost per disability-adjusted life year (DALY) averted associated with each FGD unit.

Reducing SO₂ emissions from coal-fired power plants offers additional benefits that we do not quantify. These include improvements in visibility (which yield aesthetic and recreation benefits) and reduced acidic deposition. Acidic deposition can reduce soil quality (through nutrient leaching), impair timber growth, and harm freshwater ecosystems (USEPA 2011).

## METHODS

### Estimating the Health Impacts of SO₂ Emissions from Power Plants

Our analysis focuses on 72 coal-fired power plants (shown in map 13.1) which in March 2009 constituted 90 percent of the coal-fired generating capacity

**Map 13.1** Coal-Fired Power Plants: All Plants in Dataset

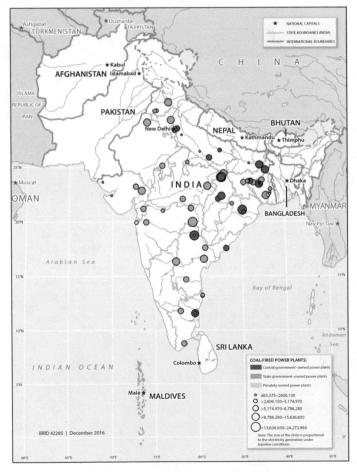

connected to the grid in India. The size of each circle on the map is proportional to the electricity generated by each plant. State governments owned 45 of the plants, the central government owned 22, and private entities owned 5. Table 13.1 describes the operating characteristics of these plants in terms of installed capacity, electricity generated, and other characteristics. We analyze the impact of plant emissions in 2008–09, the year for which we have information on the sulfur content of coal.[1]

Total coal-fired generating capacity in India doubled between March 2009 and March 2015 (CEA 2015), from 76 gigawatts (GW) to 164.6 GW.[2] Accordingly, our analysis underestimates the health impacts of current SO₂ emissions from the power sector. We note, however, that the plants we analyze remain subject to pollution control laws, and most plants would find it difficult to meet these laws without installing FGD units.

To calculate the SO₂ emissions of each plant, we must know the plant's annual electricity generation, the amount of coal burned per kWh, and the sulfur content of the coal burned.[3] We estimate the cost-effectiveness of FGD units using the Central Electricity Regulatory Commission of India's benchmark operating conditions.[4] These assume that each plant operates at 85 percent of capacity (the median operating capacity for the 72 plants was 79 percent in 2008–09). We use benchmark conditions because actual operating conditions are likely to fluctuate from year to year.

Coal consumption per kWh is based on actual coal consumption per kWh in 2008–09. On average, coal burned per kWh is much higher at Indian power plants than at coal-fired power plants in the United States (0.77 kg/kWh versus 0.47 kg/kWh) (Malik 2013). This difference is due in part to the lower heat content of Indian coal, but it is also due to inefficiencies in plant operation (Chan, Cropper, and Malik 2014). The sulfur content of coal (averaging 0.53 percent sulfur by weight) comes from a survey of Indian power plants conducted by the authors. This finding corresponds closely to figures reported by Lu and others (2013), Garg and others (2002), and Reddy and Venkataraman (2002). Based on benchmark conditions, the 72 plants emit approximately 3 million tons of SO₂ annually.

CAMx, an Eulerian photochemical dispersion model, was run to estimate the impact of each plant's SO₂ emissions on ambient air quality.[5] The model, which includes gas-to-aerosol conversion for SO₂ to sulfates, supports plume rise calculations for each power plant using three-dimensional meteorological data.[6] The model was run separately for each plant, simulating 365 days of emissions, to calculate the increase in annual average fine particle concentrations corresponding to the plant's emissions. The model was run at a 0.25°grid resolution

**Table 13.1** Operating Characteristics of Power Plants in the Dataset
*Summary Statistics—Actual Operations*

| | Average | Standard deviation | Median | Minimum | Maximum |
|---|---|---|---|---|---|
| Nameplate capacity (MW) | 948 | 674 | 840 | 63 | 3,260 |
| Generation (GWh) | 6,393 | 5,446 | 5,305 | 103 | 26,601 |
| Capacity utilization (%) | 75 | 20 | 79 | 11 | 100 |
| Sulfur content of coal (%) | 0.53 | 0.19 | 0.5 | 0.21 | 2.00 |
| $SO_2$ emissions (tons/yr) | 37,727 | 31,857 | 30,423 | 778 | 188,010 |

*Note:* Number of observations = 72 power plants. Data based on actual operations for the year 2008–09. GWh = gigawatt hour; MW = megawatt; $SO_2$ = sulphur dioxide.

and combined with 2011 population data to calculate the population-weighted increase in annual average $PM_{2.5}$ concentrations associated with the plant.

Epidemiological research has found consistent associations between premature mortality and $PM_{2.5}$. Pope and others (2002) report significant impacts of exposure to $PM_{2.5}$ in cities in the United States on all-cause, cardiopulmonary, and lung cancer mortality. This work formed the basis of early studies of the global burden of air pollution (Cohen and others 2004). More recent studies of the Global Burden of Disease (GBD) (Lim and others 2013) use meta-analyses of epidemiological studies from several sources to quantify the impact of a wider range of $PM_{2.5}$ exposures on cardiovascular and respiratory deaths, as well as deaths from lung cancer and ALRI (Burnett and others 2014). The 2013 GBD estimates that 587,000 deaths in India in 2013 were attributable to ambient air pollution (GBD 2013 Risk Factors Collaborators 2015).

Premature mortality associated with the increase in annual average $PM_{2.5}$ concentrations for each plant was calculated as the product of baseline deaths (by cause) and the fraction of deaths attributable to sulfates. The fraction of deaths attributable to sulfates for each disease is given by $1-\exp(\beta^*\Delta C)$, where $\beta$ is the change in the relative risk attributable to a one microgram per cubic meter change in $PM_{2.5}$, and $\Delta C$ is the population-weighted change in ambient $PM_{2.5}$ concentrations associated with $SO_2$ emissions from the plant. The $\beta$ coefficients were calculated using the IERs for ischemic heart disease, stroke, lung cancer, COPD, and ALRI developed by Burnett and others (2014) and reported by the Institute for Health Metrics and Evaluation (IHME).[7] For each disease, the change in relative risk ($\beta$) was evaluated at the population-weighted annual average exposures for India used in the 2010 Global Burden of Disease (Brauer and others 2012).[8] Baseline deaths by age and cause were obtained from the IHME.[9]

We also calculate the years of life lost (YLL) associated with mortality attributable to $SO_2$ emissions. We estimate that, on average, each death is associated with

25.54 YLL, a figure close to that reported in the 2013 GBD. DALYs lost because of $PM_{2.5}$ are the sum of YLL and years lived with disability (YLD). In the 2013 GBD, 97 percent of DALYs associated with ambient air pollution are YLL. We have not calculated the YLD associated with $SO_2$ emissions; therefore, our estimates of the health benefits of emissions reductions understate total health benefits.

### Estimates of Health Effects Associated with $SO_2$ Emissions

Our calculations suggest that approximately 15,500 deaths in 2013 were attributable to $SO_2$ emissions from the 72 plants, with stroke (7,600) and ischemic heart disease (4,200) accounting for the majority of deaths. Table 13.2 reports the distribution of deaths and DALYs (by cause) for the 72 plants. These deaths, in the aggregate, are associated with approximately 400,000 YLL.[10] If the plants in our study were to operate under benchmark operating conditions at capacity factors of 85 percent, the deaths attributable to $SO_2$ emissions would increase to approximately 17,900 per year, with an associated 457,000 YLL.

The number of deaths per plant varies from more than 1,300 to fewer than 20. The 30 plants with the highest number of deaths account for 78 percent of the total deaths and 56 percent of the total generation capacity. The 20 plants with the highest number of deaths account for 65 percent of total deaths. Deaths per plant are correlated with total emissions (r = 0.38) and also with the size of the exposed population. Population density in India is highest in the north of India, which is also the part of India with the highest levels of ambient $PM_{2.5}$. Therefore, it is not surprising that the 30 plants with the highest number of deaths (map 13.2) are located in northern India.

### Costs and Benefits of FGD Units

An FGD unit is an end-of-pipe technology that removes $SO_2$ from combustion gases before they exit the smokestack. Flue gases are treated with an alkaline

**Table 13.2** Deaths and DALYs Associated with SO₂ Emissions, by Plant

| Cause | Deaths | | | DALYs | | |
|---|---|---|---|---|---|---|
| | **Mean** | **25%ile** | **75%ile** | **Mean** | **25%ile** | **75%ile** |
| COPD | 18.5 | 5.5 | 20.1 | 351 | 104 | 392 |
| Stroke | 106 | 31.4 | 115 | 2,230 | 660 | 2,490 |
| IHD | 58.8 | 17.4 | 63.8 | 1,350 | 399 | 1,510 |
| ALRI | 29.9 | 8.9 | 32.5 | 1,510 | 449 | 1,690 |
| Lung cancer | 2.3 | 0.68 | 2.6 | 60.1 | 17.8 | 67.1 |
| All causes | 216 | 64 | 241 | 5,500 | 1,630 | 6,150 |
| All causes, benchmark conditions | 249 | 77.3 | 301 | 6,360 | 1,974 | 7,690 |

*Note:* ALRI = acute lower respiratory infection; COPD = chronic obstructive pulmonary disease; DALY = disability-adjusted life year; IHD = ischemic heart disease; SO₂ = sulphur dioxide.

**Map 13.2** Coal-Fired Power Plants: Top 30 Sulfate Deaths

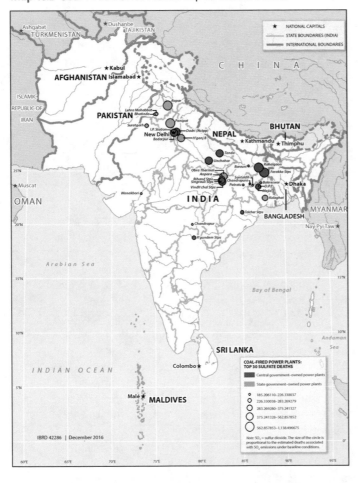

substance that reacts with the acidic SO₂ to form a by-product that is removed before flue gases are emitted. In a wet limestone FGD (wFGD) unit, gases are treated with limestone slurry, which is sprayed on the gas in an absorber unit. Gypsum, which can be sold commercially, is produced as a by-product. Approximately 85 percent of the scrubbers installed in the United States are wet scrubbers (USEPA 2004).[11] Another rapidly expanding technology is seawater FGD (swFGD) units. These units use the alkalinity of seawater to remove SO₂ from the flue gases; the by-product is water, which is then treated and discharged back into the sea. Seawater FGD units are capable of reducing SO₂ emissions up to 95 percent, depending on the technology used.[12]

Both scrubber technologies are in use in India. The Indian Supreme Court required the installation of an FGD unit at the Dahanu plant in Maharashtra. FGD units are also in operation at the Trombay and Udupi plants (table 13.3).[13] Both Dahanu and Trombay have swFGD units. Seawater FGD units have lower capital costs and much lower variable costs than wFGD units, but they can be installed only in coastal areas. We assume that FGD units installed at plants in coastal areas are swFGD units, and that FGD units installed at all other locations are wFGD units.

The estimates of FGD unit costs are based on tariff orders issued by State Electricity Regulatory Commissions (SERCs) for power plants that currently operate an FGD unit or for plants that are planning to install one in the near future (table 13.3). We also use information from tariff determination norms and calculations of benchmark capital costs used by the Central Electricity Regulatory Commission (CERC 2009).[14]

Table 13.4 shows the assumptions used to construct the cost estimates. We assume a capital cost of US$84,000/MW for a swFGD unit (MERC 2009, 2011) and a cost of US$109,000/MW for a wFGD unit, based on 250 MW units.[15] For smaller units, we assume that the elasticity of capital costs with respect to installed capacity is −0.3 (Cichanowicz 2010). The greater costs for wFGD units reflect the expenditures for reagent handling and by-product disposal facilities. In contrast, swFGD units discharge their water by-product back into the sea and do not require as much capital investment.

**Table 13.3** FGD Units in India, Planned and Operational

| Location | Company | State | Status of FGD unit | Capacity | Manufacturer | Type |
|---|---|---|---|---|---|---|
| Trombay | TATA Power | Maharashtra | Operating | Unit 5: 500 MW | ABB | Seawater |
| Trombay | TATA Power | Maharashtra | Operating | Unit 8: 250 MW | — | Seawater |
| Ratnagiri | JSW | Maharashtra | Under construction | 1,200 MW (4 units × 300 MW) | Alstom | Seawater |
| Udupi | LANCO | Karnataka | Operating | 1,200 MW (2 units × 600 MW) | Ducon | Wet limestone |
| Dahanu | RELIANCE | Maharashtra | Operating | 500 MW | Ducon | Seawater |
| Bongaigaon | NTPC | Assam | Under construction | 750 MW | BHEL | Wet limestone |
| Vindhyachal, stage V | NTPC | Madhya Pradesh | Planned | 500 MW | BHEL | Wet limestone |
| Mundra, stage III | ADANI | Gujarat | Planned | 1,980 MW | — | Seawater |

*Note:* FGD = flue-gas desulfurization; MW = megawatt; — = not available.

**Table 13.4** Operating Characteristics for Cost Calculations: Baseline Assumptions

| | Benchmark |
|---|---|
| Capacity utilization (%) | 85 |
| Capital discount rate (%) | 8 |
| Plant life (retrofit) (yrs) | 20 |

| | FGD Unit Type | |
|---|---|---|
| | **Wet limestone** | **Seawater** |
| Capital costs (US$/MW) | $109,091 | $84,364 |
| Fixed operating costs (US$/MWh) | $0.473 | $0.364 |
| Electricity costs (US$/kWh) | $0.0636 | $0.0636 |
| Auxiliary consumption (%) | 1.5 | 1.25 |
| FGD unit efficiency (%) | 90 | 90 |
| Retrofit cost factor (%) | 30 | 30 |

*Note:* The capital costs above are derived from information for the Dahanu (seawater FGD unit) and Bongaigaon (wet FGD unit) power plants. In both cases, the costs reflect installation of an FGD unit in a new plant and not a retrofit. Costs are increased by 30 percent to reflect the higher costs of retrofitting a scrubber. FGD = flue-gas desulfurization; kWh = kilowatt hour; MW = megawatt; MWh = megawatt hour.

As a comparison, these figures are slightly lower than wFGD unit prices in the United States prior to the post-2006 spike in prices.[16] Capital and operating costs per plant are summarized in table 13.5. We note that the cost per ton of $SO_2$ removed implied by our calculations is, on average, US$613 (2013 US$).

To calculate the health benefits of installing an FGD unit, we assume that the FGD unit will remove 90 percent of $SO_2$ emissions. Because of the linearity of sulfate formation and the approximate linearity of relative risk for a small change in concentrations, this reduction in emissions implies a 90 percent reduction in deaths attributable to $SO_2$ emissions. An important question is the period over which this reduction would occur. Apte and others (2015) assume no lag between emissions reductions and the associated reductions in deaths. USEPA (2011) assumes that 80 percent of the reduction in $PM_{2.5}$ mortality is achieved within five years of the reduction in emissions. We view our calculations as representing the benefits of a scrubber that has been in operation for at least 5 years and therefore assume that 80 percent of the reduction in mortality has been achieved in calculating lives saved and DALYs averted.

## RESULTS

Our benchmark calculations suggest that requiring all 72 plants in our study to install scrubbers would save 12,890 lives and 329,000 DALYs annually, at an average cost of US$131,000 per life saved or US$5,140 per DALY averted (table 13.6).[17] The cost per life saved (CPLS) of installing a scrubber, however, varies greatly across plants, from US$24,700 to US$1,244,000, depending on the magnitude of the plant's emissions and the size of the exposed population. If plants are ranked by their CPLS, retrofitting scrubbers at the 30 most cost-effective plants would save approximately 9,200 lives at an average cost of US$67,000 per life saved or US$2,600 per DALY averted.[18] Requiring scrubbers at the 30 plants with the highest deaths associated with $SO_2$ emissions would save more lives and DALYs (10,060 and 257,000, respectively) at a higher average CPLS of US$96,000. This finding is not surprising: lives saved (the denominator when calculating CPLS) is increasing in the number of deaths associated with plant when operating without an FGD unit; hence, CPLS is negatively correlated with deaths attributable to baseline $SO_2$ emissions for each plant ($r = -0.43$).[19]

**Table 13.5** Capital and Operating Costs of FGD Unit Installation per Plant
*Summary Statistics: Benchmark Operations*

| | Average | Standard deviation | Median | Minimum | Maximum |
|---|---|---|---|---|---|
| SO$_2$ emissions (tons/yr) | 42,678 | 30,344 | 36,405 | 2,704 | 169,192 |
| FGD unit capital costs (US$, millions) | 133 | 95.4 | 119 | 10.9 | 462 |
| Operating costs, fixed (US$, millions) | 3.3 | 2.4 | 3.0 | 0.22 | 11.5 |
| Operating costs, variable (US$, millions) | 6.7 | 4.8 | 6.0 | 0.4 | 23.2 |
| Total annual FGD unit cost (US$, millions) | 23.5 | 16.9 | 21.1 | 1.77 | 81.7 |

*Note:* Number of observations = 72 power plants. Calculations based on benchmark capacity utilization of 85 percent. FGD = flue-gas desulfurization. SO$_2$ = sulphur dioxide.

**Table 13.6** Cost-Effectiveness of FGD Unit Installation, US$

| | Total lives saved | Total cost (millions) | Cost per Life Saved, by Plant | | | Total DALYs averted | Cost per DALY Averted, by Plant | | |
|---|---|---|---|---|---|---|---|---|---|
| | | | Median | Minimum | Maximum | | Median | Minimum | Maximum |
| All plants | 12,890 | $1,691 | $167,000 | $24,700 | $1,244,000 | 329,000 | $6,540 | $967 | $48,713 |
| 30 plants with lowest CPLS | 9,196 | $615 | $62,490 | $24,707 | $137,474 | 235,000 | $2,447 | $967 | $5,383 |
| 30 plants with most deaths | 10,061 | $965 | $111,980 | $24,707 | $381,676 | 257,000 | $4,385 | $967 | $14,944 |
| 30 largest plants (MW) | 7,910 | $1,164 | $251,980 | $33,439 | $1,244,127 | 202,000 | $9,866 | $1,309 | $48,713 |

*Note:* Calculations based on benchmark operating conditions (capacity factor of 85 percent), assuming an FGD unit removes 90 percent of flue gases. The number of lives saved (or DALYs averted) is the number saved five years after installation, holding population and death rates at 2013 levels. CPLS = cost per life saved; DALY = disability-adjusted life year; FGD = flue-gas desulfurization; MW = megawatt.

However, identifying plants with the lowest CPLS may be difficult from a policy perspective. A more likely option would be to require the largest plants to scrub their emissions. The 30 largest plants in terms of installed capacity account for 61 percent of sulfate deaths. Requiring them to be retrofitted with FGD units would save approximately 7,910 lives and 202,000 DALYs, at an average CPLS of US$147,000 (US$5,760 per DALY averted). This approach clearly delivers fewer health benefits per dollar spent than requiring the plants associated with the largest number of deaths and DALYs to scrub their emissions. Although economies of scale exist in scrubber installation, and although deaths are positively correlated with plant size, the effectiveness of a scrubber also depends on the size of the exposed population; the largest plants are not necessarily those with the largest exposed populations.[20]

To maximize the number of lives saved for a given amount spent, plants with the lowest CPLS would be retrofitted first. These are not necessarily the largest plants. The benefits of installing a scrubber depend on the size of the exposed population, which depends on plant location. The 30 plants with the lowest CPLS associated with SO$_2$ emissions are primarily located in densely populated northern India, primarily in Uttar Pradesh, West Bengal, Punjab, Haryana, and Jharkhand.

Our estimates are sensitive to assumptions about scrubbing costs, as well as to assumptions about health impacts. Our baseline discount rate of 8 percent is a social discount rate, equal to the rate of interest on government bonds in India. If this is replaced by the weighted private cost of capital, which we estimate to be 11.2 percent, the CPLS would increase by 14.3 percent, from US$131,000 to US$150,000.[21] Reducing capacity factors from the benchmark level of 0.85 to 0.68 would increase the CPLS by approximately 20 percent. At the same time, our estimate of the impact of a cessation lag is quite conservative. We effectively assume that only 80 percent of the ultimate mortality benefits of scrubbing will be received. Eliminating the cessation lag would reduce the CPLS by 20 percent.

We also note that retrofitting power plants with scrubber units would increase the cost of electricity. In Cropper and others (2012), we estimate that a swFGD unit would increase the levelized cost of electricity by approximately 9 percent. A wFGD unit could increase the cost by up to 15 percent.

## DISCUSSION

Compared to coal mined in the rest of the world, domestic coal in India has high ash content but low sulfur content. Since 1984, regulations have limited particulate matter emitted directly from coal-fired power plants; however, before December 2015, no regulations existed that would limit secondary particle formation by restricting emissions of $SO_2$ or $NOx$.[22] Plants are, however, subject to minimum stack height requirements and plants generating 500 MW of electricity or more are required to leave space to allow for an FGD unit retrofit in the future. Plants generating between 210 and 500 MW of electricity must have stacks at least 220 meters in height; units that generate more than 500 MW of electricity must have stacks at least 275 meters in height. Taller stacks decrease ambient $SO_2$ concentrations by causing the particulate matter they emit to be dispersed over a larger area, but they do not eliminate exposure, especially in densely populated areas.

In December 2015, the Ministry of Environment, Forests and Climate Change issued limits on $SO_2$ emissions.[23] Plants built before 2017 that generate more than 500 MW of electricity are restricted to $SO_2$ emissions of 200 milligrams per cubic meter ($mg/Nm^3$); plants that generate less than 500 MW are restricted to $SO_2$ emissions of 600 $mg/Nm^3$.[24] A plant burning coal that contains 0.5 percent sulfur by weight emits approximately 1,350 $mg/Nm^3$, thus violating current standards. Retrofitting the plant with an FGD unit would permit the plant to achieve the Ministry's standards.[25] Currently, three plants in India have installed FGD units—Dahanu (Maharashtra), Trombay (Maharashtra), and Udupi (Karnataka). According to the Central Electricity Authority, eight FGD units either are in operation or are in the planning stages (table 13.3).

Our analysis suggests that the emphasis placed on $SO_2$ controls is warranted. The historic approach—relying on tall stacks—mirrors the approach taken in the United States in the 1980s to achieve local air quality standards. Although Indian coal has lower sulfur content than coal mined in the eastern United States, a greater amount of coal is used to produce a kWh of electricity in India because of the low heating value of Indian coal. In addition, the increase in imported coal with higher sulfur content will potentially increase the average sulfur content of coal used in Indian power plants. The large numbers of people exposed combined with the magnitude of $SO_2$ emissions from coal-fired power plants makes $SO_2$ a key pollutant of concern from a health standpoint.

## CONCLUSIONS

Our analysis suggests that retrofitting existing plants with FGD units could yield significant health benefits. Requiring all 72 plants in our sample to retrofit FGD units would save almost 13,000 lives (330,000 DALYs)

annually at an average cost of US$131,000 per life saved (US$5,140 per DALY averted). However, considerable heterogeneity exists in the CPLS across plants. Targeting the retrofitting regulation to plants with lower CPLS would be more cost-effective.

For any of the policy options considered, a relevant question is whether the CPLS is less than the value of the associated mortality reductions, measured in terms of what people are willing to pay for them. In the United States and other Organisation for Economic Co-operation and Development (OECD) countries, the value of mortality risk reductions is measured by the value per statistical life (VSL)—the sum of what people would pay for small risk reductions that sum to one statistical life saved.[26] Both the United States and OECD countries have adopted official values for the VSL that are used in benefit-cost analyses of environmental policies. Whether FGD units pass the benefit-cost test requires an estimate of the VSL for India.

Estimates of the VSL for India could be based on empirical studies conducted in India or could be transferred from United States and OECD values, taking into account differences in incomes. Empirical estimates of the VSL in India range widely, from US$57,000 (Bhattacharya, Alberini, and Cropper 2007) to US$407,000 (Madheswaran 2007).[27] Transferring the USEPA's VSL from the United States to India at current exchange rates (using an income elasticity of one) implies a VSL of US$250,000.[28] This suggests that a program to retrofit FGD units on all 72 power plants in our study would pass the benefit-cost test, on average. FGD unit installation also would pass the benefit-cost test on an individual plant basis at most of the plants in the study, including the 30 plants with the lowest CPLS.[29]

Because big plants are easier to target, regulations that would require the retrofitting of FGD units at the largest plants (those with the largest installed capacity) might be possible. The CPLS averaged over the 30 largest plants in our sample is US$147,000, suggesting that this regulation would, on average, pass the benefit-cost test. However, targeting the installation of FGD units to plants with the highest number of deaths would save more lives per dollar spent.

## ACKNOWLEDGMENTS

We thank Resources for the Future and the World Bank for funding, and Zachary Lazri and Anna Malinovskaya for excellent research assistance. We dedicate this chapter to Shama Gamkhar, our coauthor, who died before it was completed. We also thank Russ Dickerson, Jeremy Schreifels, and two anonymous referees for helpful comments.

# NOTES

World Bank Income Classifications as of July 2014 are as follows, based on estimates of gross national income (GNI) per capita for 2013:

- Low-income countries (LICs) = US$1,045 or less
- Middle-income countries (MICs) are subdivided:
  a) lower-middle-income = US$1,046 to US$4,125
  b) upper-middle-income (UMICs) = US$4,126 to US$12,745
- High-income countries (HICs) = US$12,746 or more.

1. The Indian fiscal year runs from April 1 of each year through March 31.
2. Average installed capacity of all coal-fired plants in March 2015 was 1,067 MW, and median installed capacity was 950 MW, which is slightly larger than for our 72 plants.
3. Total emissions of $SO_2$ are calculated using the sulfur content of coal and coal consumption, as well as assumptions about the volume of flue gases per ton of coal burned.
4. The CERC's benchmark operating conditions are used in tariff setting by the central government (CERC 2009). We also use these benchmark conditions in calculating the annualized cost of operating an FGD unit.
5. See http:// www.camx.com.
6. The meteorological data (wind, temperature, pressure, relative humidity, and precipitation) are derived from the global reanalysis database of the National Center for Environmental Prediction (NCEP) and processed through the Weather Research and Forecasting (WRF) meteorological model at a one-hour temporal resolution.
7. See http://ghdx.healthdata.org/record/global-burden -disease-study-2010-gbd-2010-ambient-air-pollution -risk-model-1990-2010.
8. Specifically, we evaluated the change in relative risk at the population-weighted ambient concentration of $PM_{2.5}$ within a 100 kilometer radius surrounding each plant, computed using the supplementary material from Brauer and others (2012). Concentrations ranged from 15 to 46 µg/m³, with a mean of 27 µg/m³.
9. We use death rates by age and cause reported in the 2013 Global Burden of Disease. https://cloud.ihme.washington .edu/index.php/s/b89390325f728bbd99de0356 d3be6900?path=%2FIHME%20GBD%202013%20 Deaths%20by%20Cause%201990-2013.
10. YLL are calculated for each cause of death by multiplying the number of deaths by the average number of life years lost based on the age distribution of deaths. YLL are then summed across all five causes of death.
11. Dry scrubber technologies (including spray dry scrubbers and circulating fluidized bed scrubbers) have lower capital costs than wFGD units and lower removal rates. These are much less commonly used than wFGD units (Carpenter 2014), and we have no cost data on their operation in India. Therefore, we do not analyze them as a control option.
12. USEPA's AP-42 database indicates that a swFGD unit can achieve up to 95 percent $SO_2$ removal; equipment suppliers claim $SO_2$ removal efficiencies of up to 99 percent with additives in the flue gas stream.
13. The only plants in table 13.3 that are in our sample are the Trombay, Udupi, and Vindhyachal plants.
14. The CERC is responsible for tariff determination for all central government–owned power plants and those selling inter-state power. The guidelines established by the CERC are also used by individual state SERCs in their tariff calculations. All costs in Indian rupees (Rs^k) have been converted to US$ using an exchange rate of US$1 = 55Rs^k and are thus in 2013 US$.
15. Personal communication with an NTPC (India's largest power utility) engineer. NTPC is involved in setting up a new plant in Bongaigaon, Assam, that will have a wFGD unit installed. The FGD unit is being provided by an Indian company, BHEL. According to online sources, BHEL reports a rule of thumb cost estimate for a wFGD unit of US$90,700/MW. We use the more conservative estimate.
16. https://www.eia.gov/electricity/annual/html/epa_09_04 .html. See also Muller (2016).
17. The average CPLS of requiring all plants to scrub their emissions is the total cost listed in table 13.6 (US$1.69 billion) divided by the lives saved. Similarly, the average cost per DALY averted is US$1.69 billion divided by the DALYs averted (329,000).
18. A ranking based on CPLS is identical to a ranking based on cost per DALY. A simplifying assumption underlying the calculations (as in the 2013 GBD) is that the age distribution of the population and death rates by age and cause are uniform throughout the country.
19. Twenty-one of the plants with the lowest CPLS are also the plants with the largest number of deaths associated with $SO_2$ emissions.
20. The 13th largest plant in the sample, based on installed capacity, has the highest CPLS (US$1,244,000). The plant is located in the south of India and has a smaller exposed population than plants in northern India.
21. Our estimate of the private cost of capital is based on a debt-equity ratio of 70–30, the private rate of return on capital allowed by the CERC (15.5 percent), and the assumption that the plant can borrow at a rate of 9.3% (the Bank of India base rate at the time of writing).
22. Prior to December 2015, emission limits for total suspended particulates called for units below 210 MW to emit no more than 350 mg/Nm³ and units greater than 210 MW no more than 150 mg/Nm³. The use of coal with ash content exceeding 34 percent is prohibited in any thermal power plant located more than 1,000 km from the pithead or in urban, sensitive, or critically polluted areas. http://cpcb.nic.in/Industry_Specific_Standards.php.
23. *Gazette of India*, December 8, 2015. Ministry of Environment, Forests and Climate Change Notification. S.O. 3305(E). Environment (Protection) Amendment Rules, 2015.

24. Plants built after 2017 may emit no more than 100 mg of $SO_2$ per $Nm^3$. These plants certainly would require FGD units; however the cost of installing scrubbers when plants are built is lower than the cost of retrofitting them.

25. A referee notes that the 600 mg/$Nm^3$ standard could be achieved by installing a dry scrubber, which would have lower capital costs than a wFGD unit.

26. To illustrate, if each of 10,000 people were willing to pay US$100 over the coming year to reduce their risk of dying by 1 in 10,000 during this period, on average, one statistical life would be saved and the VSL would equal US$100 × 10,000 or US$1,000,000.

27. Both values were obtained by converting Indian rupees ($Rs^k$) to US$ using the average exchange rate for 2007 and then converting to 2013 US$ using the Consumer Price Index.

28. USEPA's official VSL is US$7.4 million (2006 US$), implying a VSL to per capita income ratio of 159:1 (USEPA 2011). Applying this ratio to per capita income in India in 2014–15 (US$1,570) yields a VSL of US$250,000.

29. Forty-seven of the 72 plants have a CPLS of less than US$250,000; 64 have a CPLS of less than US$407,000.

## REFERENCES

Apte, J. S., J. D. Marshall, A. J. Cohen, and M. Brauer. 2015. "Addressing Global Mortality from Ambient $PM_{2.5}$." *Environmental Science and Technology* 49: 8057–66.

Bhattacharya, S., A. Alberini, and M. Cropper. 2007. "The Value of Mortality Risk Reductions in Delhi, India." *Journal of Risk and Uncertainty* 34 (1): 21–47.

Brauer M., M. Amann, R. T. Burnett, A. Cohen, F. Dentener, and others. 2012. "Exposure Assessment for Estimation of the Global Burden of Disease Attributable to Outdoor Air Pollution." *Environmental Science and Technology* 46: 652–60.

Burnett, R. T., C. A. Pope III, M. Ezzati, C. Olives, S. S. Lim, and others. 2014. "An Integrated Risk Function for Estimating the Global Burden of Disease Attributable to Ambient Fine Particulate Matter Exposure." *Environmental Health Perspectives* 122 (4): 397–403.

Carpenter, A. 2014. "Water-Saving FGD Technologies." *Cornerstone.* http://cornerstonemag.net/tag/dry-scrubbers.

CEA (Central Electricity Authority). 2015. *Growth of Electricity Sector in India from 1947–2015.* New Delhi: Government of India.

CERC (Central Electricity Regulatory Commission). 2009. *Tariff Determination Methodology for Thermal Power Plants.* New Delhi: Government of India.

Chan, H. S., M. L. Cropper, and K. Malik. 2014. "Why Are Power Plants in India Less Efficient Than Power Plants in the United States?" *American Economic Review Papers and Proceedings* 104 (5): 586–90.

Chikkatur, A. P., and A. D. Sagar. 2007. "Cleaner Power in India: Towards a Clean-Coal-Technology Roadmap." *Belfer Center for Science and International Affairs Discussion Paper* 6: 1–261.

Cichanowicz, J. E. 2010. "Current Capital Cost and Cost-Effectiveness of Power Plant Emissions Control Technologies." Prepared for Utility Air Regulatory Group.

Cohen, A. J., H. R. Anderson, B. Ostro, K. D. Pandey, M. Krzyzanowski, and others. 2004. "Mortality Impacts of Urban Air Pollution." In *Comparative Quantification of Health Risks: Global and Regional Burden of Disease Due to Selected Major Risk Factors*, volume 2, edited by M. Ezzati, A. D. Lopez, A. Rodgers, and C. U. J. L. Murray. Geneva: World Health Organization.

Cropper, M., S. Gamkhar, K. Malik, A. Limonov, and I. Partridge. 2012. "The Health Effects of Coal Electricity Generation in India." Discussion Paper 12–25, Resources for the Future, Washington, DC.

Garg, A., M. Kapshe, P. R. Shukla, and D. Ghosh. 2002. "Large Point Source (LPS) Emissions from India: Regional and Sectoral Analysis." *Atmospheric Environment* 36 (2): 213–24.

GBD 2013 Risk Factor Collaborators. 2015. "Global, Regional, and National Comparative Risk Assessment of 79 Behavioral, Environmental and Occupational, and Metabolic Risks or Clusters of Risks in 188 countries, 1990–2013: A Systematic Analysis for the Global Burden of Disease Study 2013." *The Lancet* 386 (10010): 2287–323.

Guttikunda, S. K., and P. Jawahar. 2014. "Atmospheric Emissions and Pollution from the Coal-fired Thermal Power Plants in India." *Atmospheric Environment* 92: 449–60.

Lim, S. S., T. Vos, A. D. Flaxman, G. Danaei, K. Shibuya, and others. 2013. "A Comparative Risk Assessment of Burden of Disease and Injury Attributable to 67 Risk Factors and Risk Factor Clusters in 21 Regions, 1990–2010: A Systematic Analysis for the Global Burden of Disease Study 2010." *The Lancet* 380 (9859): 2224–60.

Lu, Z., D. G. Streets, B. de Foy, and N. A Krotkov. 2013. "Ozone Monitoring Instrument Observations of Interannual Increases in $SO_2$ Emissions from Indian Coal-Fired Power Plants during 2005–2012." *Environmental Science and Technology* 47: 13993–4000.

Madheswaran, S. 2007. "Measuring the Value of Statistical Life: Estimating Compensating Wage Differentials among Workers in India." *Social Indicators Research* 84: 83–96.

Malik, K. 2013. "Essays on Energy and Environment in India." PhD dissertation, University of Maryland, College Park, MD.

MERC (Maharashtra Electricity Regulatory Commission). 2009. "MERC Order for RInfra-G for APR of FY 2009-10 and Determination of Tariff for FY 2010–11." Case 99 of 2009, Maharashtra Electricity Regulatory Commission, Mumbai.

———. 2011. "MERC Order for Truing Up of FY 2009-10 and APR of FY 2010–11." Case 122 of 2011, Maharashtra Electricity Regulatory Commission, Mumbai.

Ministry of Environmental Protection, People's Republic of China. 2014. *List of $SO_2$ Scrubbers in Coal-Fired Power Plants.* http://english.mep.gov.cn.

Muller, N. Z. 2016. "Environmental Benefit-Cost Analysis and the National Accounts." NBER Working Paper, Cambridge, MA.

Pope, C. A., III, R. T. Burnett, M. J. Thun, E. E. Calle, D. Krewski, and others. 2002. "Lung Cancer, Cardiopulmonary Mortality, and Long-Term Exposure to Fine Particulate Air Pollution." *Journal of the American Medical Association* 287 (9): 1132–41.

Reddy, M. S., and C. Venkataraman. 2002. "Inventory of Aerosol and Sulphur Dioxide Emissions from India: I—Fossil Fuel Combustion." *Atmospheric Environment* 36 (4): 677–97.

Schmalensee, R., and R. N. Stavins. 2013. "The $SO_2$ Allowance Trading System: The Ironic History of a Grand Policy Experiment." *Journal of Economic Literature* 27 (1): 103–22.

USEPA (United States Environmental Protection Agency). 2004. *Air Pollution Control Technology Fact Sheet.* Washington, DC: USEPA.

———. 2011. *The Benefits and Costs of the Clean Air Act from 1990 to 2020.* Washington, DC: USEPA.

# DCP3 Series Acknowledgments

*Disease Control Priorities,* third edition *(DCP3)* compiles the global health knowledge of institutions and experts from around the world, a task that required the efforts of over 500 individuals, including volume editors, chapter authors, peer reviewers, advisory committee members, and research and staff assistants. For each of these contributions we convey our acknowledgment and appreciation. First and foremost, we would like to thank our 32 volume editors who provided the intellectual vision for their volumes based on years of professional work in their respective fields, and then dedicated long hours to reviewing each chapter, providing leadership and guidance to authors, and framing and writing the summary chapters. We also thank our chapter authors who collectively volunteered their time and expertise to writing over 170 comprehensive, evidence-based chapters.

We owe immense gratitude to the institutional sponsor of this effort: The Bill & Melinda Gates Foundation. The Foundation provided sole financial support of the Disease Control Priorities Network (DCPN). Many thanks to Program Officers Kathy Cahill, Philip Setel, Carol Medlin, Damian Walker and (currently) David Wilson for their thoughtful interactions, guidance, and encouragement over the life of the project. We also wish to thank Jaime Sepúlveda for his longstanding support, including chairing the Advisory Committee for the second edition and, more recently, demonstrating his vision for *DCP3* while he was a special advisor to the Gates Foundation. We are also grateful to the University of Washington's Department of Global Health and successive chairs King Holmes and Judy Wasserheit for providing a home base for the *DCP3* Secretariat, which included intellectual collaboration, logistical coordination, and administrative support.

We thank the many contractors and consultants who provided support to specific volumes in the form of economic analytical work, volume coordination, chapter drafting, and meeting organization: the Center for Disease Dynamics, Economics & Policy; Center for Chronic Disease Control; Centre for Global Health Research; Emory University; Evidence to Policy Initiative; Public Health Foundation of India; QURE Healthcare; University of California, San Francisco; University of Waterloo; University of Queensland; and the World Health Organization.

We are tremendously grateful for the wisdom and guidance provided by our advisory committee to the editors. Steered by Chair Anne Mills, the advisory committee ensures quality and intellectual rigor of the highest order for *DCP3*.

The National Academies of Sciences, Engineering, and Medicine, in collaboration with the Interacademy Medical Panel, coordinated the peer-review process for all *DCP3* chapters. Patrick Kelley, Gillian Buckley, Megan Ginivan, Rachel Pittluck, and Tara Mainero managed this effort and provided critical and substantive input.

World Bank Publishing provided exceptional guidance and support throughout the demanding production and design process. We would particularly like to thank Carlos Rossel, Mary Fisk, Nancy Lammers, Rumit Pancholi, Deborah Naylor, and Sherrie Brown for their diligence and expertise. Additionally, we thank Jose de Buerba, Mario Trubiano, Yulia Ivanova, and Chiamaka Osuagwu of the World Bank for providing professional counsel on communications and marketing strategies.

Several U.S. and international institutions contributed to the organization and execution of meetings that supported the preparation and dissemination of *DCP3*.

We would like to express our appreciation to the following institutions:

- University of Bergen, consultation on equity (June 2011)
- University of California, San Francisco, surgery volume consultations (April 2012, October 2013, February 2014)
- Institute of Medicine, first meeting of the Advisory Committee to the Editors (March 2013)
- Harvard Global Health Institute, consultation on policy measures to reduce incidence of noncommunicable diseases (July 2013)
- National Academy of Medicine, systems strengthening meeting (September 2013)
- Center for Disease Dynamics, Economics & Policy (Quality and Uptake meeting, September 2013; reproductive and maternal health volume consultation, November 2013)
- National Cancer Institute, cancer consultation (November 2013)
- Union for International Cancer Control, cancer consultation (November 2013, December 2014)
- Harvard T. H. Chan School of Public Health, economic evaluation consultation (September 2015)
- University of California, Berkeley School of Public Health, and Stanford Medical School, occupational and environmental health consultations (December 2015).

Carol Levin provided outstanding governance for cost and cost-effectiveness analysis. Stéphane Verguet added valuable guidance in applying and improving the extended cost-effectiveness analysis method. Elizabeth Brouwer, Kristen Danforth, Nazila Dabestani, Shane Murphy, Zachary Olson, Jinyuan Qi, and David Watkins provided exceptional research assistance and analytic assistance. Brianne Adderley ably managed the budget and project processes, while Jennifer Nguyen, Shamelle Richards, and Jennifer Grasso contributed exceptional project coordination support. The efforts of these individuals were absolutely critical to producing this series, and we are thankful for their commitment.

# Volume and Series Editors

## VOLUME EDITORS

### Charles N. Mock

Charles N. Mock, MD, PhD, FACS, has training as both a trauma surgeon and an epidemiologist. He worked as a surgeon in Ghana for four years, including at a rural hospital (Berekum) and at the Kwame Nkrumah University of Science and Technology (Kumasi). In 2005–07, he served as Director of the University of Washington's Harborview Injury Prevention and Research Center. In 2007–10, he worked at the World Health Organization (WHO) headquarters in Geneva, where he was responsible for developing the WHO's trauma care activities. In 2010, he returned to his position as Professor of Surgery (with joint appointments as Professor of Epidemiology and Professor of Global Health) at the University of Washington. His main interests include the spectrum of injury control, especially as it pertains to low- and middle-income countries: surveillance, injury prevention, prehospital care, and hospital-based trauma care. He was President (2013–15) of the International Association for Trauma Surgery and Intensive Care.

### Olive Kobusingye

Olive Kobusingye is an accident and emergency surgeon and injury epidemiologist. She is on faculty at Makerere University School of Public Health where she heads the Trauma, Injury, and Disability (TRIAD) Project and coordinates graduate training in those disciplines. Before Makerere, Olive was the Regional Advisor on Violence, Injuries, and Disabilities at the World Health Organization's regional office for Africa (AFRO). She is the founding Executive Director of the Injury Control Center–Uganda, and founding Secretary General of the Injury Prevention Initiative for Africa. She established the first hospital trauma registries in Sub-Saharan Africa and codeveloped the Kampala Trauma Score, now used in many low-income countries. Her research interests include injury surveillance, injury severity measurement, emergency trauma care systems, road safety, and drowning.

### Rachel Nugent

Rachel Nugent is Vice President for Global Noncommunicable Diseases at RTI International. She was formerly a Research Associate Professor and Principal Investigator of the DCPN in the Department of Global Health at the University of Washington. Previously, she served as Deputy Director of Global Health at the Center for Global Development, Director of Health and Economics at the Population Reference Bureau, Program Director of Health and Economics Programs at the Fogarty International Center of the National Institutes of Health, and senior economist at the Food and Agriculture Organization of the United Nations. From 1991–97, she was associate professor and department chair in economics at Pacific Lutheran University.

### Kirk R. Smith

Kirk R. Smith is Professor of Global Environmental Health at University of California, Berkeley School of Public Health. He is also founder and coordinator of the campus-wide Masters Program in Global Health and Environment. Previously, he was founder and head of the Energy Program of the East-West Center in Honolulu. He serves on a number of national and international scientific advisory committees, including the Global Energy Assessment, National Research Council's Board

251

on Atmospheric Sciences and Climate, the Executive Committee for WHO Air Quality Guidelines, the Intergovernmental Panel on Climate Change, and the Global Burden of Disease. He is a member of the U.S. National Academy of Sciences and holder of the Tyler and Heinz Prizes for environmental achievement.

## SERIES EDITORS

### Dean T. Jamison

Dean T. Jamison is Emeritus Professor in Global Health Sciences at the University of California, San Francisco, and the University of Washington. He previously held academic appointments at Harvard University and the University of California, Los Angeles. Prior to his academic career, he was an economist on the staff of the World Bank, where he was lead author of the World Bank's *World Development Report 1993: Investing in Health*. He serves as lead editor for *DCP3* and was lead editor for the previous two editions. He holds a PhD in economics from Harvard University and is an elected member of the Institute of Medicine of the U.S. National Academy of Sciences. He recently served as Co-Chair and Study Director of *The Lancet's* Commission on Investing in Health.

### Rachel Nugent

See the list of Volume Editors.

### Hellen Gelband

Hellen Gelband is an independent global health policy expert. Her work spans infectious disease, particularly malaria and antibiotic resistance, and noncommunicable disease policy, mainly in low- and middle-income countries. She has conducted policy studies at Resources for the Future, the Center for Disease Dynamics, Economics & Policy, the (former) Congressional Office of Technology Assessment, the Institute of Medicine of the U.S. National Academies, and a number of international organizations.

### Susan Horton

Susan Horton is Professor at the University of Waterloo and holds the Centre for International Governance Innovation (CIGI) Chair in Global Health Economics in the Balsillie School of International Affairs there. She has consulted for the World Bank, the Asian Development Bank, several United Nations agencies, and the International Development Research Centre, among others, in work conducted in over 20 low- and middle-income countries. She led the work on nutrition for the Copenhagen Consensus in 2008, when micronutrients were ranked as the top development priority. She has served as associate provost of graduate studies at the University of Waterloo, vice-president academic at Wilfrid Laurier University in Waterloo, and interim dean at the University of Toronto at Scarborough.

### Prabhat Jha

Prabhat Jha is the founding director of the Centre for Global Health Research at St. Michael's Hospital and holds Endowed and Canada Research Chairs in Global Health in the Dalla Lana School of Public Health at the University of Toronto. He is lead investigator of the Million Death Study in India, which quantifies the causes of death and key risk factors in over two million homes over a 14-year period. He is also Scientific Director of the Statistical Alliance for Vital Events, which aims to expand reliable measurement of causes of death worldwide. His research includes the epidemiology and economics of tobacco control worldwide.

### Ramanan Laxminarayan

Ramanan Laxminarayan is Director of the Center for Disease Dynamics, Economics & Policy in Washington, DC. His research deals with the integration of epidemiological models of infectious diseases and drug resistance into the economic analysis of public health problems. He was one of the key architects of the Affordable Medicines Facility–malaria, a novel financing mechanism to improve access and delay resistance to antimalarial drugs. In 2012, he created the Immunization Technical Support Unit in India, which has been credited with improving immunization coverage in the country. He teaches at Princeton University.

### Charles N. Mock

See the list of Volume Editors.

# Contributors

**Safa Abdalla**
School of Medicine, Stanford University, Palo Alto, California, United States

**Rajeev B. Ahuja**
Department of Burns and Plastic Surgery, Lok Nayak Hospital and Maulana Azad Medical College, New Delhi, India

**Spenser S. Apramian**
Stanford University, Palo Alto, California, United States

**Abdulgafoor M. Bachani**
Department of International Health, Johns Hopkins University, Baltimore, Maryland, United States

**Mark A. Bellis**
Centre for Public Health, Liverpool John Moores University, Liverpool, United Kingdom

**Alexander Butchart**
World Health Organization, Geneva, Switzerland

**Linda F. Cantley**
School of Medicine, Yale University, New Haven, Connecticut, United States

**Claire Chase**
Water and Sanitation Program, World Bank, Washington, DC, United States

**Maureen L. Cropper**
Energy Research Center, University of Maryland, College Park, Maryland, United States

**Mark R. Cullen**
School of Medicine, Stanford University, Palo Alto, California, United States

**Nazila Dabestani**
Department of Global Health, University of Washington, Seattle, Washington, United States

**Kristie L. Ebi**
Department of Global Health, University of Washington, Seattle, Washington, United States

**Xiagming Fang**
College of Engineering, China Agricultural University, Beijing, China

**G. Gururaj**
National Institute of Mental Health and Neurosciences, Bangalore, India

**Sarath Guttikunda**
Division of Atmospheric Sciences, Desert Research Institute, Reno, Nevada, United States

**Jeremy J. Hess**
Division of Emergency Medicine, University of Washington, Seattle, Washington, United States

**Susan D. Hillis**
U.S. Centers for Disease Control and Prevention, Atlanta, Georgia, United States

**Connie Hoe**
Bloomberg School of Public Health, Johns Hopkins University, Baltimore, Maryland, United States

**Guy Hutton**
WASH Section, United Nations Children's Fund, New York, New York; formerly at the Water and Sanitation Program, World Bank, Washington, DC, United States

**Adnan A. Hyder**
Department of International Health, Johns Hopkins University, Baltimore, Maryland, United States

**Rebecca Ivers**
The George Institute for Global Health, Sydney, New South Wales, Australia

**Dean T. Jamison**
Global Health Sciences, University of California, San Francisco, San Francisco, California, United States

**Puja Jawahar**
Urban Emissions, New Delhi, India

**Lisa Keay**
The George Institute for Global Health, Sydney, New South Wales, Australia

**Carol Levin**
Department of Global Health, University of Washington, Seattle, Washington, United States

**David Mackie**
Department of Intensive Care, Red Cross Hospital, Beverwijk, the Netherlands

**Kabir Malik**
World Bank, Washington, DC, United States

**David Meddings**
Department for Management of Noncommunicable Diseases, Disability, Violence and Injury Prevention, World Health Organization, Geneva, Switzerland

**James A. Mercy**
U.S. Centers for Disease Control and Prevention, Atlanta, Georgia, United States

**Nam Phuong Nguyen**
World Health Organization, Vietnam Country Office, Hanoi, Vietnam

**Robyn Norton**
The George Institute for Global Health, Sydney, New South Wales, Australia

**Zachary Olson**
Berkeley School of Public Health, University of California, Berkeley, California, United States

**Ian Partridge**
School of Public Affairs, University of Texas, Austin, Austin, Texas, United States

**Margie Peden**
Department for Management of Noncommunicable Diseases, Disability, Violence and Injury Prevention, World Health Organization, Geneva, Switzerland

**Ajay Pillarisetti**
Berkeley School of Public Health, University of California, Berkeley, California, United States

**Fazlur Rahman**
Centre for Injury Prevention, Health Development and Research, Dhaka, Bangladesh

**Mark L. Rosenberg**
The Task Force for Global Health, Decatur, Georgia, United States

**John A. Staples**
Department of Medicine, University of Washington, Seattle, Washington, United States

**Stéphane Verguet**
Department of Global Health and Population, Harvard T. H. Chan School of Public Health, Boston, Massachusetts, United States

**Catherine L. Ward**
Department of Psychology, University of Cape Town, Cape Town, South Africa

**David A. Watkins**
School of Medicine, University of Washington, Seattle, Washington, United States

**Paul Watkiss**
Paul Watkiss Associates, Oxford, United Kingdom

# Advisory Committee to the Editors

**Anne Mills, Chair**
Professor, London School of Hygiene & Tropical Medicine, London, United Kingdom

**Olusoji Adeyi**
Director, Health, Nutrition and Population Global Practice, World Bank, Washington, DC, United States

**Kesetebirhan Admasu**
Former Minister of Health, Addis Ababa, Ethiopia

**George Alleyne**
Director Emeritus, Pan American Health Organization, Washington, DC, United States

**Ala Alwan**
Regional Director Emeritus, World Health Organization, Regional Office for the Eastern Mediterranean, Cairo, Arab Republic of Egypt

**Rifat Atun**
Professor, Global Health Systems, Harvard T. H. Chan School of Public Health, Boston, Massachusetts, United States

**Zulfiqar Bhutta**
Chair, Division of Women and Child Health, Aga Khan University Hospital, Karachi, Pakistan

**Agnes Binagwaho**
Former Minister of Health, Kigali, Rwanda

**Mark Blecher**
Senior Health Advisor, South Africa Treasury Department, Cape Town, South Africa

**Patricia Garcia**
Minister of Health, Lima, Peru

**Roger Glass**
Director, Fogarty International Center, National Institutes of Health, Bethesda, Maryland, United States

**Amanda Glassman**
Chief Operating Officer and Senior Fellow, Center for Global Development, Washington, DC, United States

**Glenda Gray**
Executive Director, Perinatal HIV Research Unit, Chris Hani Baragwanath Hospital, Johannesburg, South Africa

**Demissie Habte**
Chair of Board of Trustees, International Clinical Epidemiological Network, Addis Ababa, Ethiopia

**Richard Horton**
Editor, *The Lancet*, London, United Kingdom

**Edward Kirumira**
Dean, Faculty of Social Sciences, Makerere University, Kampala, Uganda

**Peter Lachmann**
Professor, University of Cambridge, Cambridge, United Kingdom

**Lai Meng Looi**
Professor, University of Malaya, Kuala Lumpur, Malaysia

**Adel Mahmoud**
Senior Molecular Biologist, Princeton University, Princeton, New Jersey, United States

**Anthony Measham**
World Bank (retired)

**Carol Medlin**
Independent Consultant, Washington, DC, United States

255

# Reviewers

**Roberto Bertollini**
Scientific Committee on Health, Environmental, and Emerging Risks of the European Commission, Luxembourg

**H. Ron Chan**
University of Manchester, Manchester, United Kingdom

**Carolyn J. Cumpsty-Fowler**
Center for Injury Research and Policy, Bloomberg School of Public Health, Johns Hopkins University, Baltimore, Maryland, United States

**Kathie L. Dionisio**
National Exposure Research Laboratory, U.S. Environmental Protection Agency, Research Triangle, North Carolina, United States

**Jay P. Graham**
Milken Institute School of Public Health, The George Washington University, Washington, DC, United States

**James Hammitt**
Harvard T. H. Chan School of Public Health, Boston, Massachusetts, United States

**Rema Hanna**
Harvard Kennedy School, Cambridge, Massachusetts, United States

**Stephen Hargarten**
Injury Research Center, Medical College of Wisconsin, Milwaukee, Wisconsin, United States

**Marcus R. Keogh-Brown**
Department of Global Health and Development, London School of Hygiene & Tropical Medicine, London, United Kingdom

**Patrick Kinney**
Department of Environmental Health Sciences, Columbia University, Mailman School of Public Health, New York, New York, United States

**Barry Kistnasamy**
South African Department of Health, Johannesburg, South Africa

**Sharon Levi**
Beterem-Safe Kids Israel, Petah Tikva, Israel

**Leslie Morris-Iveson**
Consultant, Oxford, United Kingdom

**Daniel Pope**
Department of Public Health and Policy, University of Liverpool, Liverpool, United Kingdom

**Saidur Rahman**
Bangladesh University of Health Sciences, Dhaka, Bangladesh

**Gordon S. Smith**
School of Medicine, University of Maryland, College Park, Maryland, United States

**Jukka Takala**
Workplace Safety and Health Institute, Singapore

**Leonardo Trasande**
School of Medicine, New York University, New York, New York, United States

**Elizabeth Ward**
Violence Prevention Alliance, Kingston, Jamaica

**Yuan Xu**
Institute of Environmental, Energy, and Sustainability, The Chinese University of Hong Kong, Hong Kong SAR, China

**Hisham Zerriffi**
Faculty of Forestry, University of British Columbia, Vancouver, British Columbia, Canada

# Policy Forum Participants

*The following individuals provided valuable insights to improve this volume's key findings through participation in the Disease Control Priorities–World Health Organization, Regional Office for the Eastern Mediterranean policy forum on Road Traffic Injury Prevention and Trauma Care. The forum was held in Sharjah, the United Arab Emirates, on February 22, 2016, and was organized by Dr. Ala Alwan, Regional Director Emeritus and member of the DCP3 Advisory Committee to the Editors.*

**Bahar Idris Abu Garda**
Federal Minister of Health, Khartoum, Sudan

**Faisal Al-Anaizi**
Director of Injury Prevention Programme, Ministry of Health, Riyadh, Saudi Arabia

**Mohamed Saad AlKharji**
Head of Traffic Department, Ministry of Interior, Doha, Qatar

**Wahid Al-Kharusi**
Ambassador Emeritus, Muscat, Oman

**Reda'a Al Menshawy**
Minister of Health, El-Beida, Libya

**Yasser Al Naimi**
Consultant, Hospital Sector, Ministry of Health, Abu Dhabi, United Arab Emirates

**Omran bin Mohammad Al Omran**
Director General of Road Services Department, Ministry of Transport, Riyadh, Saudi Arabia

**Hussain Abdul Rahman Al-Rand**
Assistant Undersecretary, Health Centers and Clinics, Ministry of Health, Abu Dhabi, United Arab Emirates

**Mohamed Awadh Alrawas**
Director General of Traffic Affairs, Royal Oman Police, Muscat, Oman

**Ala Alwan**
Regional Director Emeritus, World Health Organization, Regional Office for the Eastern Mediterranean, Cairo, Arab Republic of Egypt

**Raed Arafat**
Deputy Health Minister, Ministry of Health, Bucharest, Romania

**Osama Bahar**
Major, Directorate of Traffic Services, Ministry of Interior, Manama, Bahrain

**Nasir Baoum**
Minister of Public Health and Population, Sana'a, Republic of Yemen

**Gayle DiPietro**
Global Road Safety Program Manager, The International Federation of Red Cross and Red Crescent Societies, Geneva, Switzerland

**Ahmed ElAnsary**
Head of Ambulance and Emergency Medical Services, Ministry of Health and Population, Cairo, Arab Republic of Egypt

**Gururaj Gopalakrishna**
Professor and Head, Department of Epidemiology, World Health Organization Collaborating Centre for Injury Prevention and Safety Promotion, Centre for Public Health, National Institute of Mental Health and Neurosciences (NIMHANS), Bangalore, India

**Mohammad Jalili**
Associate Professor of Emergency Medicine and Vice Chancellor of Education, Tehran University of Medical Science, Tehran, Islamic Republic of Iran

**Junaid Razzak**
Director, Telemedicine Program, and Senior Advisor for Global Health, Department of Emergency Medicine, Johns Hopkins University School of Medicine, Baltimore, Maryland, United States; Joint Appointment, Department of International Health, Johns Hopkins Bloomberg School of Public Health; Visiting Faculty, Department of Emergency Medicine, Aga Khan University, Karachi, Pakistan

**Ramzi Salamé**
Executive Director, Interministerial National Road Safety Council, Beirut, Lebanon

**Essam Sharaf**
Former Prime Minister and Minister of Transport; Professor of Road Engineering, Cairo University, Cairo, Arab Republic of Egypt

# Index

*Boxes, figures, maps, notes, and tables are indicated by b, f, m, n, and t respectively.*

Cameron, J., 203
Cameroon, violence against women in, 74
Canada
    climate change in
        related costs, 162
        related labor productivity improvements, 162
    costs of intimate partner violence in, 79*t*, 81
    electronics industry in, 110
    lung cancer studies in, 139
    Youth Relationship Project, 83
cardiovascular disease, 141, 141*f*
Caribbean. *See* Latin America and the Caribbean
cataracts, 139, 140*t*
Centers for Disease Control and Prevention (CDC), 58
CEREAL (Centro de Reflexión y Acción Laboral, or
        Centre for Reflection and Action on Labour
        Issues), 114
Chad, diarrheal disease burden in, 164
chemical contamination, 4
    essential interventions to address, 17*t*
    exposure to chemicals and toxins, 4, 29, 30*t*, 119–21
        essential interventions to address, 17*t*
        prevention, 120–21
        types of hazards, 120
Chiabai, A., 161, 162
child abuse
    Children and Violence Evaluation Challenge Fund, 83
    costs and cost-effectiveness of interventions, 88*t*
    costs associated with, 76, 78–79*t*
    DALYs among youth ages 10 to 24 years, 74
    interventions, 83
        essential interventions to address, 16*t*, 19
    as risk factor for youth violence and intimate
        partner violence, 82
    street children, increased risk of, 75
child health
    acute lower respiratory infection (ALRI), 138, 139*f*,
        141, 223
    child safety caps on medications, 64
    diarrheal illnesses responsible for deaths, 31
    drowning and, 29, 59
        interventions, 61*t*
        prevention programs, 62
    falls, risk of, 59, 66
        interventions, 61, 61*t*, 66
    India, household air pollution case study, 223
    noncommunicable diseases, increased risk of due to
        violence during childhood, 76
    poisoning cases, 28, 60
    water, sanitation, and hygiene-related illnesses,
        31, 177, 178
        children in poor households, increased health
            risk of as justification for targeting, 190

improvements, effect of, 183
    vulnerability of children, 177
child labor, 30, 108, 116
Children and Violence Evaluation Challenge Fund, 83
child sexual abuse, 74
Chile
    costs
        of intimate partner violence in, 79*t*
        of road traffic injuries in, 38
        of violence against women in, 81
    labor productivity, climate change's impact on, 163
China
    benefit-cost analysis of clean energy in, 14, 225
    coal-fired power plants in, 239
    diarrheal disease burden in, 164
    household air pollution trends in
        coal stoves with chimneys, introduction of
            (National Improved Stove Program), 136, 139,
            144, 148
        impact on outdoor pollution, 147
    labor productivity, climate change's impact
        on, 162, 163
    occupational injuries in
        electronics industry, 110
        health care sector, 117
        health services coverage for, 109
        manufacturing sector, 106*t*
        migrant workers' risk, 108, 109
        participatory discussions with health care
            providers to prevent, 116
        textile, clothing, and footwear industry, 111
    road traffic injuries, costs of, 38
    tobacco taxes in, 224
    water, sanitation, and hygiene (WASH) services in
        cost-effectiveness, 191
    water insecurity in Northern China, 180
Chisholm, D., 44, 202
cholera, 178
chronic obstructive pulmonary disease (COPD),
        138–39
CIRCLE (Climate Impact Research and Response
        Coordination for a Larger Europe) study,
        161, 163
civil conflict. *See* collective violence and conflicts
climate change, 153–70
    adaptation, 154, 163–64
        methods to estimate costs of, 160
        need for cost estimations, 166
    agriculture sector, 164
    air conditioning and, 164
    challenges related to estimating costs and
        benefits, 166
    climate-resilient health systems, 157–58, 159*t*

essential interventions to address, 16t
evidence for prevention, 62
prevention challenges in LMICs, 62–63
LMICs vs. HICs, 3, 4t, 63
mortality trends in, 9, 12f, 56–58, 56f
age group, gender, and country type, 58t
income and regions, 56t, 57t
LMICs (all ages and genders), 27t, 29
males and age groups, 57t, 58
Working Group on Child Drowning in LMICs, 62

**E**

East Asia. *See also specific countries*
financial and economic consequences of inadequate
WASH in, 181
household air pollution in, 143
road traffic mortality rate in, 35
textile, clothing, and footwear industry in, 111
Eastern Mediterranean. *See also specific countries*
burns, mortality rates from, 58
burns in, 29
diarrheal disease burden in, 164
poisoning mortality rate in, 58
unintentional injuries (nontransport) in, 57t
Ebi, K. L., 161
Economic Commission for Latin America and the
Caribbean (ECLAC), 162
economic evaluation for informed decision
making, 13–14b. *See also* cost-effectiveness of
interventions
benefit-cost analysis (BCA), 13–14b, 200
benefit-cost ratios (BCRs), 14, 203, 203t
cost-effectiveness analysis (CEA), 13–14b, 200
extended cost-effectiveness analysis (ECEA),
13–14b
health and financial risk, 13b
specific health outcome, 13b
Ecuador
clean fuel initiatives in, 149
intimate partner violence, costs of, 80t
violence against women in, 74
education
burns and heat exposure, 63
cost-effectiveness of training programs in
preventing low-back pain, 14–15
interpersonal violence, teaching life skills to children
and adolescents to prevent, 83, 84t
poisoning, community-based educational
interventions for, 63
preschool enrichment programs, 83
water, sanitation, and hygiene (WASH) services in
schools, 176, 178, 180, 184
Egbendewe-Mondzozo, A., 162

Egypt, health care sector's occupational risks in,
105t, 117
electronics industry, 110–11
Elliot, G., 201
El Salvador
interpersonal violence, costs of, 76, 78t
violence against women in, 74
emissions. *See* air pollution; household air pollution
environmental risks. *See also* air pollution; household
air pollution; water, sanitation, and hygiene
age-standardized mortality, 9f
burden of, 33
drowning, 59
economic evaluation of interventions, 10–15,
202–4t, 202–5
approaches to inform decisionmaking, 13–14b
costs of interventions, 205–7
environmental risk transition, 6
essential interventions to address, 15–19, 17–18t
global environmental health risks, 7–9
decline in, 8, 11f
greenhouse gas emissions, 8, 11f. *See also* air
pollution
intersectoral partnerships to address, 199
modern environmental health risks, 7
morbidity and mortality trends, 6, 31t
traditional environmental health risks, 6–7
water, sanitation, and hygiene, risks for inadequate
services, 180–81
epilepsy, 59
ergonomic problems, 4, 29–30, 30t
ergonomic problems and interventions, 4, 15, 29–30,
30t, 115
Ethiopia
diarrheal disease burden in, 164
manufacturing sector's occupational risks in, 105t
European Commission on societal burden of road
traffic injuries, 38
European Survey of Enterprises on New and Emerging
Risks, 118
European Working Conditions Survey, 99, 100
Europe/European Union
burns in, 29
mortality rates from, 58
climate change's impact
Climate Impact Research and Response
Coordination for a Larger Europe (CIRCLE)
study, 161, 163
costs of, 162
on labor productivity, 163
diarrheal disease burden in, 164
global supply chains of, 108
lung cancer studies in, 139

health care sector, 117
injury care and return to work, 112
machine safety, 118
migrant workers' safety training, 117
participatory approaches, 115–16, 116t
planning, monitoring, and evaluation data, 113
primary prevention, 112
protective covering and equipment, 107, 112
psychosocial risk management, 118–19
regulation and enforcement, 113–14
responsible parties for, 199
safety climate and safety culture, 114–15
safety incentive programs, 115
slip, trip, and fall prevention, 116–17
worker training, 114
workplace violence, 118
LMICs vs. HICs, 4, 5t
manufacturing sector, 102–3, 105t
migrant workers, 98–99, 107–9
mortality trends in, 9, 12f, 29–30
age-standardized mortality, 8–9f
deaths possible to avert through interventions, 20, 20t
LMICs, by all ages and genders, 30t
LMICs, by type of risk, 104f
NGOs regulating working conditions, 109–10, 114
noise exposure, 4, 30, 30t, 121
outsourcing of hazardous jobs, 4, 97, 98, 99t, 110
psychosocial exposures, 99–100
risk management of, 118–19
recession of 2007–09, effect of, 97
regulation of occupational health, 109–10
repetitive motion, 99, 110
small and medium enterprises (SMEs), 98, 106, 113
temporary vs. permanent workers, 98
textile, clothing, and footwear industry, 111–12, 111t
trade unions' role, 104
wholesale and retail trade, 103
work–life conflict and adverse outcomes, 100
work organization and shifts, 100, 118
OECD countries. See high-income countries
open defecation, incidence of, 31, 174, 185
organic solvents, exposure to, 120
Ortiz, R. A., 162
outdoor worker productivity, impact of climate change, 162–63
outsourcing of hazardous jobs, 4, 97, 98, 99t, 110
Ozdemir, R., 63

**P**
Pakistan
children in poor households, increased health risk of, 190

diarrheal disease burden in, 164
poisoning interventions, economic analysis of, 66
road safety interventions, economic analysis of, 44
safety warnings on medications and consumer products in, 64
Pandey, K., 161
Pant, K. P., 225
Paraffin Safety Association of Southern Africa, 63–64
Paraguay
clean fuel initiatives in, 149
climate change-related costs in, 162
Paraguay–Argentina migration corridor, 107
violence against women in, 74
Parry, M., 161
particulate matter exposure
generally. See air pollution
in households. See household air pollution
in workplace, 4
Pattanayak, S. K., 205, 224
pedestrian injuries. See road traffic injuries
Peru
costs of interpersonal violence in, 76, 77t
physical violence in the workplace in, 105t
Water and Sanitation Program's Global Scaling Up Handwashing Projects, 184
pesticides, exposure to, 118, 120
Philippines
health care sector's occupational risks in, 106t
water, sanitation, and hygiene (WASH) services in
cost-effectiveness, 191
water pollution, 181
Pierfederici, R., 161
poisoning
behavioral strategies for prevention of, 63–64
burden of injuries, 56f, 66
child poisoning cases, 60
child safety caps on medications, 64
community-based educational interventions, 63
costs and cost-effectiveness of interventions, 65t, 66
DALYs trends in, 57t, 58
LMICs (all ages and genders), 28, 28t
environmental strategies for prevention of, 64
gender differences, 60
interventions, 61t, 63–64, 67
essential interventions to address, 16t, 18
LMICs vs. HICs, 4t
mortality trends in, 9, 13f, 58
income and regions, 57t
LMICs (all ages and genders), 27t, 28
males and age groups, 57t, 58
pesticide poisoning of agricultural workers, 118
risk factors for, 60

study results, 216–18
variables in study, 214
wealthy accruing larger share of benefit, 218
violence. *See* collective violence; interpersonal violence; women, violence against
vitamin D supplementation, 64

## W

water, sanitation, and hygiene (WASH), 4–5, 171–98
  arsenic in groundwater, 177
  benefit-cost analysis of, 14, 189–90, 190*t*, 203, 204*t*
  benefits of services, 188, 189*t*
  children in poor households, increased health risk of as justification for targeting, 190
  climate change and, 192
  cost-effective analysis of, 190–91, 191*f*, 200, 203
  costs of universal access and improved services, 186–88, 187*f*, 188*t*, 205, 206–7*t*
  DALYs in LMICs from, 31–32, 190
  definitions, 172–73
  dehydration, 177
  diarrheal disease and, 177–78
  diseases transmitted through inadequate services, 177–78
  distribution of services, 175–77
  effectiveness and costs of technologies and practices, 181–84, 182*f*, 208
  environmental consequences of inadequate WASH, 180–81
  financial and economic consequences of inadequate WASH, 181
  global monitoring of, 172, 173*t*
  Global Public-Private Partnership for Handwashing (PPPHW), 184
  health consequences of inadequate WASH, 177–79
  helminth infections, incidence of, 31, 178–79, 183
  interventions, 181–84
    approaches to improve effectiveness of service delivery, 185–86
    behavioral change and promotion of, 184
    community-driven development (CDD) programs, 186
    Community-Led Total Sanitation (CLTS), 184
    deaths possible to avert through interventions, 20, 20*t*
    demand-based approaches, 184
    effectiveness of service delivery models, 184–86
    essential interventions to address, 17*t*, 19
    nutrition interventions promoting hygiene, 186
    public regulation, 208
    results-based approaches, 185, 193*n*11
    results for, 183, 183*t*, 208
    safety-net programs, 186
    School-Led Total Sanitation (SLTS), 184
    supply-side approaches, 184–85
  Joint Monitoring Programme's (JMP) focus, 172, 174*f*, 175, 190
  LMICs vs. HICs, 4–5, 5*t*
  menstrual hygiene management, 180
  microfinance linked to household sanitation, 185
  Millennium Development Goal (MDG) targets, 5, 31–32, 171, 172, 174, 175, 186, 191, 199
  morbidity and mortality attributable to lack of, 31–32, 31*t*
  on-plot sanitation, 179–80
  reporting system for institutions, 175–76
  research needs, 192
  risks linked to income, 6–7, 9*f*
  scope of services, 171, 172*t*
  social welfare consequences of inadequate WASH, 179–80
  status of, 172–76
  sustainability of, 191
  Sustainable Development Goals (SDGs), 171, 172, 192
  undernutrition and, 179
  universal access and improved services, 186–88, 187*f*, 191–92
  vulnerability of children and, 177
  willingness-to-pay (WTP) studies, 188, 208
water pollution, consequences of, 180–81
water supply, 173–74. *See also* water, sanitation, and hygiene
  supply-side approaches to rural areas, 185
  treatment of, 182
  virtual water trade, 180, 193*n*6
Watkiss, P., 163
weather variables. *See* climate change; natural disasters
Western Asia. *See also specific countries*
  informal sector's occupational risk in, 106
  women as workers in, 101
Western Pacific. *See also specific countries*
  benefit-cost analysis of clean energy in, 14, 225
  diarrheal disease burden in, 164
  road traffic deaths as leading cause of mortality for people 15–49 years, 213
  unintentional injuries (nontransport) in, 57*t*
willingness-to-pay approach, 37, 38
  India, coal-fired power plants case study, 245, 247*n*26
  water, sanitation, and hygiene, 188, 208
Wilson, A., 202
women. *See also* gender
  access to water and, 31, 173, 177, 179–80

burns, incidence of, 29
menstrual hygiene management, 180
women, violence against, 74, 75. *See also* interpersonal violence
    acid attacks on women, 29
    costs of, 81, 207
    interventions to promote gender equality, 84*t*, 86
    rape or sexual assault, 72, 180
Working Group on Child Drowning in LMICs, 62
work–life conflict and adverse outcomes, 100
workplaces
    safety. *See* occupational injuries
    water, sanitation, and hygiene (WASH) services in, 180
World Bank
    on diarrheal disease and malaria in climate-change scenario, 161
    Global Partnership on Output-Based Aid (GPOBA), 185
    on household air pollution, 136
    International Benchmarking Network for Water and Sanitation Utilities (IBNET), 181
    Program-for-Results Financing (PforR), 185, 193*n*11
    on WASH initiatives
        child mortality reduction, 190
        costs of universal access to WASH services, 186–87
        output-based aid, 185, 193*n*11
        Water and Sanitation Program, 185
*World Development Report* (1993), 2
World Health Assembly
    resolution to improve trauma and emergency care services, 40
    violence as public health priority for, 71
World Health Organization (WHO)
    on alcohol and health, 83
    on burns data and surveillance, 58

on climate-change related child mortality, 178
on climate-resilient system, 157
Global Health Estimates database, 26, 35, 58
*Global Status Report on Road Safety*, 20, 48, 49–50*n*1
on household air pollution, 136, 144
Indoor Air Quality Guidelines, 133, 150*n*4
on interpersonal violence, 71–72
on kerosene use as household fuel, 150*n*3
on occupational health
    integration with primary health care, 104
    regulations for, 109
on pesticide poisoning, 118
on road traffic injuries responsible for life years lost, 37
*Strengthening Road Safety Legislation*, 47
WHO-CHOICE methodology to determine cost-effectiveness of interventions, 14, 44, 65, 202, 203
World Mental Health Survey, 75
*World Report on Child Injury Prevention*, 62–63
*World Report on Road Traffic Injury Prevention*, 42

**Y**
youth
    road traffic injuries, young people as most affected age group, 37
    violence. *See* interpersonal violence

**Z**
Zambia, violence against women in, 74
Zimbabwe
    child abuse in, 74
    occupational injuries in
        health care sector, 106*t*
        migrant workers, 107
        miners' risk, 105*t*
    violence against women in, 74

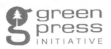

# Percent Reduction in Premature Mortality 2003–2013

**Legend:**

- ■ Less than or equal to 10.00%
- ■ 10.01%–15.00%
- ■ 15.01%–19.00%
- ■ 19.01%–22.49%
- ■ Greater than or equal to 22.50%
- ■ No data

Premature mortality is defined as death before age 70. The map groups countries by percentage reduction in premature mortality rates in the decade from 2003. Ole F. Norheim and others propose a goal for 2030 of a 40 percent reduction in premature mortality from what would have resulted at 2010 death rates ("Avoiding 40% of the Premature Deaths in Each Country, 2010–30: Review of National Mortality Trends to Help Quantify the UN Sustainable Development Goal for Health," *The Lancet*, September 19, 2014, doi:10.1016/S0140-6736(14)61591-9). Countries in green had rates of reduction in 2003–2013 high enough to meet that 40 percent goal.